$\mathcal{P}$EDIATRIC NURSING

$\mathcal{P}$EDIATRIC NURSING

McGraw-Hill

Health Professions Division
M c G R A W - H I L L   N U R S I N G   C O R E   S E R I E S

New York St. Louis San Francisco Auckland Bogotá Caracas Lisbon
London Madrid Mexico City Milan Montreal New Delhi San Juan
Singapore Sydney Tokyo Toronto

EDITORS

MARTHA VELASCO-WHETSELL, Ph.D.,
R.N., A.R.N.P.
School of Nursing
Florida International University
North Miami, Florida and
Endicott College
Graduate School
Mexico City, Mexico

DOUGLAS A. COFFIN, Ph.D., A.R.N.P.
School of Nursing
Florida International University
North Miami, Florida

LOURDES M. LIZARDO, Ed.D., R.N.,
A.R.N.P.
School of Nursing
Florida International University
North Miami, Florida

MARIA L. V. LIZARDO, M.S.N., A.R.N.P.
Miami, Florida

BARBARA J. MacDOUGALL, M.S.N.,
A.R.N.P.
Bay Point Schools
Miami, Florida

TOMAS M. MADAYAG, Jr., Ed.D., R.N.,
A.R.N.P.
School of Nursing
Florida International University
North Miami, Florida

MEG SELENE MARCUS, M.S.N., R.N.,
A.R.N.P.
Adjunct Clinical Professor
School of Nursing
Florida International University
North Miami, Florida;
Pediatric Nurse Practitioner
Voluntis Medical Care Group, Inc.
Miami, Florida

McGraw-Hill

A Division of The **McGraw-Hill** *Companies*

PEDIATRIC NURSING

Copyright © 2000 by The McGraw-Hill Companies, Inc. All rights reserved. Printed in the United States of America. Except as permitted under the United States Copyright Act of 1976, no part of this publication may be reproduced or distributed in any form or by any means, or stored in a data base or retrieval system, without the prior written permission of the publisher.

1 2 3 4 5 6 7 8 9 0 DOW DOW 9 9

ISBN 0-07-070009-5

This book was set in Sabon by V&M Graphics, Inc.
The editors were John Dolan and Susan Noujaim.
The production supervisor was Richard Ruzycka.
The project was managed by Hockett Editorial Service.
The cover designer was Joan O'Connor.
The index was prepared by Christina Palaia, Emerald Editorial Services.
R.R. Donnelley and Sons was printer and binder.

This book is printed on acid-free paper.

Library of Congress Cataloging-in-Publication Data

Pediatric nursing review / editors, Martha Velasco-Whetsell ... [et al.].
      p.   c.m.
    Includes bibliographical references and index.
    ISBN 0-07-070009-5 (alk. paper)
    1. Pediatric nursing.   I. Velasco-Whetsell, Martha
    [DNLM: 1. Pediatric Nursing.   WY 159 P3738 2000]
RJ245.P426   2000
610.73'62—dc21
DNLM/DLC
for Library of Congress   99-32630
                              CIP

CONTENTS

Color plates appear between pages 422 and 423.

CONTRIBUTORS

Douglas A. Coffin, Ph.D., A.R.N.P.
School of Nursing
Florida International University
North Miami, Florida

Opal P.M. Hamilton, M.S.N., A.R.N.P.
Pediatric Special Care Unit
Jackson Memorial Hospital
Cooper City, Florida

Jacquelyn T. Hartley, Ph.D., R.N.
School of Nursing
Florida International University
North Miami, Florida

Cynthia G. Hunt, R.N., M.S.N.
Miami, Florida

Lourdes M. Lizardo, Ed.D., R.N., A.R.N.P.
School of Nursing
Florida International University
North Miami, Florida

Maria L. V. Lizardo, M.S.N., A.R.N.P.
Miami, Florida

Barbara J. MacDougall, M.S.N., A.R.N.P.
Bay Point Schools
Miami, Florida

Tomas M. Madayag, Jr., Ed.D., R.N., A.R.N.P.
School of Nursing
Florida International University
North Miami, Florida

Meg Selene Marcus, M.S.N., R.N., A.R.N.P.
Adjunct Clinical Professor
School of Nursing
Florida International University
North Miami, Florida;
Pediatric Nurse Practitioner
Voluntis Medical Care Group, Inc.
Miami, Florida

Lucille Piea, M.S.N., A.R.N.P.
Fort Meyers, Florida

Teresa L. Rudes
School of Nursing
Florida International University
North Miami, Florida

Martha Velasco-Whetsell, Ph.D., R.N., A.R.N.P.
School of Nursing
Florida International University
North Miami, Florida and
Endicott College
Graduate School
Mexico City, Mexico

This book is dedicated to the memory
of
Douglas A. Coffin

$\mathcal{P}$REFACE

In designing the pediatric nursing review textbook, we set out to produce a comprehensive pediatric nursing textbook that will help the nursing students provide quality, comprehensive nursing care to their pediatric patients. One of the main components of the book is to teach students the ability to reason or to think critically and clinically about the gathered information obtained from patients.

The main purpose of this textbook is to address the questions that are commonly asked by nursing students in the daily routine of their nursing care. All the chapters address basic pathophysiology, general pediatric principles, and practical management issues.

Another purpose of this textbook is to make the reader aware that children have needs that are unique and different from adults. These needs not only require special provisions from the health care system, but also critical provisions for growth and development, and include levels of communication that are based in the cognitive development of the child.

This textbook also addresses the child's and family's mode of interaction, being keenly aware that this communication changes as the child grows and the family also grows as a unit.

One of the forces behind the production of this textbook is my own experience as a nursing student, practicing nurse, faculty member, and, most important, as a parent. In the early years of my career, I was very involved in perfecting my nursing skills in the hospital. It was not until years later that I realized that the major component of my nursing care was intuitive in nature, or based on what the hospital procedures were. As I entered graduate school, I realized that the reality of pediatric nursing is not the knowledge of the skill, but the knowledge of theories, especially developmental theories. Developmental theories, when applied to the nursing care of children, clarify many concepts and become the cornerstone for the success of nursing management.

Pediatric Nursing summarizes the treatment guidelines from national health advisory boards, current nursing journals, and current reference books. Extensive efforts have been made to include the most current available research and literature in all the chapters. This textbook was also written with input and support from several nurses across the country. We appreciate the comments and time from our nursing colleagues who helped with the revisions for the production of this textbook.

In writing this textbook we realized that nurses enter the profession because they care for people, and more important, pediatric nurses enter the specialty because they love children. Therefore we wrote a textbook that will provide comprehensive and current information relevant to the practice of pediatric nursing and that will aid in a more successful nursing practice.

Acknowledgments

First, I am very grateful to my husband, Douglas, and my son, Vinson H, for making me believe that I could write this textbook and for reminding me that my biggest strength is my love for teaching. I would also like to thank my colleagues Doctors Coffin, Madayag, and Lizardo; and Ms. MacDougall, Ms. Marcus, and Ms. Lizardo for their hard work and dedication to the production of the book. A very special thanks to a brilliant editor and friend, Terry Rudes, who provided counsel and kept me focused. I will always be grateful to John Dolan at McGraw-Hill, for believing in the group, to Susan Noujaim, also at McGraw-Hill, for her invaluable knowledge and professionalism, and to Rachel Youngman of Hockett Editorial Service for shepherding the book through production. Finally, I want to also thank Kay Stanley for her help and encouragement. In the process of the production of this text all of us came close to may wonderful people; we cannot mention them all, but we are most grateful.

OVERVIEW

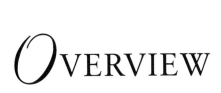

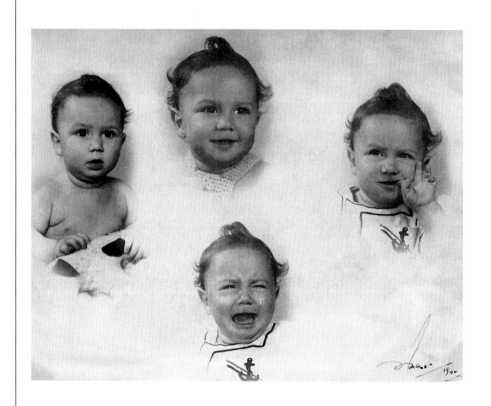

C H A P T E R   1

EFFECTIVE STUDYING HABITS AND THINKING DISPOSITIONS

INTRODUCTION

Effective study skills and learning dispositions are the basis for effective learning. Effective study skills provide you with an opportunity to approach learning tasks systematically and independently. By always using good study habits, you are learning to work smarter. Yet it takes more than just good study habits to be successful in college and in taking tests.

The majority of college success and successful test taking is due to self-motivation and time management. Anyone who says that he/she is successful at taking tests without studying or could finish college without any effort is not being completely honest. Success in college, at work, and in test taking requires effort.

This means you must be willing to set aside time to study. Setting aside time may also mean recognizing the value in meeting specific short-term objectives to achieve specific long-term goals. Effective time management will permit adequate time for school, work, and a social life or at least enough free time to do other enjoyable activities.

Motivation is the primary key to success in college, in work, and in life. There are many helpful hints that can be provided to any learner to enhance motivation. Yet neither this portion of the book, a faculty member, nor others can be a motivator for learning. This book is only a resource. It is the reader's own responsibility to develop and use sound study habits, to seek out resources and assistance when needed, and to successfully manage his/her time. The reader, as a learner, must want to do well enough to put forth the effort.

ℱIVE MAJOR STUDY PROBLEMS AND WAYS TO AVOID THEM

Five major study problems have been found by students:

1. Not studying enough—relying on cramming.
2. Wasting time when studying—having read several pages only to discover that you can't remember what you just read, nor any of the other material, for that matter.
3. Having trouble getting ready to study—have to feed the kids, have to do the laundry, cook dinner, etc.
4. Unable to find a good place to study—using the kitchen table.
5. Not using a good learning strategy—just memorizing.

The following is a list of suggestions to help you avoid these problems.

1. Establish a Schedule

Take your current schedules into account when allocating time for studying. Designate the most difficult classes and/or materials for the beginning of your study sessions when energy levels and concentration ability will be at their peak.

Make sure to allot time for recreation and social activities, too. Schedule them as rewards for successful completion of scheduled studying times. Once it is established, follow the schedule. Readjust the schedule if you have over- or underestimated the time needed. Recognize that daily reorganization may be needed to accommodate conflicts that arise, always being mindful of short- and long-term priorities.

Conflict in priorities, or trying to accomplish too many goals at one time, suggests the need for rethinking and then reranking priorities and goals against a more realistic set of objectives. Normally, what is needed is to establish specific and measurable objectives that will accomplish a specific goal. For example, after reading a chapter, complete all the multiple choice study questions at the end of the chapter to enhance learning.

2. Start Studying for Short Periods, and Slowly Build Up to Longer Periods

The majority of study skills programs suggest reading only in 10- to 15-minute increments as a freshman, then building up to 45 minutes at a time as a graduate student. As in physical exercise, one needs to work toward longer and longer periods of intense studying. Be realistic. Recognize that, if your concentration wavers, stop for a while. Why waste time? Do something else and then come back to studying.

3. Take Short Breaks

Studying is, or should be, an intense mental activity. The average person's attention span for a single task is about 20 minutes. So cramming for more than 20 minutes makes little sense. What makes better sense is studying small portions of materials at a time, taking a break, and then returning for an additional time. This has been demonstrated to be a more effective strategy than cramming. Make study breaks mandatory and use them. Even if the material is interesting and enjoyable, it is wise to get up and take a break. How long should the break be? Give yourself enough time to relax, rest your eyes and brain, and regain your attention span for studying.

4. Reward as Reinforcement

Knowing that there is a reward at the end of completing a task such as studying is very reinforcing. Be realistic about rewards, however, and make sure any reward immediately follows the desired behavior rather than coming at some future time. This is important, since the closer the reward is to the behavior, the more reinforcing it is.

5. Find a Good Place to Study

Location is a form of reinforcement, so it is better to make the study setting like the testing atmosphere. For instance, sitting at a desk in a hardback chair is preferable to lying in a bed. Using the library is preferable to using a desk at work during a lunch break.

6. Use the Same Location for Studying

Association is a strong reinforcement. Learning to associate one particular location with studying will facilitate concentration and learning. When you are in your study location, it will be associated with learning and concentration. Over time, it becomes easier and easier to settle quickly into studying, concentrating, and learning.

7. Make Sure the Study Location Is Quiet

It is important to find and use a well-lit study area. But of equal importance is that the site is quiet and without distractions. Some learners can tolerate a radio or stereo blaring, or have the TV on, but for most learners, any of these factors is enough to disturb concentration and inhibit the ability to learn effectively. The location, therefore, should be quiet and free of such distractions.

8. Eliminate Obvious Distractions

The more obvious distractions are friends calling on the telephone, or friends, family, or neighbors dropping by for a visit. However, unread newspapers, magazines, journal articles, and other unfinished projects should also be placed out of sight. Only materials needed to complete the task at hand should be present, and nothing else. Textbooks from other courses, notebooks for other classes, or any materials not associated with the task at hand can serve as conscious or unconscious distractions. These distractions end up being reminders about other things that have yet to be completed, possibly causing wasted time in worrying. Eliminating the distractions will improve study skills.

9. Memory and Recall Are Context Dependent

Studying in a physical situation similar to the one in which the test will be given increases the chances of information recall. This is why studying in bed or in an easy chair does not work. If at all possible, review materials in the classroom where the test will be given.

10. Memory and Recall Are State Dependent

One should study in an emotional mood similar to that experienced during tests, i.e., with an increased sense of awareness and alertness, with higher levels of concentration and focus, and even, perhaps, with a little tension. Higher levels of concentration and activation during study periods will increase the chances of recalling the materials during test taking. However, if getting too psyched up or too anxious during tests is a problem, information recall will be inhibited because studying and test-taking moods will not be the same. Remember that too much anxiety is like too little—either way, memory is influenced. If too much anxiety during test taking is the case, learn to relax and calm down in testing situations in order to match the study mood to the test mood. Use relaxation techniques if needed.

11. Increase Reading Effectiveness

There are several methods for increasing reading effectiveness. Two will be discussed. Choose the one that will be the most effective. It is important to remember that there is a purpose for your reading. With textbooks and other college materials, it may take several readings to fully comprehend material. This may be especially true if the subject is unfamiliar to you or of little interest.

$\mathcal{S}$Q4R METHOD

The SQ4R method (survey, question, read, write, recite, and review) is a reading and studying system preferred by many educators. Reading research indicates that it is an extremely effective method for both comprehension and memory retention. It is effective because it is a system of *active* reader involvement.

Step 1: Survey

Before you actually read a chapter or review particular notes or other materials, take a few minutes to survey the material. Briefly check the headings and subheadings in order to understand how the author's organizational pattern of ideas is to be discussed or covered. Scan all the visual or graphical material used in the chapter. Read the introductory and summary paragraphs. This previewing or surveying enables you to anticipate what the chapter or the material is all about.

Step 2: Question

Create interest in the material by asking questions, such as: What are the main points or concepts covered? Read with your questions in mind, and attempt to figure out and list the most important points or concepts. Another means of creating questions is to convert topical headings and subheadings into questions. Attempt to answer the questions by paraphrasing the author's words. Remember to use the evidence (facts) found in the material to support your answers. Using either technique gives a clearly defined purpose for reading and helps maintain interest in the material.

Step 3: Read

Read the chapter or material actively for meaning. Go through any paragraph before underlining; then underline only key words, concepts, and phrases to help you recall the main points. Be selective. Don't highlight unimportant points or miss anything that can help with comprehension. Summarize main concepts in the margins. The more actively you are involved in the reading process, the more you will retain.

Step 4: Write

After you have answered the questions constructed from headings, or from asking the main point of each chapter or paragraph, write the answer down.

Summing up such information in your own words aids in retaining the information. Restructure the information so that it makes the most sense. Be sure to use the evidence found in the materials to support your answers.

Step 5: Recite

After every few pages, close the book and recite aloud the main points to the questions proposed in Step 2. Try to recall the basic details of the author's intent. Use the evidence (facts) found in the text to support the answers to the questions and verify the answers by checking the text. If memory fails, read through the portion of text again. Knowing the information rather than memorizing it will make recall on a test easier, so take as much time as needed to answer the questions. Be patient. Studying this way may take more time, but the information will be clearer and retention will be longer.

Step 6: Review

Finally, review the chapter or material every so often to fix it in your mind. Verbalize the sequence of main ideas and supporting facts to aid in retention. Keep rereading the margin notes and the underlined material. Numerous reviews are more effective than one cramming session the night before a test. Review the information once again after reading and then every couple of days to keep it fresh for the test.

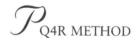

$\mathcal{P}$Q4R METHOD

The PQ4R method (preview, question, read, reflect, recite, and review) is also preferred by many educators. It is very similar to the SQ4R method. Reading research indicates that it too is an extremely effective method for both comprehension and memory retention. It is effective because it is a system of active reader involvement.

Step 1: Preview

Survey the chapter to determine the general areas to be discussed. Identify those sections to be read as units and then apply the next four steps to each of the sections.

Step 2: Questions

Make up questions about each of the sections. Often the easiest means of creating questions is to transform section headings into questions. It may be helpful to work with a classmate in creating questions or at least have a classmate review them.

Step 3: Read

Read the section carefully with the question in mind. After reading the section, pose the question aloud. Cover the section and try to answer the question adequately.

Step 4: Reflect

Read and reflect upon what is being said. As in a conversation or in a lecture, attempt to understand the material as it is presented in the text. Try to think of examples while reading and relate them to prior knowledge.

Step 5: Recite

After finishing a section or a unit, try to recall the information. Try answering questions created for each section or unit. Inability to recall enough details or facts to answer the questions adequately requires rereading that portion or unit.

Step 6: Review

After completing the entire unit or chapter, mentally recall its main points and major concepts. Once again, answer the questions posed for each portion of the unit or chapter.

$\mathcal{S}$EVEN POINTS TO REMEMBER ABOUT YOUR CLASSES

1. Go to Class

Class attendance is crucial. Research demonstrates a positive correlation between class attendance and grades. Higher attendance is associated with higher grades. Instructors believe that their lecture material is as important as the textbook. Missing a class means missing what the professor emphasizes or says is important. And that information will more than likely end up on the test.

2. Participate in Class

To learn from a lecture and from a classroom environment, it is important to become involved by participating in the classroom discussions. Asking questions for clarification and maintaining good eye contact with the instructor during a lecture is important for increasing your concentration and involvement. Asking questions indicates active involvement in what has been said and trying to anticipate what is going to be said next. Of equal importance is having read the material to be covered in the lecture prior to attending the class. This also aids in retention and makes following the lecture material easier, while providing a basis for asking clarification questions.

3. If a Class Must Be Missed, Let Someone Know

If a class must be missed, let the professor know ahead of time if possible. It is helpful to know a reliable classmate who can take notes and pick up any handouts. However, be sure to establish such a relationship with your classmate ahead of time.

4. Take Good Notes

Proper note taking is a skill just as important as good reading and active listening. It is important not to be a human tape recorder. Do not attempt to write everything down; it isn't necessary. Be concise; sum up the lecture material in writing and relate the lecture to what was read. Write down unfamiliar terms, concepts, or relationships, and then look them up. Be sure to maintain your notes consistently in the same notebook, number and date your pages, and keep the notebook in good condition.

5. Use the Textbook

The textbook is often the primary source of lecture and test materials and often a professor will follow the book closely. In such cases it may be helpful to take the book to class and highlight important topics or terms that the professor emphasizes, as well as writing notes in the margins. It is also important to ask for examples, clarification, or a different form of explanation of text that is unclear. Be sure to use more than the written text. Look at the illustrations and attempt to understand the logic behind them.

6. Meet and Talk with the Professor

When having difficulties with the material or the course, it is important to speak with the professor as soon as possible. Often he/she can assist or make suggestions to get the resources or help needed. However, don't wait until the last minute. Few professors have sympathy for a student who waits until a week or two before the end of a semester, or a day before an exam, to discuss the possibility of failing the course, or lack of understanding the course materials.

7. Form or Join a Study Group

Forming or joining a study group is one way to review for a test. However, make it clear that the purpose of the study group is to review and study for an examination, not to teach or relearn the material. The major problem with some study groups is that they turn into chat sessions with little productive work done. To refocus the group and get it back to task is often difficult; recognize that some members of the group may have another agenda. One strategy to use, if the group goes off onto another track, is to ask for a short break, and then bring them back together with a focused question about the material. Remember to reward a successful study session with a pizza and good conversation.

The key to achieving any goal is giving yourself permission to be "average." Permitting yourself to do what you fear appears to lessen the fear and its impact. Paradoxically, once you relax without the burden of achieving a perfect score, you will probably find that you will score higher than average anyway.

$\mathcal{H}$ow to take essay exams

There are several basic rules to keep in mind when taking essay examinations. Begin preparing for essay examinations by reading the instructor's course description and syllabus. Write down whatever assumptions, biases, and teaching objectives are stated or implied in these materials. Determine how the various course topics relate to one another, and to the course objectives, and note any repeated themes. Think about any potential essay questions suggested by this information and then write them down.

Read the assignments and listen to lectures and discussions with the purpose of determining how the course content supports the major themes and answers the major questions generated from the course description and course objectives. Modify and refine these themes and questions throughout the course as additional information is gained.

At some point before the test, normally a week or more before the essay examination, quickly review all notes and the chapter headings from the readings. From this review, generate a list of major topics for the course material covered so far. For each major topic, create a summary sheet of all the relevant factual data that relate to that topic. In addition, determine any logical relationships among the topics. These relationships often predict essay test questions. For example, in a course on advanced nursing practice, you find that multiple advanced nursing practice roles have changed over time. The instructor may require that the students compare and contrast these roles against current trends in health care. Generate a list of possible essay questions and then consider answering as many of these questions as time permits.

There are several things to be done when taking the essay test.

1. Before Writing, Make Sure You Understand the Question

If a question is vague or not understood, ask for clarification. It is very important to have a grasp of what is being asked. Carefully read all the essay questions before beginning to answer any of them. Clarify any confusion about meaning with the instructor; do not assume what a question means. Budget your time according to the point value of each question, allowing time for proofreading and any unexpected emergencies such as going blank for awhile.

Underline key words and phrases such as "compare," "explain fully," "justify your reasons for," "define," and make sure you understand what, specifically, you are being asked. Obviously, begin with the easiest questions. This reduces anxiety and facilitates clear thinking.

2. Do an "Information Dump" for Each Question

Look over the questions and write down all the specific points as quickly as possible for each of them. Write down names, dates, statistics, and any other pertinent information you recall. Do not worry about the order of the material or whether it is "relevant." An "information dump" frees your mind of details, and it should help you settle down. Do this for all the questions before beginning to write.

3. Do an "Outline" on the Information Dump

Before beginning to write, take a couple of minutes to plan your answer. Make a brief outline of intended points to be used from your "information dump." This helps streamline your thoughts and should help make your answers seamless.

4. Be Concise

On an essay exam chances are there will be no time to meander. Decide on main points and get right to them. Do not waffle around and pad the essay with unnecessary words, ideas, and/or paragraphs. Cut the essay answer to the bone. Avoid the use of jargon words, unless they naturally fit into the context of the exam.

Provide specific as well as general information in your responses by including examples, substantiating facts, and relevant details from the "information dump." Use the technical vocabulary of the course rather than jargon.

5. Write Carefully

Always go through the exam to check for spelling and grammar mistakes. Make your handwriting as legible as possible to avoid confusion about the content of the answers. Leave enough space for additions to each answer by writing on every other line and on only one side of each page.

6. Read Through Your Essays

Make sure your conclusions are supported by the information you provided. The introduction should be either a question that the conclusion answers, or a statement that the conclusion backs up, depending on either reasoning from specified evidence (facts) to a specific conclusion (theory or tentative hypothesis), or reasoning to evidence (from a theory or tentative hypothesis to specific facts). If the introduction and conclusion do not jibe, do some rewriting. Do not panic. There should be plenty of time to write a tight, well-planned essay.

7. Relax and Brainstorm if Your Mind Goes Blank

Brainstorming helps clear the mind of doubts or blanks. Recall pages from your texts, particular lectures, and classroom discussions to trigger recall. Write down the ideas as they come up without considering their relevance or worth.

8. Do Not Exceed Your Allotted Time Period

When self-imposed time limits are reached for a question, move on to the next item. Remember that a partially answered question is worth more than one that has no answer.

How to take objective exams

Like essay examinations, objective examinations require understanding the nature of what is being asked. There are a few general approaches that are useful when preparing for and taking objective examinations.

How to Prepare for Objective Tests

Objective tests measure the student's ability to remember many facts and figures, and to understand the course materials. Often these tests are designed to make a student think independently, i.e., critically. Do not count on simply recognizing the right answer. Instead, it is better to prepare for high-level critical reasoning and for making finer and finer levels of discrimination to determine the best answer from, perhaps, several good answers.

The most common forms of objective tests are multiple choice, true-false, and matching items. Doing well on these types of questions requires not only mastery of the information but also the ability to interpret the test maker's intentions. Mastery of the information is attained if you can recall specific terms, facts, names, and other key words; distinguish the ways that ideas, facts, theories, or other observations differ from each other; categorize ideas, facts, theories, or other observations according to the ways they are similar; and answer the questions and solve the problems in the text and create your own questions or problems.

How to Take Objective Tests

1. Listen to or Read the Instructions Carefully For objective exams, it is important to listen carefully to the professor's instructions. If something seems unclear, ask for an explanation. Do not lose points by misunderstanding what the questions are asking or how you should respond.

2. Preview the Whole Exam before Starting Plan test time and be aware of the time. One method is to take off your watch and put it on top of the desk. Be sure to allow for more time for high-point-value questions and to reserve enough time at the end to review. Go through the entire exam to get a sense of the structure and to figure out where the most difficult sections are. After figuring out the structure, answer all the familiar questions first. Before writing on an exam, be sure that this is okay with the instructor. If the test is in sections, start with the highest value section and then work your way to the lowest value set of questions.

Work quickly, check your time usage, and adjust your time accordingly. On multiple-choice exams, generally, two answers are correct (one being the best choice of the two), one is doubtful, and one is flat-out wrong. Choose the best option.

3. Do Not "Read" into or Argue with the Question Try to keep it simple. Go with the obvious choice. Do not set up an internal dialogue as to how "stupid" the questions are, or how poorly they are written, or that the answer is too easy, therefore it must be a trick, or fret about material that is unfamiliar. Such self-talk can lead to increased anxiety and a mood that does not support taking a test. Choose the answer the test maker intended and stay within the scope of the course.

4. Mark the Questions You Need to Return To In surveying the test, mark the more difficult questions with a dot, so you know to go back to them. Most examinations are timed. Use the allotted time wisely and answer the easier questions first. Be aware of the time, mark the difficult questions, and then move on. When finished, go back and attempt to answer the harder questions. Answering the easier questions may provide information for answering the more difficult ones. Again, stay within time constraints for each question, moving on when time expires. Once all questions are answered, in the time remaining, go over the test at least once more, making sure the answers chosen are the most correct. If there is a separate answer sheet, make sure that the answer marked corresponds to the correct question.

Critically Thinking about Multiple-Choice Questions

The most commonly used objective questions are multiple choice. Such questions consist of two parts: the stem or the statement or question; and the choices, also known as the distracters. For the distracters there are normally three to five options from which you choose the one that will complete the stem question or statement. From a five-option set of distracters there is a 20% opportunity to guess correctly. Although multiple-choice questions may be constructed to test memory and recall facts and relationships, they are more often constructed to test comprehension and the ability to solve problems. Critical reasoning ability is a very important skill for doing multiple-choice examinations.

Carefully and critically read the stem of the multiple-choice question or statement as if it were an independent, free-standing statement. Anticipate the phrase that would complete the thought, then evaluate each answer against the anticipated answer. It is important to read each answer carefully, even if the first choice matches the answer that you anticipated, because an even better answer may be found.

Another evaluation method is to read the stem together with each answer choice as if it were a true-false statement. If the answer makes the statement a false one, then cross it out. Check all the choices that complete the stem as a true statement. Try to suspend your judgment about the choices that are true until all the choices have been evaluated. Beware of words like "not," "but," and "except." Mark these words because they specify the direction and the limits of the answer. Also watch for such words as "never," "always," and "only." These must be interpreted as meaning always, not just 99% of the time. These choices are frequently incorrect because there are few statements that have no exceptions.

If there are two or more options that appear to be the correct answer, compare them to determine the differences between them. Relate these differences with the stem to deduce which of the choices is the better one. The best choice is the one that provides the most complete information.

If there is an encompassing answer, for example, "all of the above" or "none of the above," and you are unable to determine that there are at least two correct choices, select the encompassing choice. Use hints that are found in other questions when attempting to answer more difficult questions. At best, make an educated guess by eliminating inappropriate options.

Critically Thinking about True-False Questions

Although not popular on national examinations, true-false questions are used in objective tests. The true-false question has only two options and you therefore have a 50-50 chance of guessing correctly. Typically test makers tend to focus on details within the stem of the true-false question. In order for a statement to be true, it must be true 100% of the time. Therefore, it is critical to evaluate the truth of the what, who, when, where, and how for each statement. Beware of words that qualify and give specific meanings. Words like "some," "usually," and "not" frequently denote true statements. But be careful to interpret each statement as a special case. Words such as "always" and "never" should be interpreted as meaning without exception. If an exception comes to mind, then the statement is false. Test makers often mismatch items or names with inappropriate events or definitions to test the student's mastery of the information and his/her alertness.

Analyzing Returned Objective Tests

After taking an objective test, it is important to analyze the questions you missed. If the test is not returned in class, it is worth asking the professor for the chance to review the test with him/her during office hours. When reviewing the test, recognize that this is an evaluation of performance.

Read all comments and suggestions on the examination. Look for the origin of the questions. Did they come from class notes or the book? From the class or from the lab? Look at the questions missed. Verbalize the rationale for the correct answer. Try to figure out why the correct answer was a better choice than the one you selected. Did you read the question incorrectly? Were there any areas tested that you didn't prepare for? What was the reason for the lack of preparation? Did you misinterpret any questions?

Check the level of difficulty or the level of detail of the test questions. Were most of the questions you missed asking for precise details, or were they about main ideas, concepts, or principles? Did most of the questions appear to come directly from the material covered in the lecture or the book? Did the test maker expect students to be able to analyze and evaluate the information? Was the test too long and not completed? Did anxiety or other factors inhibit your ability to complete the test or answer certain questions?

GENERAL TIPS: TEST PREPARATION, NOTE TAKING, AND USING THE TEXTBOOK

Test Preparation

1. Know What to Expect Get all the information possible about the test before you study. Find out what type of test it will be (multiple-choice questions, essay, short answers, etc.) and what material it will cover. Also, know how specific the test will be. Is it a general-concept test, or one looking for particular names, dates, and numbers? Knowing what to expect is key to preparing emotionally and intellectually. Knowing can eliminate many of the potential sources of anxiety, too.

2. Review Often It is a good idea to review your class notes right after writing them and again just before the next class. Understand the concepts illustrated. Review any pictorial information, such as concept trees, to enhance understanding of the material.

3. Exam Review Start studying for the exam early. Allow at least a week before taking it, to balance studying with other needs. Divide large amounts of material into smaller portions, and then study the most difficult sections first. Go over that material again just before the test, so it is fresh. To fix the material in memory, practice recalling the information or try explaining the material to someone else.

4. Study for Main Ideas and Concepts Learn the main ideas and concepts and their relationships first. This provides a framework on which to hang supporting ideas and details. Study to recall and to deepen understanding of the material, not just for recognition. Prepare as if the test were short answer. Short answers require a deeper understanding of the material than recall.

5. Be Well Rested Generally, it is not advisable to stay up all night cramming the night before a test. Learning diminishes with fatigue and the ability to think clearly is enhanced with rest. If staying up studying is unavoidable, take frequent breaks to keep alert.

6. Stay Relaxed Excessive anxiety will reduce thinking ability. Get to class early and use those minutes to unwind and relax. Set a positive mental attitude about the test. Self-talk, such as, "Oh no, just another stupid test!" sets the stage for negative emotions and responses. Chances are, given adequate preparation time, the test will seem less intimidating.

7. Identify with the Test Writers The writers of the examination have a perspective. What is it? If it is a national examination, then the test must be broad enough to capture a consensus among the test writers about solutions to nursing problems in various clinical settings.

8. Think Average Rather than Specific Detail Normally, nurses come to a national examination or to a graduate school with a highly specialized health sciences background. This is needed for work but can be a problem when taking a test. Because of this specialization, nurses may have too much detail and specialized content in mind when reading a test item, and can then read into a question detail that, perhaps, is not there. Remember that, for the most part, the perspective of any examination is basic, general, and certainly noncontroversial nursing care. Any approach to a clinical situation that is experimental or still under debate is not the best choice, even if it is true for a particular clinical environment. The best choice is the safest and most conservative answer since the perspective in most nursing examinations is based on safe care.

Note-Taking Techniques

The most comprehensive note-taking systems require attention. Paying attention in class allows for legible, meaningful notes. Don't try to write down every word that is said because a lot of information in a given lecture will not help in actually learning the material. If you have problems determining the specific relevant points in a particular class, always ask the professor to summarize and clarify them.

The 2-6 Method The 2-6 method refers to a way of organizing that helps the student to take legible, meaningful notes. It involves dividing the space on note paper. Make 2 columns, using the red line on the left of the notepaper as the border. Then start taking notes in class, using the wider 6 column on the right of the red line for the notes and the smaller 2 column on the left of the red line as a highlighting system. Write down main headings and important points on the left, including material that might appear on a test. When finished, you should have a comprehensive page of information, quickly scannable for important points.

Using the Textbook as a Learning Resource

There are many ways to mark a textbook. A textbook is a learning resource and an instructional medium. Thinking as you read is an active process, much like a conversation. It requires alertness and focus rather than allowing the mind to wander.

After buying the textbook, become familiar with its structure. Read the table of contents to discover how the book has been organized conceptually. Most authors will outline the basic structure of the book and in the preface describe how each section or portion of the book relates to the overall concept. Then look over the back of the book and each of its divisions. Does it have a comprehensive index? Are major words in the index recognizable? Does it contain a glossary of terms? Is there an overview at the beginning of each chapter? Is there a summary at the end of each chapter? Are there sample questions and exercises at the end of each chapter? All of these items can be used when studying for an exam.

There are certainly many ways to highlight or emphasize what has been said in a conversation so the listener understands that what has been said is important to the speaker. A similar approach to a textbook is essential to getting the most from it. Here is a combination of approaches. Use whatever works best.

Circle key words, concepts, and phrases. Underline major points. In the margin, place some sort of symbol, such as * (asterisk) to emphasize a key section or point of the text. Place a number in the margin for each item in a process, series, or protocol. For example, if there are five items in a process, each item should have a corresponding number in the margin.

In the margin, note questions, relationships, and major points; summarize complex arguments; or identify important points. Remember to use all margins, not just the side ones.

Develop a color-coding system rather than just underlining everything in one color. Note the color-coding system in the textbook so you will remember it. Red can stand for important points or concepts, blue for supporting arguments, and green for detail or facts. But remember that too much detail in a coding system creates more confusion than it clears up. Add relationships, propositions, or phrases to graphics, decision trees, and flowcharts, if none are provided.

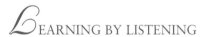

LEARNING BY LISTENING

A student can think four times faster than an instructor can speak. To effectively compensate for the difference between the rate of presentation and the speed of thinking requires using energy to concentrate fully, to listen actively, and to interpret what has been said, using prior knowledge. Note taking enhances listening, and using a systematic approach to both note taking and reviewing your notes may add immeasurably to understanding and retaining the content of a lecture. Knowing how to listen actively and to take lecture notes is the key to learning from lectures.

Taking lecture notes requires an active rather than passive set of listening skills, and is an acquired skill. It is a skill that requires concentration and a focused attention. There are several steps to improving your listening skills.

Step 1: Ask, "Why Am I Listening?"

Why is what the lecturer is saying important? Granted, you are required to be in the classroom, but that is not the reason for listening. The material being presented has some importance. You need it to get a passing grade in the course; to write a good essay or term paper; or because it has general or specific utility in your work, career, or for some other reason. It should be the motivating factor for actively listening to the lecture.

Step 2: Choose a Strategic Place in the Classroom

One rarely turns his/her back on someone during a conversation. It is equally important where you sit in a classroom so as to face and actively listen to the lecturer. Where you sit can either be a help or a distraction from actively listening. The front center section is normally the best spot for listening and note taking. Avoid places where there are distractions, such as near open doorways, open windows, or where you must strain to hear, see, or listen to the lecturer. Avoid sitting near people who want to talk more than listen.

Step 3: Come Prepared to Listen and to Take Notes

Bring to class the materials needed to take notes. Have a notebook that will sit flat and that can be turned easily. Wide-lined paper is easier to write on, allows room to add materials, and can be organized later. Keep a couple of pens or pencils handy and be sure that they are in working order. Keep a good supply of such materials on hand.

Be sure to label class notes with the date, page number, and time for organization later. Include any handouts and other materials from the lecture so that when studying, they will be available to refer to easily. Keep all course materials in the same notebook. Often a three-ring notebook is the easiest way of organizing course materials. Simply place the materials in the order received and keep the materials well organized and readily available for studying.

Step 4: Listen to the Speaker

Appearances and mannerisms can be distracting. Refocus and concentrate on what is being said, rather than attending to packaging or quirks.

Step 5: Listen Actively for the Organization of Material

Actively listen and look for main ideas or concepts during a lecture. Actively listen for how these ideas or concepts are related to each other and to the overall course objectives. Be aware of when the lecturer digresses from the main ideas of the lecture, and figure out how or if the digression supports what has been said. If not understood, ask how the digression material relates to what has been discussed so far.

Step 6: Actively Take Notes

Taking notes helps keep one actively involved in the lecture. Write down only the key points, including those that are already known or understood. During review, the notes will help in remembering the lecture.

Step 7: Concentrate, Concentrate

Keep actively involved in the lecture and not on distractions in the classroom. Look at the lecturer, try to maintain eye contact, and try to anticipate what is going to be said next. If distracted, bring concentration and focus back to the lecture as quickly as possible. Ask the professor to repeat any point that is unclear or missed, either at the end of the lecture or when there is an appropriate moment.

Step 8: Transform Concerns or Thoughts into Questions

Ask, "What is going to be covered today?" "How will the lecturer cover the topic in Chapter 3?" "What should I get out of this lecture in particular?" "Will she fully explain the concept that we heard last time and I don't really understand that well?" With such thoughts, you create interest. These and other questions can be asked before, during, or after a lecture.

Step 9: Maintain Focus and Concentration

Keep both mind and eyes focused on the speaker. Listen actively to what is being said. Focus attention on key elements and important details. Listen for the speaker's way of organizing the materials, and relate key points or concepts to one another. Be alert to tone, gesture, and repetition, especially surrounding key points, concepts, and ideas. Often a speaker will provide hints on what to expect in an examination with such statements as, "This would be useful to remember," or "This would be material for a quiz."

Step 10: Review, and Then Review Again

Is there a pattern emerging from today's lecture? Clarify anything that is unclear by asking questions at the end of the lecture. Look for implications beyond what has been said. Relate what has been said to what is already known from other classes.

Step 11: After Class

Attempt to clear up any questions raised by the lecture by asking either the teacher or a classmate. Fill in any missing details or misunderstood terms from the text or other sources. Edit class notes by labeling the main or key points. Add any recall cues and write questions to be answered through further reading. Use various colored pens to highlight key points and main ideas found in the lecture. If you make notes of personal ideas and reflections about the material, keep them separate from those of the speaker.

Step 12: Periodically Review Notes

Glancing over the notes from time to time is important, especially for recalling cues and to see how much is remembered before rereading the notes. The idea is to identify the emergence of themes, main concepts and their relationships with other details, and methods of presentation over the course of several lectures. Lecturers have different styles of presentation, and it is important to learn to recognize material and how it is organized and presented.

*D*ISPOSITIONS THAT SUPPORT GOOD THINKING

Historically, good thinking has been defined solely in terms of cognitive ability or skill. Many **critical thinking** courses or interventions are based on the notion of simply improving the student's cognitive skills, such as learning formal logic or problem-solving techniques. Good thinking does indeed require **cognition** and skill, but also much more. A passion for truth and a set of attitudes, values, and habits of mind all play a key role in good thinking. These habits of mind play an even larger part when combined with cognitive ability, such as using formal logic or learning and thinking skills strategies, since such habits are the governing values that help the learner use **thinking skills**. Good thinking, therefore, not only requires cognitive ability and skills, it also requires that the learner have the right set of thinking dispositions.

What is a **thinking disposition**? It is a pattern of behaviors that include cognition, motivation, and actions. For example, expert clinical nurses, those who demonstrate good clinical reasoning, have the tendency to identify and investigate clinical problems, to probe their own and others' assumptions, to seek sound reasons, and to be reflective while in action. Novice nurses similarly have the same cognitive ability and skills as the experts but often are not disposed to use them, even when invited to do so.

What kinds of dispositions should a student attempt to develop? According to the literature there are a number of dispositions that demonstrate a pattern of good thinking. One disposition is to be broad and adventurous rather then narrow and restricted in one's thinking. This disposition's tendency is based on the desire to be open-minded, to explore alternative views. Open-mindedness means to be alert toward narrowing one's thinking, and to seek the ability to generate multiple options rather than just one.

Another disposition is toward wondering and problem finding. It is a disposition that supports a zest for inquiry and for being alert for anomalies and puzzles. At its core is the ability to formulate questions and then to investigate carefully. From this disposition, one is led to a disposition to build explanations and understanding. Central to this disposition is the desire to explore the parts and purposes of things, and then to seek connections and explanations. At its core is the desire to actively use one's knowledge, based on the ability to build complex conceptualizations.

Critical thinking. The disposition to reason to and from evidence. The disposition to provide evidence in support of one's conclusions and to request evidence from others before accepting their conclusions. The process of determining the authenticity, accuracy, and worth of information or knowledge claims. To be reflective, mindful, and reasonable in one's thinking, which is focused on deciding what to believe or to do. To demonstrate a consistent pattern of mindful behavior that includes meta-cognition and motivation when engaged in learning or problem solving.

Cognition. The mental operations involved in thinking; the biological and neurological processes of the brain that facilitate thought.

Thinking skills. The set of basic and advanced skills (strategies) and subskills that govern (mediate) a person's mental processes: knowledge (declarative, procedural, and conditional), disposition (cognitive, motivational, and behavioral), and cognitive and meta-cognitive operations (ability to integrate and differentiate information).

Thinking disposition. The tendency toward a particular pattern of cognitive, motivational, and behavioral interactions.

A tendency toward wanting to use one's knowledge actively can also dispose one to make plans and to be strategic. Central to this disposition is the drive to formulate and set goals, and then to make and execute plans of actions to meet those goals. At its core is the ability to envision outcomes and to be alert to the lack of direction or purpose in one's thinking or actions. In order to remain alert against lack of direction or purpose, one must be disposed toward being intellectually careful, precise, organized, and thorough. Central to this disposition is the ability to remain alert to possible error or inaccuracy in one's thinking. At its core is the desire and ability to process information precisely.

The ability to seek and to process information precisely requires the disposition of seeking and evaluating reasons. The pattern of thinking within this disposition is one of questioning the given, of demanding justification, and remaining alert to the need for evidence. At its core is the ability to weigh and assess reasons and to recognize the difference between opinion and fact.

The last disposition is to be **meta-cognitive**. It is a pattern of thinking in which one is aware and can monitor the flow of one's own thinking and its products. It is to be aware that one is a thinker, and of the process by which one thinks. At its core is the ability to exercise executive control over thinking processes. Central to this disposition is the ability to reflect while in action.

Meta-cognition. The process of planning, assessing, and monitoring one's thinking; the pinnacle of mental functioning.

$\mathcal{C}$ONCLUSION AND CRITICAL POINTS

As we move from the twentieth century into the twenty-first, the ability to engage in careful, reflective thought is viewed as a fundamental characteristic of an educated person. It is fundamental because we have left the Industrial Age and have moved through the Information Age, into a post-Information Age. The cognitive, motivational, and behavioral ability to engage in careful, reflective thought is now viewed as a requirement for responsible citizenship and even as an essential skill for an increasingly wide range of jobs. Critical thinking is an essential characteristic needed to produce sound clinical reasoning in nursing.

This chapter has reviewed only a small portion of the research and literature surrounding thinking, learning, and study skills deemed necessary tools in a society characterized by rapid change, many alternatives of actions, and many individual and collective choices and decisions. A textbook is only a tool. It cannot create critical thinking or positive study habits. Critical thinking is not widespread and rote memorization still plays a central role in most students' subject-centered learning models. Most students do not score well on tests that measure the ability to recognize assumptions, evaluate arguments, and appraise inferences. However, the authors of this book firmly recognize that it is possible to increase one's creative and critical thinking capabilities through instruction and practice. To that end, the following chapters have been written with a view to improving critical/creative thinking.

$\mathcal{G}$LOSSARY

cognition   the mental operations involved in thinking; the biological and neurological processes of the brain that facilitate thought.

critical thinking   the disposition to reason to and from evidence. The disposition to provide evidence in support of one's conclusions and to request evidence from others before accepting their conclusions. The process of determining the authenticity, accuracy, and worth of information or knowledge claims. To be reflective, mindful, and reasonable in one's thinking, which is focused on deciding what to believe or to do. To demonstrate a consistent pattern of mindful behavior that includes meta-cognition and motivation when engaged in learning or problem solving.

meta-cognition   the process of planning, assessing, and monitoring one's thinking; the pinnacle of mental functioning.

thinking disposition   the tendency toward a particular pattern of cognitive, motivational, and behavioral interactions.

thinking skills   the set of basic and advanced skills (strategies) and sub-skills that govern (mediate) a person's mental processes: knowledge (declarative, procedural, and conditional), disposition (cognitive, motivational, and behavioral), and cognitive and meta-cognitive operations (ability to integrate and differentiate information).

$\mathcal{B}$IBLIOGRAPHY

BELLANCA, J. *The Cooperative Think Tank*. Chicago: Skylight Publishing, 1990. Chap. 5.

BUZAN, T. *The Mind Mapping Book*. London: BBC Books, 1993.

BUZAN, T. *Use Your Head*. London: BBC Publications, 1974. Chap. 4.

KESSELMAN-TURKEL, J., AND PETERSON, F. *Study Smarts*. Chicago: Contemporary Books, 1981. Chap. 9.

PAUK, W. *How to Study in College*. Boston: Houghton Mifflin, 1989. Chap. 3, 10.

SMITH, S., SHORE, L., AND BRITTAN, R. *Best Methods of Study*. New York: Barnes and Noble, 1955. Chap. 16.

SOTIRIOU, P. *Integrating College Study Skills*. Belmont, CA: Wadsworth, 1989. Chap. 11.

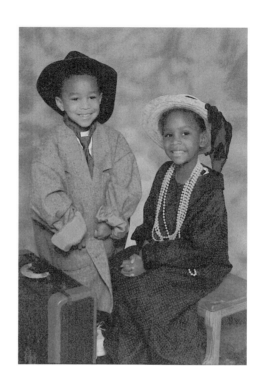

$\mathcal{P}$EDIATRIC ASSESSMENT

$\mathcal{I}$NTRODUCTION

This chapter introduces the essential components of a comprehensive pediatric assessment: taking a history and doing a physical assessment. Taking a patient's history and performing a physical assessment are necessary components in the problem-solving process used to make a diagnosis or to determine a patient's health status. The nurse must be able to reason or to think critically and clinically about the gathered information to generate a possible problem list and plan of care.

$\mathcal{D}$ATA COLLECTION, DATA PROCESSING, AND PROBLEM LISTS

The components of the history and pediatric assessment are very similar to those of a general adult assessment. Key differences or additions to a general assessment sequence will be indicated in the discussion. Although most of the techniques used to examine adults are applicable to infants, children, and adolescents, some methods are unique to the examination of infants (the first year of life), young children (1 to 4 years of age), older children (5 to 12 years of age), or adolescents (12 to 20 years of age).

Data gathering and processing are the chief critical thinking and reasoning processes used during physical assessment. In the data processing step the patient's database is transformed into a problem list that is a list of possible diagnoses. The transformation requires thinking critically about the data as evidence, and then using that evidence in support of one's conclusions as to the patient's chief problem. This transformation process is carried on throughout the collection of patient data. It continues when weighing every item in the history, during the physical examination, and in the laboratory studies. The transformation process is one of reasoning from evidence to some sort of conclusion. All the items gathered are critically evaluated in terms of their significance to the chief complaint, as well as to the various initial educated guesses as to its etiology or causes. Significance, in this context, is related to whether the information is considered a positive or a negative clue.

Positive or Negative Clues

A positive or negative clue can be defined as that bit of clinical information that guides or directs thinking while solving a clinical problem. Positive clues are considered significantly related to the chief complaint. Positive clues are grouped into meaningful and related clusters of data that suggest possible future diagnoses. Elevated temperatures at night, night sweats, and a history of several months of traveling in a Third World country, for example, are grouped together as possibly related with a tentative diagnosis of TB. Each of these clues is considered positively related to the diagnosis as well as the etiology. Clues found in the physical examination are considered positive when they are both present and are abnormal findings. Examples in the physical examination of positive clues are such things as elevated temperature, higher than normal respiratory rate, and weight considered greater or lesser than the norms for the child's age and sex. Positive clues in history taking can be hostile or aggressive behaviors, lack of age-appropriate immunizations, food or drug allergies, and poor feeding patterns. Diagnoses, then, are explanations that account for the positive clues, the data gathered from the history, and the physical assessment. The diagnosis or diagnoses should account for all of the positive clues and data gathered.

The absence of certain history or physical assessment clues may cancel one or more possible diagnoses for the chief complaint. Negative clues, then, are those items in the history, physical examination, or laboratory findings that are considered normal, or are not present. For example, negative clues might be that there is no cough; the neck veins are not distended; one hears no heart murmurs; and the chest x-ray demonstrates a clear lung field. Negative findings exclude certain possible explanations for a chief complaint simply by their nonexistence. In order to make diagnoses, one should have the associated positive clues in the history and physical examination, otherwise there is insufficient evidence or facts to support the diagnosis at the time.

Positive clues are as important as negative clues. When taken together, positive and negative clues balance the meaning of individual signs and symptoms in a particular clinical picture. Consider a young child who is having difficulty in breathing and is complaining of shortness of breath.

Upon assessment the nurse finds that the child has a mild fever, dry mucous membranes, a harsh barking cough, and appears mildly distressed. This clinical picture looks very different from a child who presents gravely ill with a moderate to high fever, complaining of difficulty in breathing, shortness of breath, and with inspiratory retractions and cyanosis. The positive clues for the first child indicate the child has a viral croup. This diagnosis is linked to the fact that this distress is seasonal, occurring in the late fall and early winter, and is highly associated with the child's clinical signs and symptoms. The second child presents with similar complaints but has a vastly different clinical picture. The positive clues of high fever, inspiratory retractions, and cyanosis indicate that the nurse is dealing with epiglottitis.

Negative clues serve best to rule out a tentative explanation for the chief complaint or a possible diagnosis. The fact that something does not exist as a clue or is absent may be considered a strong indicator that a particular disease in question does not exist in the patient. Pertinent negative findings or facts are often included on a history or physical assessment since they aid in one's decision making. Pertinent negative findings exclude the possibility of related hypotheses or explanations for the chief complaint's existence and force one to think of another explanation for the findings. Negative findings make the final diagnosis more probable, or more accurate, since the competing reasons or explanations have been excluded or at least considered less probable.

PROBLEM SOLVING, CLUES, AND THE NURSING PROCESS

The nursing process is a problem-solving process used to discover what is wrong with the patient and also to deal with issues of wellness and normalcy. The nursing process is considered a consistent and systematic approach to clinical problem solving or to clinical assessment. A comprehensive patient assessment is one part of such a systematic approach. The ability to use such a systematic approach is based upon the nurse's knowledge of normal growth and development, normal physiologic parameters, disease processes, their pathophysiology, and their signs and symptoms. Once the nurse develops the knowledge base and uses critical thinking and problem-solving skills, he/she is able to tackle the task of asking the correct questions and knowing where and when to search for additional clues.

A comprehensive assessment therefore requires critical thinking as well as good clinical reasoning and problem-solving skills. By being critically aware, the nurse can tell whether certain evidence provides the positive or negative clues needed to guide assessment. More often than not, positive and negative clues guide the choice of additional history questions to be asked or physical maneuvers to be done. The principal clues that a nurse seeks in a comprehensive assessment can be found primarily in the history and validated in the physical examination and diagnostic studies.

The clustering and rearranging of clues into meaningful groupings is part of the gathering and data-processing part of assessment. The key is *mean-*

ingful grouping of signs and symptoms that are related to one system, or one another. For example, nausea, vomiting, diarrhea, fever, and diffuse abdominal tenderness are related. One would then relate these to the GI tract.

Often students feel that only positive clues are significant and overlook essential negative clues. But, as stated before, negative clues are just as important when thinking critically about clinical evidence or when trying to decide on a course of action. The absence of clues is as important as their presence when thinking about underlying causes and processes. All information, positive or negative, must be critically evaluated in light of what is known. Because clues are the basic elements upon which many of the subsequent diagnostic steps will depend, their various types and properties will be reviewed throughout this chapter. Essential negatives for each portion of the history taking and physical examination will be included.

$\mathcal{S}$EQUENCE OF A COMPREHENSIVE ASSESSMENT

It is important to develop a consistent approach to a comprehensive assessment. The chief purpose of fact finding and data gathering is to arrive at a nursing diagnosis. Without accurate, timely, and comprehensive data, making an accurate diagnosis is not possible.

The general outline of a comprehensive examination begins with data collection organized on the patient's history, followed by a physical examination. A comprehensive history and physical are necessary for first-time visits and for yearly follow-ups. A general understanding of the patient's health history and medical status provides a foundation for moving into a more specific physical examination. During the history-taking process the nurse is able to develop a sense of trust with the caregiver and the patient. Here the nurse can take the time to answer questions, provide answers, teach, and show interest. History taking, unfortunately, is often the least perfected and most neglected nursing skill. Too often too few questions are asked, and then the physical examination is cursory.

The approach to history taking should allow the parent/caregiver to talk freely and to express concerns about any issues involving the child's health. The nurse should be able to show sympathy, politeness, humility, and a smile. Introduce yourself, telling the caregiver and the patient why you are there and what you want to do. Be as informal and relaxed as possible, but not overly familiar. Allow the parent/caregiver to express concerns and thoughts in his/her own words. Use silence and active listening, without making comments or clarifications of what is being said. This can promote a more open and friendly climate for the nurse, parent, and patient.

The nurse's observations during the interview often reveal additional information that otherwise would be unavailable. It is therefore essential to maintain a calm, open, observant, and low-key approach to the history-taking process. The interview should not be hurried. Allow the parent/caregiver or patient to provide the information.

At the beginning, ask mainly open-ended questions that encourage the patient or parent/caregiver to talk. For example, "Tell me more," "What about that?" "And then?" "Yes?" and "Bobby had pain?" are all invitations for the caregiver and/or the patient to continue. Specific closed-ended questions should come later. For example, questions like "Did the pain make you vomit?" or "make him vomit?" and "What was the color of Bobby's stools?" require simple answers. It is best not to ask questions that require a simple yes or no but rather ones that will provide data. Remember that you are gathering facts that will serve as evidence to support your educated guesses as to what is going on with the patient. You are attempting to solve a mystery through interviewing the chief source of information, the patient or the parent/caregiver. The facts should guide whatever questions you ask and physical examination procedures you do.

COMPREHENSIVE HISTORY

The following guidelines are provided as a means to sequence assessment and to develop a sense about what types of clinical clues to key in on while assessing the patient. This chapter does not replace a more thorough client assessment book but should reinforce that source of information. The focus of this section is on the general health assessment of the infant, child, or adolescent. At each stage of the assessment important differences from a generic assessment will be noted. At the end of each stage of the assessment critical thinking cues and clinical clues will be included.

The physical assessment that follows is broken down into general systems of the body. Even though we look at systems the assessment process should not be fragmented, but rather continuous, since the human body functions as a whole. The assessment begins the moment you first meet the infant, child, or adolescent patient and start to observe him/her. The health assessment normally begins with the collection of general information, followed by more specific information.

General Information

Record the patient's name (including nickname), the parents' names, home telephone number, and number where the parent or parents may be reached during working hours. Note the patient's age (in months and years), date of birth, marital status of parents and adolescents, occupation of parents and adolescents, sex, race, primary language spoken, and language understood. Include the date of the last visit to a health care agency and the source of referral if this is the first visit.

Normally health agencies have standard forms used for health assessments, which may require other general information. It is important to have enough identifying information noted on each page of the record so that the pages do not get misfiled. Document the historian's identification, such as whether or not the source is the patient or the patient's parent or guardian. Your judgment as to the accuracy and reliability of the historian's information should also be noted.

Clinical Clues/Critical Thinking Cues Important clues during this stage of information gathering center on the informant's manner of providing information. Uneasiness about providing details, inability to provide specifics, changing stories when asked for specifics, vague responses, and other such behaviors should alert you to potential problems, especially child abuse. Observe the quality and quantity of interaction between parents (if present), parents and patient, and with the nurse. If both parents are present, note who is the primary source of information concerning the health status, and if there are any disagreements concerning important events and data. The health interview for the adolescent is most critical for the development of trust between the health professional and the patient. It should be completed with the parents out of the room. The boundaries of confidentiality should be established early in the interview, so that the adolescent feels free to discuss sensitive issues. Health care providers need to be familiar with the laws of confidentiality involving adolescents.

Chief Complaint

This is the reason the patient or family sought health care. It should be stated in the patient's own words or paraphrased. Restatement of the information should be done only if you think that it makes the complaint more clear. It should be a complaint, such as a statement of symptoms, not a premature diagnosis, even if the patient or parent provides a diagnosis; for example, "vomiting since Monday" rather than "appears to have the flu."

Clinical Clues/Critical Thinking Cues It is important to note who has identified the chief complaint. In some cases a schoolteacher, a grandparent, a neighbor, or a physician may have expressed concern and requested the visit. Agreement between parents and other such referral sources is important to have and to record.

History of the Present Illness

Here you list and describe current symptoms of the chief complaint and their chronological appearance in reverse order (start with current symptoms and work backward to onset). Note and add to the list the absence (negative clues) of certain symptoms you might expect from the pattern of complaint. The narrative should answer questions related to where, what, when, and how much of symptoms. Ask either the parent or child to clarify the associated manifestations. Include any significant negatives expressed, such as, "The child denies feelings of fatigue during exercise," or "The mother states that the child does not appear to become fatigued with exercise." Use direct questions to focus on specific details/facts. Direct questions clarify and help interpret the symptoms.

If more than one complaint is stated, each new problem should be addressed in a separate paragraph. Include the following details of symptom occurrence:

1. Time intervals: time of day, duration, and changes in symptoms over time.
2. Character or quality: severity, location, and nature.
3. Association with certain events: during eating, activity, rest, sleep, etc.
4. Treatments: any and all attempts and their outcomes.
5. Interference with daily living.

Clinical Clues/Critical Thinking Cues Parents and the patient may need help in learning to identify and sort out details. What may be of importance to you may have no significance to the parent or patient. Ask for details and clarification of what is said in order to encourage the disclosure of data. When asking for details and clarification, persistent denial in the face of unexplained, inconsistent data or vaguely defined injuries alert you to possible child abuse.

Past Medical History (Infant, Child, and Teenager): General State of Health

This section should include appetite (poor, fair, good), recent weight losses or gains (if unexplained), fatigue, and stressors. Do not include information that already may have been gathered under chief complaint or present illness. List and describe the following with dates of occurrence and any specific information available:

1. All hospitalizations and illnesses, such as surgery, injuries, and disabilities, and major childhood illnesses.
2. Any previous health care contacts, such as past health examinations, immunizations, and laboratory studies with their dates and results.

Clinical Clues/Critical Thinking Cues When asking for details and clarification, persistent denial in the face of unexplained, inconsistent data or vaguely defined injuries should alert you to possible child abuse. A pattern of emergency room visits and a lack of consistency in care, such as obtaining required immunizations, may alert you to potential abuse or neglect.

Birth History (Including Prenatal and Neonatal History)

When discussing the birth history, include the prenatal and neonatal history as well. It is possible to make separate selections or subselections for these histories, especially if the assessment is focused on a neonatal health assessment; however, you can make one selection for the 1-month-old or older infant, child, and teenager.

For prenatal history ask questions about maternal health, sexually transmitted diseases (STDs), maternal purified protein derivative (PPD) status, medication taken, abnormal bleeding, weight gain, duration of the pregnancy, attitude toward the pregnancy, birth, birth order, duration of labor, type of delivery, complications, birth weight, and conditions of the infant at birth. The neonatal history should focus on respiratory distress, cyanosis, jaundice, seizures, poor feeding, patterns of sleeping, and length of stay in nursery.

Clinical Clues/Critical Thinking Cues An accurate and in-depth birth history (prenatal and neonatal histories included) is important, especially if there are developmental delays or neurological problems, and if the child is less than 2 years of age.

Feeding History (Infant and Child)

Include type of feeding (bottle, breast, solid foods), frequency of feedings, quantity of feeds, responses to feedings, and any specific problems with feeding (such as colic, regurgitation, lethargy, allergic reactions). Ask about parental concerns. For children, assess their self-feeding abilities, food preferences, general appetite, and amounts of food taken.

Clinical Clues/Critical Thinking Cues Development delays, such as reluctance to move to solid foods, demanding a bottle instead of solid food, or not feeding self should alert the nurse to potential developmental, behavioral, or parenting issues. At this point in the assessment this is an area where diet and nutrition teaching can be done.

Growth and Development

If possible the health care records of the patient should be obtained. If not the parents should be asked to recall the patient's approximate height and weight at 1, 2, 5, and 10 years of age, and when the first tooth eruption/ loss occurred. This information is important in order to prevent future problems or to predict patterns of growth and development.

Clinical Clues/Critical Thinking Cues Is the patient within norms for growth for his/her age group? If not, the contributing factors should be the focus of specific questions. If the patient is obese or underweight, this should alert the nurse to potential health risks as well as neglect. If the patient is extremely tall or short for the age group, this should also alert the nurse to investigate potential risks.

Development History (Infant and Child)

Assess at what age the child was able to roll over, sit alone without support, crawl, walk, speak his/her first words and first sentence, and dress without help.

Clinical Clues/Critical Thinking Cues A complete and thorough growth and development history (physical and social) is important in planning any form of intervention. Any intervention needs to be appropriate to the patient's level. Concurrently, the assessment also focuses on screening for developmental and neurological problems. The social assessment focuses on the potential need for guidance.

Behavior and Social History

Though associated with developmental history, this section is separated because the focus is on behaviors, especially social ones. Include the age that the child began toilet training; when the child was able to achieve both night and day control or his/her current level of control; and any problems associated with enuresis, encopresis, and self-toileting abilities. What terminology does the child use when discussing toileting? Note amount and patterns of sleep, both during the day and at night. Are there any bedtime rituals? Does the child use any security objects (such as a favorite toy), express any particular fears, or have any recurring nightmares? Note speech production, especially as to quality and quantity of speech, lisping, stuttering, and intelligibility. Note the child's level of awareness of his/her sexuality, interaction with the opposite sex, level of inquisitiveness about sexual information and sexual activity, and the type of information provided to the child by a caregiver. Also note school progress, grade level, level of academic achievement, and adjustment to school.

Note any particular habits, such as nail or lip biting, thumb sucking, pica, head banging, or others that appear unusual (excessive hitting, biting, and other habits expressed toward others). What forms of discipline do the parents use? What methods of discipline do the parents favor, such as time out, rewarding appropriate behavior, or use of verbal and physical threats? Has any mental health screening been done in conjunction with behavioral problems, such as for attention deficit disorders?

What is your assessment of the patient's personality and temperament? Does the child appear congenial, overly aggressive, display temper tantrums, or act overly shy and withdrawing? What is the child's relationship to other children and family?

Ask children and teenagers if they ever feel sad or down. If they say yes, ask if they ever think of harming or killing themselves. The health care provider should know that there is a difference between suicidal ideation, suicide attempt, and suicide. It is not uncommon for adolescents and older children to experience occasional suicidal thoughts. Expressions of suicidal preoccupation need to be taken seriously, and the assessment should be done by an appropriate professional.

Clinical Clues/Critical Thinking Cues Behavioral and social development clues provide important diagnostic and intervention information. Hearing-impaired children, children who experience abnormal fears, and children who have aggressive behaviors will have very different temperaments. Children who have chronic conditions are often more intense, more withdrawn, and more negative in mood than healthy children. Children, especially boys, who come from homes that value aggressiveness, violence, and other forms of impulsiveness often tend to bully, be argumentative, and have temper tantrums. Such children often have short attention spans and learning disabilities, and will act out, especially in stressful situations. Girls who come from violent homes are more often withdrawn and depressed and tend to cling and be perfectionists. Infants and children born to women with drug- and alcohol-related problems tend to have low impulse control, learning disabilities, and sleep difficulties.

Immunization History

Record specific details of immunizations (dates, types, and reactions). If the parent has any records of previous immunizations they should be copied and filed in the child's record. If the child has not been immunized, note the reasons. It is important to note the patient's reactions to various immunizations, especially allergic reactions. Note any desensitization procedures, such as the measles-mumps-rubella (MMR) vaccine. Screening tests, such as the tuberculin test, blood examinations, and other laboratory studies in conjunction with immunizations should be noted as well. If the parent reports that the immunization records have been lost, advise him/her that most likely copies of those records are in the school the child has attended.

When discussing immunizations the nurse should find out if anyone in the family is immunosuppressed. Some vaccines can be dangerous to a family member who is immunosuppressed.

Clinical Clues/Critical Thinking Cues If the patient was born outside the United States, or has lived or vacationed for long periods of time outside the United States, additional desensitization procedures may have been performed. Certain immunizations or medications are required for travel to developing nations as well. It is important, therefore, to ask such questions in order to obtain a comprehensive list of all immunizations done and for what reasons.

Current Medications

Include any over-the-counter as well as prescription drugs, their dose, frequency, and the time of the last dose. Include the reason for giving the medication, and whether the child had any side effects or intolerance to the medication.

The goal of the assessment of allergies is the prevention of an allergic reaction. The assessment should obtain information on all the allergic reactions that the patient has, such as fever or headaches, hives, and so on. These reactions are usually caused by allergens such as drugs, food, dust, and animals.

Clinical Clues/Critical Thinking Cues It is important to know the patient's medication usage as well as his/her allergies. Reactions to medications, especially allergic reactions, should be recorded, clarified, and interpreted. Mark the patient chart appropriately and prominently to indicate the allergy. Some reactions considered allergic by the parent or patient are, in fact, not allergic but simply a side effect. Often one can intervene with teaching about such misinterpretations. Overdependence on prescription drugs, especially antibiotics, for viral or other conditions that do not require such drugs needs to be clarified with parents.

History of Past Illnesses, Injuries, or Operations

In obtaining information about previous illness, the focus should be on recognizing recurrent illnesses and/or injuries and their resolution—where (location), what (quality), and how long (time) they lasted. Ask about typical childhood diseases and illnesses. What kinds of operations were performed, when, and what was the outcome? Find out the name of the hospital and its location. Record specific dates of operations.

Family History

Information about the health of family members may be recorded in the form of a genogram. A genogram is a graphic representation of a family system. It may cover several generations. It facilitates recognition of areas that require change. Genograms are an efficient way of gathering a great deal of information in a small amount of space. They can also be used as teaching tools with the family. Genograms offer an overall picture of the life of the family over several generations, including roles that various family members play. Areas that need change can be easily identified as well as areas that produce support and help for the family.

Family Members This section should include parents, grandparents, aunts and uncles, siblings, spouse, and children. For deceased family members, note the age at time of death and cause of death, if known.

Major Health and/or Genetic Disorders Include any history of hypertension; cancer; cardiac, respiratory, renal, cerebrovascular, or thyroid disorders; asthma or other allergic manifestations; blood dyscrasias; psychiatric difficulties; and tuberculosis, diabetes mellitus, hepatitis, immunosuppression, or other familial disorders.

Personal/Social History of the Family The information included in this section varies according to the concerns of the patient and/or guardian/parent, and the influence of the health problem on the patient's life as a family member. The focus of the family's personal and social history is that the family is a dynamic interactive system, and the patient is best understood in the context of those interactions.

Similar to the idea of homeostasis within the body, which means to keep a balance in all the body systems, family members covertly or overtly act to maintain a balance in their relationships. Family homeostasis is largely revealed through the repetitious, circular, and predictable communication patterns established among the members. Whenever the homeostasis is threatened or is in precarious balance, members will exert large amounts of effort to maintain it. According to this view of family dynamics, parents, other family members, and the patient cannot be considered the family unit when assessed separately since such assessment lacks the observation of the dynamics of the interactions that produce a family homeostasis. The nurse should focus on the quality, quantity, and type of the interactions (specific communication patterns) expressed among and between family members. Several factors are considered to influence the development and maintenance of such homeostatic communication patterns.

Cultural Background Culture has a major influence on how a family member, a parent, and a patient come to view an illness and how that concern is expressed within the family. Cultural interpretations of an illness and its relation to the patient, the family, the parent, and other such factors need to be assessed in order to produce an intervention that is acceptable and will be followed. Mainstream health care may not have been the parent's first choice; alternative or nontraditional methods may have been tried first. It is important to assess these choices.

It is important to ask the parent and patient how long they have lived in the country or in a particular area. First- and second-generation families are still attempting to incorporate into the mainstream culture. The dynamics between first-generation and second- or third-generation family members can be a source of support or distress. It is important to ask if the family identifies with a particular ethnic group or region, and if so, how such identification influences their life-style, particularly their choices in health care interventions, since such information can affect care.

It is also important for the health care professional to remember that sometimes the personal beliefs of the family affect the interpretation of illness.

Family Homeostasis, Structures, and Function The family structure and its homeostatic relationships can be related to who is at home, who works, and what the family sees as a stress. Equally, what is considered a pressing personal problem, what events are considered part of a typical day, and what is considered a source of family strength or weakness also can come from the family's structure and its attempts to maintain homeostasis. The health problem and the family's response to illness need to be assessed as to their impact on family homeostasis expressed in the family's internal and external structure, family function (specifically, communication patterns), and the family's current stage of development (in the eight stages of family development).

Internal and External Family Structure The internal structure of the family refers to the family composition. Included in the assessment of the internal structure is the rank order of the members (who is considered the head of the family, etc.), especially as to birth order and gender of the children. Subunits within a family are often marked by sex, role, interests, or age. It is important to ask if such subunits exist.

External family structure refers to those elements outside of the family. These elements are how the family relates to the community. Community relationships include school, church, friends, work, and extended family interactions.

Family Boundaries An assessment of family boundaries refers to discovering who is part of what system or subsystem within the family. Of particular importance is whether the boundaries are considered closed, open, rigid, or permeable. Rigidity of boundaries—such as who speaks to whom about what or who makes the decisions in the family—are important to know since these boundaries can influence care. It is important to discover who in the family is normally approached with concerns, especially health concerns, since he/she can influence care outcomes. The assessment of the family as to its internal and external structure is appropriate for a general practitioner, whereas family therapy falls in the realm of advanced practice and preparation.

Clinical Clues/Critical Thinking Cues Internal family structure can best be captured using a genogram that lists at least three generations of the family structure and functions (grandparents, relatives, parents, and children). The genogram is an excellent means by which to clarify and interpret information in relation to family composition and interactions. Using the genogram the nurse can ask for information to identify decision-making or problem-solving relationships. Losses or additions to families often result in crisis. It is important to note how the family interprets and reacts to such events within its functional and structural aspects.

Within the family structure, position (oldest to youngest) is thought to influence structural and functional relationships. Older children are considered more conscientious; the youngest child is often viewed as playful and less responsible. Older daughters will assume mothering roles with younger children. Note how a patient is referred to, such as the youngest or oldest, the best, the brightest, etc., which may signal that they have been assigned a particular role in the family. This role may not be a comfortable one for the parent or the patient. Sometimes the patient is assigned a role that is dysfunctional, such as surrogate parent to younger children or even surrogate spouse. Such dysfunctional roles may need more investigation.

A family that displays rigid boundaries and reports having become distanced or disengaged from other family members may need further investigation, as well as the family in which the father has assigned all family concerns to mother or oldest daughter and has become disengaged from the family. Rigid boundaries or closed boundaries influence interfamilial communication and attempting to change them may cause homeostasis-protective responses. In rigid-boundary families children are often used to communicate family matters between parents, other family members, extended family members, and even the community.

The internal and external structure of the family, choice of parenting practices, the development and use of communication channels, and various role boundaries may be influenced by ethnicity and culture. It is, therefore, important to assess cultural and ethnic influences on family structure, function, and boundaries before coming to conclusions of neglect or abuse.

Education, Mobility, and Economic Status Like culture, educational level, mobility, and economic status may play an important part in how the family interprets and reacts to an illness. Education, mobility, and economic status help mold family values. Assess work moves, job satisfaction, and transportation. The impact of illness on a family's resources (economic, social, and psychological) can be considerable. A family's homeostatic strengths and weaknesses play a part in how members interpret and respond, adaptively or not, to an illness.

Family Environment A family's environment includes home, neighborhood, school, work, and community. Within this context, the focus of the assessment is whether environmental barriers exist. For example, if one of the family members has a disability, is there handicap access within the home? What are the community services available and which services are used?

Clinical Clues/Critical Thinking Cues Various environmental stressors, such as a high level of street noise, an uncertain or poor water supply, poor sanitation, overcrowding, lack of housing, lack of playgrounds, lack of transportation (such as bus or train services), and poor handicap access can all influence a family's environmental health.

Stages of Family Development Normally the age and school placement of the oldest child can be used to decide the family's stage of development. With the birth of the first child the family moves from stage 1, which is the formation of a marriage unit, to stage 2, which is a family with an infant. The family enters stage 3 when that first child becomes a preschooler, and enters stage 4 when that first child enters school. Stage 5 is when that first child becomes a teenager, and stage 6 occurs when that first child leaves the home. The family remains in stage 6 until the last child leaves the home. Once the last child leaves, the family enters stage 7. Stage 8 is entered when the parents start retirement and ends with the death of the spouses.

Clinical Clues/Critical Thinking Cues Recognizing the family's developmental stage aids the nurse in forming questions, such as: What was the impact on the parents of the birth of their first child? Their second child? Now that the first child has started school, how do the parents feel? A family moves, with starts and stops, through each of the stages, and at each stage there are developmental issues that are normally resolved through homeostatic structural and functional mechanisms. Families that remain fixed in one stage and cannot seem to move to the next may require an intervention. For example, often one sees a family with a teenager who is still being treated like a small dependent child. Death and divorce can also influence the family's ability to move through stages.

Instrumental Functioning The focus of this portion of the assessment is on the routine and the mechanics of eating, dressing, and sleeping, or the patterns of daily life in the family. The impact of an ill infant, child, or teenager on the family's ability to have daily routines, as well as the impact of an illness on those routines, should be considered.

Clinical Clues/Critical Thinking Cues A chronically ill or acutely ill family member may alter the family's patterns of instrumental functioning. The disruption of normal habits and routines needs to be assessed.

Expressive Functioning Some families may have affective issues or may lack the ability to express both positive and negative emotions, thoughts, ideas, and feelings within the family structure. It is important to decide if the family is functioning at an appropriate expressive level. If the family is unable to effectively deal with distress and stress through emotional channels, some sort of intervention may be in order.

Clinical Clues/Critical Thinking Cues Often a family will refuse to show emotional support for an ill family member. Some members may even prevent other members from showing such support. This may indicate poor intrafamilial communication and may require some sort of intervention.

Emotional Communication Homeostatic family communication patterns include emotional communications. The nurse needs to assess the range and type of emotions that are expressed or not expressed within the family. One means of gathering these data is to ask how the family handles a particular stress, such as the death of a family pet. The nurse can ask how sadness and anger are expressed and who is considered the most expressive in the family.

Clinical Clues/Critical Thinking Cues Often emotional expressiveness or communication can be characterized as rigid and inappropriate for the given event or situation. In alcoholic families emotional responses are narrow and rigid. Boys may be encouraged to be less expressive or narrower in their verbal and nonverbal behaviors than girls. Cultural and ethnicity factors must be explored, since these factors can play a major role in what emotional communication channels are deemed appropriate within a family's structure.

Verbal Communication The level, quality, and quantity of verbal communication can be observed through the dynamic interactions between parent and child as the nurse takes the history. Verbal communication patterns can be validated by clarifying them with the individuals involved, using such statements as, "What is your mom telling you?" and then observing the response patterns that develop.

Through simply observing the communication pattern between a parent and child during the interview, one can see verbal and nonverbal communication patterns on several levels. Who is speaking, and who is listening? Who speaks for whom, and on what level? When a parent makes a statement and then looks at the child or the other parent for a nonverbal response, or when the child speaks and then validates what has been said by looking at a parent, the nurse can begin to develop an assessment of the family's communication pattern and whether it is adaptive or maladaptive (facilitates or obscures what is being communicated and how it is communicated). If a mother answers for the child, if the child is speaking and the parent frequently interrupts, or if the child interrupts the parent or ignores what has been said, the family does not have a facilitative communication pattern.

Clinical Clues/Critical Thinking Cues Dysfunctional or maladaptive communication patterns of both the sender and the receiver tend to belittle or obscure rather than to clarify what has been said. Often a triangular pattern emerges; one member communicates with another through a third member. In another pattern one person interprets the thoughts and feelings of another without validation or permission to do so. One means of intervening is to ask for clarification and validation from the person for whom the other is speaking, by asking, for example, "Mary, do you agree with what your mother just said?"

Problem Solving The problem-solving assessment focuses on the family's ability to handle its own problems as a functional unit. One means of assessing problem solving is to ask which family member notices a problem first, how decisions are then made about the problem, and how the problem is resolved.

Clinical Clues/Critical Thinking Cues Dysfunctional families tend to employ a narrow or limited set of strategies in problem solving and decision making. Often such a family continues to use inappropriate strategies even after they appear not to work or do not produce the desired outcome. The inability to reframe a problem and to consistently see a problem from one narrow perspective restricts their ability to develop and use more appropriate strategies.

Roles Roles are established patterns of behaviors over time. The focus should be on the flexibility or rigidity of the roles developed within the family and whether or not certain idiosyncratic roles are applied to specific family members. Stages of family development suggest that roles change over time. "He has always been a problem child," or "He has been a quiet kid," are indicators of role assignments that are rigid and narrowly defined.

Clinical Clues/Critical Thinking Cues Dysfunctional families often assign narrowly defined, restricted roles for various family members. These roles do not allow for flexibility and change, for either the individual or the family.

Control Homeostasis requires the manipulation and control of behaviors by family members. Such control is seen as necessary in order to maintain balance in family relationships. Assessment should focus on the types of control that are used. Such control can be psychological through the communication of feelings and thoughts. Another form is the use of physical threats and corporal punishment or reinforcement, such as the use of spankings, hugging, or holding. Another means is instrumental, such as using privileges or objects to gain control. "If you behave here in the clinic I will buy you a toy later" is an example of an instrumental form of control.

Controls are normally expressed through rules, so it is important to assess the development and use of family rules and what occurs if such rules are broken. Who is responsible for enforcing the rules? What is the level of the children's involvement in rule making and enforcement?

Clinical Clues/Critical Thinking Cues Excessive issues surrounding control and family chaos in relation to rules and their consistency in use may indicate an abusive family structure. The function of rules is to keep or to gain homeostasis. Yet rigid and narrowly defined rules that are excessively enforced or chaotically enforced indicate a potentially abusive pattern.

Alliances/Coalitions What are the balance and intensity of the relationships among and between various family members? Homeostasis requires that family members form and use alliances and coalitions in order to resolve issues of power and control. Such alliances and coalitions can be adaptive or maladaptive mechanisms. Alliances and coalitions can be observed by seeing how issues and problems that come up in the interview process are resolved in the family. Do the parents work together as a team or do they appear to ally themselves against each other using one or more of the children? Are there coalitions, such as mother and son against the father or other family members? Alliances and coalitions across generations should be noted and clarified.

Clinical Clues/Critical Thinking In sexually abusive families one often sees a father and daughter coalition that has supplanted the spousal relationship.

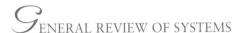

GENERAL REVIEW OF SYSTEMS

The general review of physical systems includes the following items. This review requires changes to reflect the particular age and sex of the person being assessed. Clearly some questions or portions will not be appropriate and therefore should be excluded.

1. General: weight, recent weight change, fatigue, fever.
2. Skin: rashes, lumps, sores, itching, dryness, color change, changes in hair or nails.
3. Eyes: vision, glasses or contact lenses, date of last eye examination, pain, redness, excessive tearing, double vision, spots, specks, flashing lights, glaucoma, cataracts.
4. Ears: hearing, tinnitus, vertigo, earaches, infection, discharge.
5. Nose and sinuses: frequent colds, nasal stuffiness, discharge, itching, hay fever, nosebleeds, sinus trouble.
6. Mouth and throat: condition of teeth and gums, bleeding gums, last dental examination, sore tongue, frequent sore throats, hoarseness.
7. Neck: lumps, pain, "swollen glands," goiter, pain or stiffness in the neck.
8. Breasts: lumps, pain or discomfort, nipple discharge, self-examination.
9. Respiratory: cough, sputum (color, quantity), hemoptysis, wheezing, asthma, bronchitis, pneumonia, tuberculosis, pleurisy, last chest x-ray.
10. Cardiac: congenital heart defects, high blood pressure, rheumatic fever, heart murmurs, chest pain or discomfort, palpitation, dyspnea, trouble with gaining weight, muscle weakness, hypotension, bradycardia, irritability.
11. Gastrointestinal: trouble swallowing, heartburn, appetite, nausea, vomiting, regurgitation, vomiting of blood, indigestion, frequency of bowel movements, color and size of stools, changes in bowel habits, rectal bleeding or black tarry stools, hemorrhoids, constipation, diarrhea, abdominal pain, food intolerance, excessive belching or passing of gas, jaundice, liver problems, hepatitis.
12. Urinary: frequency of urination, polyuria, nocturia, burning or pain on urination, hematuria, urgency, reduced caliber or force of the urinary stream, hesitancy, enuresis, incontinence, urinary infections, stones.
13. Genital—male: hernias, penile discharge or sores, testicular pain or masses, any STDs and their treatments, exposure to AIDS, precautions taken against AIDS and other STDs, sexual interest, orientation, function, satisfaction, and problems; contraceptive methods.
14. Genital—female: age at menarche, regularity, frequency, and duration of periods; amount of bleeding, bleeding between periods or after intercourse, last menstrual period, dysmenorrhea, premenstrual tension, discharge, itching, sores, lumps, any STDs and their treatments, exposure to AIDS, precautions taken against AIDS and other STDs, number of pregnancies, number of deliveries, number of abortions (spontaneous and induced), complications of pregnancy, contraceptive methods, sexual interest, orientation, function, satisfaction, and problems, including dyspareunia.
15. Peripheral vascular: murmurs, signs of congestive heart failure (CHF), machinery-like murmur, bounding pulses.

16. Musculoskeletal: muscle or joint pains, stiffness, arthritis, backache. If present, describe the location and associated symptoms (swelling, redness, pain, tenderness, stiffness, weakness, limitation of motion or activity).
17. Neurologic: fainting, blackouts, seizures, weakness, paralysis, numbness, tingling, tremors or other involuntary movements.
18. Hematologic: anemia, easy bruising or bleeding, past transfusions and possible reactions.
19. Endocrine: thyroid trouble, heat or cold intolerance, excessive sweating, diabetes, excessive thirst, hunger, polyuria.
20. Psychiatric: nervousness, tension, mood including depression, any suicidal ideation, memory, school performance.

$\mathcal{C}$OMPREHENSIVE PHYSICAL EXAMINATION

Although most techniques used to examine adults are applicable to infants and children, some are used only for infants (the first year of life), younger children (1 to 4 years of age), or older children (5 to 12 years). Below is a general outline of a physical examination. For a complete description consult a textbook written expressly for that purpose.

What follows is a generic overview of a physical examination. Where differences exist between the age groups above, they will be noted as to the specific age group and the particular method recommended. The physical examination of an adolescent (age 13 to 20 years) is considered essentially the same as that of an adult. Clinical clues and critical thinking cues will be provided where needed.

Preparation for the Examination

It is best not to perform a physical assessment on an infant or child in areas that he/she considers "safe." Avoid the child's bed, bedroom, and play area. Toys and other distractions should be within easy reach for the nurse and used to help facilitate the assessment. Keep fans, air conditioners, radios, telephones, beepers, and the like quiet. Noise can be a distraction and lowers your ability to concentrate on patient-produced sounds. Be sure that the examination room is comfortable and not drafty.

Make sure that all equipment is in working order before beginning the physical examination. Anything considered threatening or strange should be kept out of eyesight of the child. Warm your hands and the equipment before placing them on the child. This requires some practice in organizing, collecting, and analyzing data and writing in the appropriate area on the chart. The general assessment helps establish priorities. Obvious areas of distress, such as the child experiencing pronounced respiratory problems or abdominal pain, are a priority in the health history as well as the physical assessment.

General Guidelines for the Physical Assessment of Infant and Child

Generally one follows a head-to-toe approach while collecting the health history and the vital signs. The general assessment is done to establish priorities. Areas of distress quickly indicate systems that require immediate health history and physical assessment. Children and infants cannot fully express what is wrong with them. It is essential for the nurse to develop a means of quickly and accurately assessing what is wrong. The caregiver may be able to assist and to communicate concerns of the child that come up during the assessment. Clearly some of the complete assessment features may be omitted during daily assessment, depending on the child's age, health status, and the reasons for the health care contact. Height, head circumference, weight, deep tendon reflex, and neurologic tests need not always be done. Their omission must always be weighed against the value of the information that might have been gained in attempting to decide on the underlying cause of the complaint.

An orderly, systematic approach may not always be possible. Sometimes you have to vary the sequence to accommodate the child. Flexibility is essential, but all aspects of the examination must eventually be covered.

Often several examinations of one area must be done because of its size or because of the need for repeated measurements to assure yourself of accurate findings. This is especially true when observing and evaluating respiratory rate in an infant. It is necessary to observe the type and quality of the respiration, the presence or absence of retractions, the color of the trunk, and whether there is a heave under the nipple.

While gathering a general health history you can be taking vital signs and beginning a head-to-toe physical examination. Working quickly and calmly, talking both with the child and the parent, you can gather a great deal of data. You should perform the least distressing aspects of the examination first. What is distressing to one age group may not be for another so you must key in on the particular child's reactions to what you are doing during the assessment. It is important to use a firm but kind approach. Being overly talkative, asking for too much detail, or being short or curt with either the child or parent may result in the child becoming uncooperative. It is best to tell the child what you are about to do rather than to ask his/her permission. Never leave an infant or child unattended on an examining room table.

Age-Related Approaches to the Physical Assessment

Infant (1 to 18 Months) If the parent is willing he/she may aid you by holding the child during most of the examination, especially during the eyes and mouth assessment. Approach an infant in a quiet and gentle manner. Either you or the parent should remove all the infant's clothing, except the diaper for a male infant. If need be you can distract the infant with brightly colored toys, play peek-a-boo games, and talk quietly with the child. Vary the sequence according to the infant's activity level. Auscultate the lungs, heart, and abdomen at the beginning of the examination or when the infant is not crying or extremely active. Take a rectal temperature and perform other painful or intrusive examinations near the end or at the end of the examination.

Toddler (18 Months to 3 Years) The assessment sequence is similar to that recommended for an infant. Depending on the level of apprehension and level of activity, sequence the assessment so that you do the least intrusive assessments at the beginning and the most intrusive at the end. Allow the toddler to hold various pieces of equipment and gradually introduce and use the equipment. Throughout the assessment approach the toddler quietly and calmly, keeping physical contact low until the toddler is acquainted with you. As with the infant allow the toddler to remain near or in the parent's lap during most of the physical examination.

Preschool-Age Child (3 to 6 Years) Like the toddler, the preschooler should be allowed to stay close to the parent. You can use play to approach the child. Allow the child to handle equipment, and introduce and use equipment in a calm and professional manner. Answer any questions with short answers. If the child becomes upset or even apprehensive, complete your assessment as quickly as possible. Expose the child as little as possible by removing only that piece of clothing needed to complete a part of the assessment. Let the parent remove the clothing and allow the child to replace the clothing once that portion of the assessment is done. Be sure to use praise during the assessment when the child is cooperative, but not too much. Allow the child to hold comfort items such as a blanket or favorite toy. Those portions of the assessment that require the child to lie down should be done last.

School-Age Child (6 to 12 Years) Allow the child the choice of having the parent in the examination room. Allow the child the right to remove his/her own clothing and give him/her a gown to wear. Introduce and use equipment calmly and professionally, and allow the child to handle the equipment. At this age questions concerning the functions of the equipment can be answered.

Adolescent (12 Years and Older) Like the school-age child, the adolescent should have the choice of having the parent in the examination room. Give him/her the right to undress in private and an appropriate gown to use. Provide time for the adolescent to regain his/her self-composure before beginning the examination. Introduce equipment and procedures in a calm and professional manner, allowing the adolescent to ask questions about the purpose of the equipment or the portion of the examination being done. Findings and feedback should be at a level that the adolescent can understand. The kind and level of feedback are judgment calls that often require clarification with the adolescent and other professionals. It is important to answer any questions in a professional manner.

Measurements

Temperature Take the child's temperature in the axilla, rectum, mouth, or ears, as appropriate for his/her age and condition. Temperature may be affected by environment, exercise, stress, crying, or time of day. Hyperthermia may be an objective sign of infection, hyperthyroidism, heat exposure, collagen-vascular disease, or tumor. Hypothermia occurs with exposure to cold, inactivity, ingestion of certain drugs, and overwhelming infection.

Pulse Take the pulse with the child at rest; it may be palpated at any peripheral pulse or over the heart. Radial pulses are readily accessible for children over 2 years of age; the temporal and apical pulse areas may be the ideal sites for infants and small children. Ranges of pulse rates may vary from 70 to 170 beats per minute at birth to 120 to 140 at 1 to 2 years and 70 to 115 after 3 years. After the age of 2 variation in pulse rate when the child is awake may be about less than 20 from the pulse rate when asleep. Pulse rate increases about 10 beats per minute for each degree of temperature elevation. Exercise, excitement, and hypermetabolic states increase pulse rate; decreased activity and hypometabolic states decrease pulse rate. Irregularities in the pulse rate may arise from sinus arrhythmia or from other heart disorders.

Respiration Measure the respiratory rate by observing abdominal movement in the infant or chest wall movement in the older child. Take the respiratory rate when the child is rested or quiet. Variations in respiratory rate occur with age. Normal newborn rates are 30 to 80 breaths per minute, decreasing to rates of 20 to 40 per minute in early infancy and childhood, then 15 to 25 per minute in late childhood and adolescence. Anxiety, exercise, acidosis, infection, and hypermetabolic states increase heart rate; central nervous system problems, depressants, alkalosis, and poisons decrease respiratory rate.

Blood Pressure Choose the appropriate cuff size when determining blood pressure. The width should cover two-thirds of the upper arm or the thigh with the length of the cuff completely encircling the extremity. Consult age-specific percentiles in blood pressure measurements. A quick way of determining normal systolic blood pressure ranges for ages 1 to 7 years is to add 90 to the age in years. For ages 8 to 18 years, add two times the age in years plus 90. The normal systolic blood pressure for ages 1 to 5 years is 56 and for ages 6 to 18 years, add 52 to the age in years. Readings above the ninety-fifth percentile of age and sex taken after three separate readings should be considered abnormal.

Height, Weight, and Head Circumference Height and weight measurements are obtained with the child supine from infancy up to 2 years, then upright thereafter. Head circumference is measured in all infants and toddlers less than 2 years of age and for children with misshapen heads. Compare these measurements to height, weight, and head circumference measurement percentiles specific for gender.

Short stature may be a family pattern or may indicate chronic illness, malabsorption, hormonal problems, psychological deprivation, or syndromes associated with dwarfism. Heights greater than the ninety-fifth percentile may be from genetic inheritance or may indicate pituitary problems. Head circumference not within the fifth and ninety-fifth percentiles may indicate pathology indicative of microcephaly or macrocephaly.

Skin-Fold Measurements Measurement of skin fold is useful in determining obesity and progress in the management of this health problem. Use skin-fold calipers to measure the skin and subcutaneous tissue at the mid-upper arm.

General Appearance

Observations of the child's alertness, distress, playfulness, development, nutrition, and grooming are included in a general description of the child. Any unusual behavior, posture, or activity may alert the nurse to the presence or absence of a health problem. The child who lies quietly with hands open and stares blankly indicates serious illness. The child who is quiet when lying and cries intensely when held may indicate the presence of pain on motion. Disturbances in gait, facial expression, eye contact, and signs of distress are observations included in documenting the general appearance of the child.

Skin, Hair, and Nails

Examination of the skin, hair, and nails is done by inspection and palpation. Skin examination includes an overall visual sweep of the body, inspecting each area for color, uniformity, symmetry, thickness, hygiene, and presence of any lesions. Palpate the skin to assess moisture, temperature, turgor, and mobility.

Record the skin assessment findings and the condition of the scalp, hair, and nails. Changes in skin color may indicate normal variations, as in the bluish discoloration of mongolian spots or the brownish café-au-lait spots that may indicate possible **neurofibromatosis**. Jaundice indicates the presence of excess amounts of bile pigments in the circulation, seen in liver disease. Cyanosis is a manifestation of decreased amounts of oxyhemoglobin, which may indicate **acrocyanosis**, a benign condition in newborns, or a serious condition such as cardiac anomalies or upper airway obstruction.

Describe the characteristics of lesions, including type, size, color, blanching, texture, elevation or depression, presence of exudate, shape or configuration, pattern of arrangement, location, and distribution. These descriptions support the diagnosis of specific skin disorders.

Neurofibromatosis. A genetic disorder affecting neural tissue growth, presenting as multiple hyperpigmented areas with the appearance of multiple cutaneous and subcutaneous tumors in late childhood.

Acrocyanosis. Bluish discoloration of the hands and feet, normal for infants during the first hour of birth; can occur after that time also.

Head, Face, and Neck

Note the shape, symmetry, size, and any defects of the head, and the size and tension of the fontanels. A large head may indicate macrocephaly, hydrocephalus, or an intracranial growth. Small head size may indicate microcephaly or lack of brain development. Observation of head size is correlated with head circumference measurements.

Inspection of the face alerts the examiner to syndromes with characteristic faces. For example, Down syndrome presents with slanted eyes, **epicanthal folds**, flattened nasal bridge, low-set ears, and large tongue. Fetal alcohol syndrome has the characteristic small palpebral fissures, epicanthal folds, thinned upper lip, and small chin.

Inspect the neck for size, symmetry, movement, and pulsation. Infants normally have short necks that lengthen as the child grows older. The trachea is midline and the thyroid is normally nonpalpable. Any mass in this area is abnormal. (The thyroid can be palpable in adolescents.)

Palpate lymph nodes for size, tenderness, mobility, consistency, and temperature. Cervical lymph nodes include the preauricular, postauricular, occipital, tonsillar, submandibular, submental, anterior, posterior, and deep cervical chains, supraclavicular and infraclavicular. Other lymph nodes that should be assessed are the axillary, epitrochlear, and inguinal. Normally, lymph nodes are nonpalpable but normal variants can be less than 5 mm or up to 1 cm for inguinal lymph nodes. Larger, tender, and warm nodes may indicate infection in the areas drained by the lymph nodes. Immovable, firm, irregular, and nontender nodes may indicate HIV, Hodgkin's lymphoma, or leukemia.

> **Epicanthal fold.** Vertical fold of skin from the root of the nose to the median of the eyebrow, covering the inner canthus and caruncle.

Eyes

In infants, assess vision by observing the infant's ability to focus and follow a bright object. Older children can be evaluated using diagnostic tools to screen vision such as the Snellen Symbol Chart, Blackbird Preschool Vision Screening Test, Faye Symbol Chart, and Snellen Letter Chart.

The sclera is white, conjunctiva pink, and cornea clear. The pupils are black, equal, and reactive to light and **accommodation**. The eyelids close symmetrically and completely cover the eyeballs when the eyes are shut. Eye movements are symmetric without crossing (strabismus) or lateral movements (nystagmus). Light shone on the eyes is reflected symmetrically on the cornea. Eyebrows and eyelashes are evenly distributed and eyelids are free of lesions. Some abnormal findings include ptosis (drooping of the eyelids); whitish pupils (cataract); and red, swollen conjunctiva (conjunctivitis).

Examine the internal eye structures using an ophthalmoscope. As the examiner focuses into the retina through the pupil, the red reflex is elicited. As the ophthalmoscope draws nearer and focuses on the fundus, the arteries and veins are clearly visible, with the optic disk and physiologic cup at the nasal border and the macula at the temporal border. Poor delineation of the optic disk may indicate increased intracranial pressure. The presence of hemorrhages and blood vessel changes indicates abnormal

> **Accommodation.** Constriction of the pupil, rounding of the lens, and convergence of the eyes for near vision.

processes. Absence of the red reflex is often the result of an improperly positioned ophthalmoscope, yet it can also indicate total opacity of the pupil by a cataract or by hemorrhage into the vitreous humor.

Ears

Inspect the ears for position, placement, shape, and presence of lesions and discharge. The top of the pinna should be aligned with the outer canthus of the eye. Low-set ears, abnormal shape, and the presence of skin tags suggest the possibility of congenital syndromes, which may include mental retardation and renal anomaly.

Consider the child's safety while examining the internal ears. A younger child can be held by the parent in the supine position with both the child's hands held above the child's head. The examiner can turn the head to either side. To restrain the child in the sitting position, the parent can hold the child on his/her lap, holding the child's hands in one hand and placing the other on the child's head to immobilize it. The examiner holds the otoscope to allow for movement of the instrument with each head movement by the child. A well-lit otoscope is inserted into the infant's pinna by holding it down and back. This allows visualization of the inner ear structures of the infant, whose ear canal is straighter and shorter. As the child grows older, examination of the inner ear is done by pulling the pinna up and back.

Normal findings include a clear canal free of lesions, swelling, and redness. Small amounts of yellowish cerumen may be visible. The eardrum is pearly gray and concave, with visible landmarks such as the cone of light, the malleus, the umbo, and sometimes even the incus. Crying, as well as fever, may make the eardrums red. **Otitis media,** commonly seen in children, may present with reddish, bulging eardrums and absence of the landmarks. Drainage of clear fluid into the ear canal may indicate cerebrospinal fluid leak; bloody drainage may suggest trauma. Perforations of the eardrum may be seen as black spots on the drum with absence of the landmarks.

Otitis media. Infection of the middle ear.

Nose and Sinuses

Nasal examination of the younger child is done by tilting the nose upward with one hand while shining light into the nasal orifice. Otoscopic examination is avoided because of the fear it can trigger in the child. Note the midline septum, pink mucosa, and turbinates. A deviated nasal septum may be seen in the child who complains of nasal occlusion. Pale, boggy mucosa with prominent turbinates may indicate allergic rhinitis. Nasal polyps are pedunculated mucosal tissues seen on examination inside the nares. Patency of the nares is determined by feeling the egress of air from the nares as the child breathes.

The sinuses are not developed until the age of 6. In the older child, the frontal and maxillary sinuses are palpated and tapped for tenderness.

Tapping can be done directly with the index finger or indirectly by tapping on the index finger positioned on the sinus with the other index or middle finger.

Mouth and Throat

In the young child, assessment of the mouth and throat is the most feared part of the examination and should be done close to the end. It is best to position the child in the seated position to keep his/her tongue from obstructing your view of the throat.

Inspect the mouth and throat, noting the lips, dentition, oral mucosa, gums, palate, uvula, anterior pillars, posterior pillars, and tonsils. The mucosa should be pink and free from lesions. The tongue is freely movable. **Cheilosis** refers to fissures in the corners of the mouth and lips. Epstein pearls, yellowish-white retention cysts on the palate, are normal variants in newborns. Deciduous teeth start erupting at 6 months, and are completed with all 20 out by 2½ years. Permanent teeth erupt from 6 years of age as deciduous teeth fall off. Thirty-two permanent teeth comprise total dentition and may continue until adulthood.

Tonsils are absent in infants, grow to adult size by age 6, double the adult size by age 10 to 12 years, and atrophy to the adult size by adolescence. Enlargement of the tonsils is graded according to size in reference to the pillars and approximation of edges of both sides. Hence grade 1 refers to tonsils that are tucked in the anterior and posterior pillars; grade 2, tonsils that go beyond the pillars; grade 3, large tonsils beyond the pillars but not approximating each other; and grade 4, tonsils from either side that approximate each other.

Thorax and Lungs

Observe the chest for shape, symmetry, and respiratory excursions. In infancy the chest wall is round; by age 6 the chest wall assumes the 1:2 anteroposterior diameter seen in the adult. Abdominal breathing is characteristic of children up to age 6, after which time respirations are thoracic like those of the adult. Infants are obligate nose breathers. Observe the rate, rhythm, and characteristics of respiration.

Abnormal shapes of the thorax that influence respiration and thoracic diameters include **pectus excavatum** and **pectus carinatum**. The presence of tachypnea, sternal and intercostal retractions, flaring of the ala nasi, **stridor,** or wheezing may indicate airway obstruction, **atelectasis,** asthma, or pneumonia.

Palpation of the entire chest is done with the palms and the fingertips. Palpate for tenderness and masses. The examiner can assess tactile **fremitus** by feeling vibrations on the chest wall as the child speaks or cries. Absence of tactile fremitus may indicate airway obstruction.

Cheilosis. Reddened appearance of the lips with fissures at the angles of the lips, usually because of vitamin B deficiency.

Epstein pearls. Whitish-yellow accumulation of epithelial cells or retention cysts on the hard palate, seen in newborns; a normal manifestation that spontaneously disappears after a few weeks.

Pectus excavatum. Congenital depression of the sternum, also known as funnel chest.

Pectus carinatum. Abnormal prominence of the sternum, also known as pigeon chest.

Stridor. High-pitched blowing sound produced by obstruction of the upper airway.

Atelectasis. Collapsed or airless condition of the lungs.

Fremitus. Vibratory tremors felt by examiner on palpation over the chest while patient talks.

Percussion of the chest wall reveals **resonance** over the intercostal spaces with dullness over the scapula, liver, diaphragm, and heart. Hyperresonance is a normal finding in infants because of their thin chest wall. In older children, resonance is elicited in the intercostal spaces with normal dullness over the scapula, diaphragm, liver, and heart. Dullness where normally resonance is percussed may indicate consolidation, as in pneumonia, or fluid accumulation, as in pleural effusion. Hyperresonance, on the other hand, may indicate trapped air or pneumothorax.

Harsher and louder breath sounds may be auscultated in children because of a thin chest wall. The auscultation should be done using a pediatric stethoscope. For infants and small children, use the bell of the stethoscope. The stethoscope diaphragm may be used for older children. Bronchial breath sounds are tubular and heard over the manubrium of the sternum. Bronchovesicular breath sounds are heard over the main stem bronchi; vesicular breath sounds are heard in most of the peripheral lungs.

Abnormal breath sounds include rhonchi, which indicate the presence of secretions in the bronchi; wheezing, which indicates bronchospasm; and crackles, which indicate the presence of fluid in the alveoli. Stridor is a high-pitched piercing sound that indicates narrowing of the upper airway.

Resonance. Quality of sound produced by percussion of the chest; absence of resonance is a flat percussion note, diminished resonance is a dull percussion note.

Breasts

Adequate lighting and adequate exposure are essential for the breast examination. Inspect the breasts for symmetry, color, lesions, discharge, masses, and tenderness. When examining older children and adolescents, drape one breast while examining the other to respect the patient's modesty. Well male and female newborns may have enlarged and engorged breasts with whitish discharge (**witch's milk**) for a brief period; this is from the effect of maternal estrogen. The enlargement is less than 1.5 cm in diameter; it disappears within 2 weeks and rarely lasts beyond 3 months.

Breast development in girls is assessed using the Tanner Sexual Maturity Rating (SMR) to stage breast development from stage 1, prepubertal, to stage 5, mature.

Breast enlargement in males is termed **gynecomastia**. This is an unusual and unexpected enlargement that is readily noticeable. It is usually temporary and benign, and resolves itself spontaneously. Female adolescents may have tender swollen breasts with menstrual changes. Redness and tenderness may indicate mastitis, and masses may be seen in **fibrocystic breast disease**.

Witch's milk. Whitish discharge from newborn infant's breast, stimulated by hormones from maternal circulation.

Gynecomastia. Enlargement of mammary glands in males; sometimes may secrete milk.

Fibrocystic breast disease. Painful, palpable breast lumps that fluctuate with the menstrual cycle; involves cystic degeneration of the breasts with fluid accumulation.

Heart and Blood Vessels

Inspection of the precordium reveals visible pulsations, which are normal in thin-chested children. Lifts or pulsations under the xiphoid or on either side of the sternum indicate right ventricular hypertrophy; heaves or lateral pulsations to the anterior axillary line may indicate left ventricular hypertrophy. The point of maximum impulse or apical beat is palpable at the fourth intercostal space until the age of 7 years, after which time it drops to the fifth intercostal space at the midclavicular line.

Palpation of the heart rate reveals symmetry, contour, and rhythm between the apical and peripheral pulses. Pulse deficit refers to a difference between the apical and radial pulse due to nontransmission of some apical impulses to the peripheral circulation. This is because of nontransmission of the apical pulse to the peripheral pulse sites.

Auscultation normally reveals S_1 and S_2 without murmurs, clicks, or snaps. S_1 is synchronous with the carotid pulse, is heard loudest at the apex, and is produced by the closure of the tricuspid and pulmonic valves. S_2 is produced by the closure of the aortic and pulmonic valves and is heard loudest at the second intercostal space to the right of the sternum. S_3 is normal in some children, as are some murmurs, which are termed innocent. Characteristics of innocent murmurs include the absence of other signs of heart disease, short duration, and variation with respirations and position change; they are low-pitched and musical, with intensity less than 3/6, occur during systole, and are nonradiating. Diastolic murmurs are significant for cardiac pathology.

Abdomen

Inspect the abdomen for shape, contour, presence of pulsations, peristaltic movement, venous patterns, skin changes, and presence of hernias. Auscultate the abdomen before palpation. Normal bowel sounds are heard every 10 to 30 seconds. Increased bowel sounds are heard in pyloric stenosis and early intestinal obstruction. Absence of bowel sounds indicates pathology such as bowel obstruction. If there is absence of bowel sounds the nurse should listen for bowel sounds for 5 minutes. Otherwise auscultation should be done in all 4 quadrants to make sure that no sounds are missed.

Palpation of the abdomen can be done alternately with percussion. Light percussion of the abdomen is done to assess areas of tenderness, superficial masses, muscle guarding, and skin turgor. To palpate the ticklish child, place the child's hands under the examiner's palpating hands. Observe the child's response to light palpation, which can indicate apprehension or pain. Pain that increases on pinching the skin into a small fold may indicate **hyperesthesia**, a sign of peritonitis. The presence of guarding or taut abdominal muscles may also be a sign of peritonitis.

Deep palpation is done to assess liver, spleen, kidney, and bladder size, as well as masses that lie deeper in the abdominal cavity. Palpate an enlarged liver by starting from the lower quadrant and go up. In young children the normal liver may be palpable from 1 to 2 cm below the costal margin. Liver span can also be assessed in older children by noting changes in percussion tones from resonance at the fourth intercostal space midclavicular line (ICS MCL) to tympany at the costal margin. Interestingly, in the early years the liver tends to be larger in the female,

Hyperesthesia. Increased sensitivity to sensory stimuli such as touch or pain.

but by 4 years of age, the liver of the male becomes larger. Children at every age vary and any generalization will not hold true. What is a fact is that an enlarged liver that is tender with a firm edge may indicate liver pathology. The spleen tip may be palpable in infants and in younger children may be felt as a thumb-shaped object at the left costal margin on inspiration. An enlarged spleen is always indicative of pathology. The normal kidney may be palpable at the right costal margin. Palpation and percussion of the normal bladder reveal neither tenderness nor dullness. Tenderness may indicate cystitis and dullness may indicate bladder distension.

Genitalia

Sexual maturity ratings are assigned to document assessment of sexual development for males and females. For females sexual maturity rating is graded based on breast development and pubic hair growth. For males, genital development and growth of pubic hair are graded. Deviations from sexual characteristics according to age may indicate hormonal insufficiency or hyperactivity.

Inspection of the male genitalia reveals development of the external genitalia consistent with the child's age. Normal findings include absence of lesions, discharge, swelling, or tenderness of the penis. Note whether the child is circumcised, the location of the urethral opening, and the presence of urethral discharge with stripping. Note the distribution of pubic hair; the presence of erythema and patchy areas of baldness may indicate parasitic infestations. A tight foreskin in an uncircumcised child may impair micturition, a condition known as **phimosis**. This may require circumcision to allow for free urine flow. Infection of the glans penis (balanitis) may be seen in uncircumcised males who develop fungal, bacterial, or viral infections.

Phimosis. Stenosis of the prepuce, which prevents retraction of the foreskin over the glans penis.

The foreskin in the uncircumcised infant is usually tight; it should retract enough to permit a good urine flow. While doing the examination retract the skin gently and no more than necessary to see the urethra. Do not force the skin, because this can tear the prepuce from the glans, causing binding adhesions.

Inspect the scrotum for any lesions. Absence of one or both testicles in the scrotal sac indicates undescended testicles (cryptorchidism). When palpating the testicles in infants and younger children the examiner employs maneuvers to prevent the cremasteric reflex from pulling the scrotum back up to the inguinal canal. The reflex, which is stimulated by cold, touch, or emotional factors, can be blocked by placing two fingers over the inguinal ring and palpating downward to the scrotum with the other hand. Another maneuver that facilitates palpation of the scrotum by inhibiting the cremasteric reflex is having the child sit with flexed, abducted knees.

A tender, red, and swollen testicle may indicate epididymitis, while tender, noninflamed testicles may indicate testicular torsion. Inguinal hernias can be palpated by hooking the smallest finger on the scrotal sac and palpating for the inguinal ring. The presence of a bulge when the child strains indicates inguinal hernia.

Inspect the female genitalia for distribution of pubic hair, appearance of the external genitalia and perineum, irritation, inflammation, lesions, and discharge. The presence of urethral discharge with burning and frequency of urination and suprapubic discomfort on palpation may indicate urinary tract infection. Vaginal discharge in sexually active young children may indicate gonococcal, chlamydial, monilial, or trichomonal infection, and in sexually nonactive children may indicate child abuse. Preschool children may present with foul-smelling vaginal discharge from a foreign body in the vaginal canal.

The internal genital inspection is usually not done for younger children but may be necessary when sexual abuse or infection is suspected. An internal genital examination is indicated in sexually active adolescents. Young adolescents with menstrual problems or infections may require internal examinations regardless of sexual activity.

Visualization of the interior of the vagina and the hymenal opening in prepubertal girls can be done by anterior labial traction. Grasp the labia majora with the thumb and forefinger of each hand, gently and firmly pulling the labia forward and slightly to the side. The maneuver allows visualization of the vagina almost up to the cervix, allowing inspection for foreign bodies and obtaining vaginal cultures. An imperforate hymen bulges with coughing, while a perforate hymen does not.

Red flags for child abuse should be noted by the examiner when doing genitourinary assessments in children and adolescents. Watch for physical signs of trauma or scarring in the genital and anal areas; general signs of physical abuse or neglect; the presence of sexually transmitted diseases in oral, genital, or rectal areas in young children who are not sexually active; and anorectal problems including incontinence, pain, bleeding, lacerations, and sphincter dysfunction. Behavioral manifestations may vary from sexually explicit behaviors to depression, weight problems, insomnia, eating disorders, and poor school achievement.

Anus and Rectum

A rectal examination in infants and children is not routinely performed. The presence of symptoms such as tenderness, bleeding, or bladder and bowel symptoms, which suggest intra-abdominal or pelvic problems, requires anal and rectal examination. Explanations to the young child prior to the examination can minimize apprehension and embarrassment.

Inspection of the anal region may reveal perirectal redness, which may be seen in pinworm infestation, candidiasis, or irritation from diarrhea. Bulging of rectal mucosa from the anal opening (rectal prolapse) may result from chronic diarrhea, chronic straining from constipation, or strenuous coughing. The presence of sinuses or dimpling at the anal area may indicate the presence of a pilonidal cyst or lower spinal deformities.

For infants, patency of the anus is ascertained by inserting a lubricated rectal thermometer or catheter no more than 1 cm into the rectum. This assessment is confirmed by the passage of meconium. The rectal examination is done by placing the infant or young child on his/her back with feet held together by one of the examiner's hands and knees and hips flexed on the child's abdomen. The examiner's other hand elicits the anal reflex or "anal wink" by stroking the anal area. A quick contraction of the anus is the expected response.

To assess sphincter tone in the older child, insert a well-lubricated fifth finger into the anus. Palpate the rectal area for tenderness, masses, and presence or absence of stools. The prostate is normally nonpalpable in young and preadolescent boys. The rectal examination is included as part of the assessment for adolescent boys and girls and is done in the same manner as for adults.

Musculoskeletal Examination

Assess the extremities and back for symmetry, range of motion, movement, muscle mass, strength, joint redness, swelling, tenderness, crepitation, and deformity.

Assess the young child by observing his/her ability to pick up objects, play with toys, and move about in an unconstrained fashion without any limitation. Bone stability, range of motion, muscle strength, gait, and balance can be assessed as the child plays, jumps, and manipulates toys in the examining room.

Observe the child's spinal curvatures and symmetry of the hips and shoulders. In newborns the spine has convex dorsal and sacral curves. The lumbar curve is formed by age 12 to 18 months. Lumbar lordosis is a normal finding among younger children. Kyphosis (hunchback) may indicate habitual slouching or may be a sign of spinal tumors or tuberculosis of the spine. Scoliosis (lateral curvature of the spine) may be functional or persistent. Functional scoliosis can be voluntarily corrected by the child and disappears when the child is recumbent. Unequal shoulder height and iliac crests while the child is standing and unequal level of the scapula when the child leans forward indicate persistent structural scoliosis.

Neurologic Examination

Assessment of the neurologic system is integrated throughout the examination of the infant and the young child. Mental status and orientation give an indication of the acuteness of the child's condition. Inattention to the external environment or a fixed blank stare indicates an acutely ill child or a psychiatric problem. Uncoordination, tremors, seizures, twitching, and hyperirritability indicate serious neurologic conditions. Flexion of the neck resulting in flexion of the hip and knee (Brudzinski sign) and inability of the child to extend the leg with the hip flexed (Kernig sign) may indicate meningeal irritation.

For infants, neurologic assessment is done by testing the presence of newborn reflexes. Persistence of newborn reflexes beyond the age when they should disappear indicates neurologic dysfunction. Deficits in neurologic function can also be assessed using the Denver Development Test. Inability to perform specific activities for specific age groups may indicate neurologic dysfunction. Reflexes, coordination tests, cranial nerve assessment, and sensory tests are done for older children in the same manner as these tests are performed for adults.

SUMMARY

Health assessment of the pediatric patient involves applying the nurse's knowledge and skills in identifying normal from abnormal findings and skill in diagnostic reasoning. Following data collection, both subjective and objective data are analyzed. The steps in data analysis include identifying abnormal data and their significance, clustering the data, drawing inferences from cue clusters, proposing the possible nursing diagnoses, comparing defining characteristics for possible diagnoses, confirming or ruling out defining characteristics, testing the validity of the nursing diagnoses, and documenting conclusions.

Hypothesis generation is based on the nurse's knowledge of probable pathophysiologic or psychosocial processes explaining the abnormal findings. The history portion of the assessment process provides cues from the analysis of the symptoms related to the chief complaint. Past medical history, growth and development, cultural background, family internal and external structures, functions and boundaries, and a general review of systems provide data to support hypothesis generation. Analysis of the data obtained from the history allows the nurse to distinguish between the presence of disease, which is a biological phenomenon, and the experience of illness, which is a biopsychosocial phenomenon.

The physical assessment allows the nurse to utilize special techniques of observation, palpation, percussion, and auscultation to assess the patient's risk for specific diseases. Further confirmation is provided by diagnostic data, which provide the "gold standard" for specific diagnoses.

Differential diagnoses are ruled out on the basis of positive and negative cues from both the history and physical examination as supported by diagnostic data. The probability of a diagnosis is weighed on the basis of preponderance of evidence supporting the most likely diagnosis. The absence of sensitive cues to support a diagnosis rules out the possibility of a competing diagnosis.

The development of diagnostic reasoning skills requires an expanded background of theoretical knowledge of the various pathophysiologic and psychosocial processes in disease and wellness, practice skills in the clinical setting, and increasing experience in recognizing cues and patterns.

CRITICAL POINTS IN PEDIATRIC ASSESSMENT

Data collecting, data processing, and generating a problem list are components of the assessment process. These processes are based on critical thinking and clinical reasoning skills. Within the context of history taking and performing a comprehensive physical examination, clinical reasoning is the ability to gather, organize, and process data. Critical thinking is the ability to reason well from and to evidence while in the process of gathering, organizing, and processing the data being collected. The evidence critically analyzed comes from the history and physical examination. Evidence is what supports a diagnosis. All evidence comes from the nurse's ability to extract and process data accurately and critically from multiple resources, but chiefly from the patient.

Diagnostic reasoning skills are developed over time. They require an expanding theoretical base in the biopsychosocial aspects of disease, and clinical exposure to assessment and diagnosis. Knowledge of the patient as a person experiencing a disease process individualizes the patient's experience, making nursing diagnoses patient-specific.

Following the identification of the diagnoses is the establishment of the management plan. Priorities are set to solve the patient's health problem. Again, considerations for intervention are derived from the patient's personal circumstances, including his/her physical condition, socioeconomic resources, level of education, and previous experiences.

QUESTIONS

1. In infants, the largest part of the body is the:
   A. Neck
   B. Trunk
   C. Head
   D. Pelvic area

2. The stage used to determine sexual maturity rating is called:
   A. Tanner's
   B. Skinner's
   C. Freud's
   D. Pavlov's

3. Brain growth is reflected by:
   A. Age of child
   B. Anterior fontanel
   C. Head circumference
   D. IQ

4. The best developmental approaches to assess preschoolers include:
   A. Maintaining privacy, teaching about their bodies, and explaining equipment.
   B. Using storytelling, puppets, giving choices when appropriate.
   C. Allowing the child to sit on lap, using praise and cooperation.
   D. Ensuring privacy and confidentiality.

5. A 4-year-old comes to the clinic for a complete physical assessment. The best way to take his/her temperature is:
   A. Orally
   B. Rectally
   C. Axillary
   D. Palpating the forehead

6. Pulse rate is measured for a full minute. For children younger than 2 years, which pulse should be measured?
   A. Brachial
   B. Radial
   C. Apical
   D. Distal

7. The appropriate width of the cuff for all ages should be:
   A. 100% of the upper arm
   B. 80–90% of the upper arm
   C. 10–20% of the upper arm
   D. 50–75% of the upper arm

8. The general rule for normal systolic blood pressure for children 1–7 years is age in years + 90. For children 8–18 years, the general rule is:
   A. $2 \times$ age + 50
   B. Age $- 32 \times 5/9$
   C. $(2 \times$ age in years$) + 90$
   D. $90 + 4 \times$ age

9. The blood pressure reading is too high for the child. The reason could be:
   A. The cuff is too small.
   B. The machine is defective.
   C. The cuff is too large.
   D. The stethoscope is broken.

10. In assessing the child's skin, which of the following is considered abnormal:
    A. Hemangioma
    B. Mongolian spot
    C. Café-au-lait spot
    D. Petechia and rashes

11. In palpating and inspecting the hair of a 5-year-old, the nurse finds dull, dry, brittle hair. This may indicate:

    A. Hypothyroidism
    B. Lice
    C. Wrong shampoo
    D. Dandruff

12. The anterior fontanel is diamond-shaped and measures 4–5 cm at its widest part. This closes at:

    A. Adolescence
    B. 2 months of age
    C. 12–18 months of age
    D. Age 3

13. An infant should be able to hold his/her head erect and midline with full range of motion of the head (sideways, up, and down) at:

    A. 4 months
    B. 3 months
    C. 2 months
    D. 1 month

14. Permanent dentition begins at around:

    A. 2 years
    B. 4 years
    C. 8 years
    D. 6 years

15. Jason has eyes with wide-set position, upward slant, and thick epicanthal folds. This is suggestive of:

    A. Down syndrome
    B. Mallory-Weiss syndrome
    C. Hypothyroidism
    D. Normal finding

16. In assessing a 2-year-old with an otoscope, the nurse:

    A. Pulls the pinna up and back.
    B. Pulls the pinna down and back.
    C. Does nothing, just holds the head.
    D. Holds the head straight.

17. The normal findings in the internal ear include:

    A. Excessive cerumen
    B. Purulent discharge
    C. Pearly gray tympanic membrane
    D. Clear discharge

18. Assessing for congenital hip dysplasia is an important aspect of an infant's physical examination and is performed at each visit until 1 year of age. With the infant supine, the knees are flexed while the examiner's thumbs are mid-thigh and fingers are placed over the

greater trochanters. The leg is then abducted, moving the knees outward and down toward the table. This test is called:

    A. Barlow maneuver
    B. Ortolani maneuver
    C. Vagal maneuver
    D. Valsalva maneuver

19. The Babinski reflex disappears:

    A. After 1 month
    B. After 2 months
    C. Within 2 years
    D. When the child starts walking

20. In toddlers, limping may indicate:

    A. Scoliosis
    B. Slipped capital femoral epiphysis
    C. Congenital hip dysplasia
    D. Clubfoot

*A*NSWERS

1. *C.* At birth, the circumference of the head is greater than that of the chest.

2. *A.* Tanner's is used as a rating scale for sexual maturity; the others are all psychologists.

3. *C.* The sutures of the skull remain open to allow for brain growth and the objective measurement used is the head circumference.

4. *B.* *A* is for infants, *D* is for adolescents, *C* is for toddlers.

5. *A.* Rectal temps are too invasive for 4-year-olds, and if not used properly, perforation may occur.

6. *C.* The apical pulse should be auscultated for a whole minute. In children older than 3, the radial pulses may be palpated.

7. *D.* The cuff size should cover 50–75% of the upper arm.

8. *C.* *A* would be too low, *B* is the conversion formula of temperature, *D* would be too high.

9. *A.* When the cuff is too small for the child, the blood pressure reading will be too high.

10. *D.* Petechia and rashes. *A, B,* and *C* are all normal alterations.

11. *A.* Hypothyroidism. The classic signs are dull, dry, brittle hair.

12. *C.* The anterior fontanel closes at 12–18 months of age.

13. *C.* At 2 months of age, the infant should be able to hold his/her head erect and midline.

14. *D.* Baby teeth start falling out at age 6 and permanent dentition begins.

15. *A.* Wide-set eyes with upward slant and thick epicanthal folds suggest Down syndrome.

16. *B.* Pulls the pinna down and back because the child's ear canal is short and straight. *A* is done for adults.

17. *C.* A normal tympanic membrane is pearly gray.

18. *B.* The described maneuver is the Ortolani maneuver.

19. *C.* The Babinski reflex appears within 2 years.

20. *C.* Congenital hip dysplasia. *A* and *B* in adolescents are indicative of scoliosis. In *D*, clubfoot, the observation normally noted is intoeing.

$\mathcal{G}$LOSSARY

accommodation   constriction of the pupil, rounding of the lens, and convergence of the eyes for near vision.

acrocyanosis   bluish discoloration of the hands and feet, normal for infants during the first hour of birth; can occur after that time also.

atelectasis   collapsed or airless condition of the lungs.

cheilosis   reddened appearance of the lips with fissures at the angles of the lips, usually because of vitamin B deficiency.

epicanthal fold   vertical fold of skin from the root of the nose to the median of the eyebrow, covering the inner canthus and caruncle.

Epstein pearls   whitish-yellow accumulation of epithelial cells or retention cysts on the hard palate, seen in newborns; a normal manifestation that spontaneously disappears after a few weeks.

fibrocystic breast disease   painful, palpable breast lumps that fluctuate with the menstrual cycle; involves cystic degeneration of the breasts with fluid accumulation.

fremitus   vibratory tremors felt by examiner on palpation over the chest while patient talks.

gynecomastia   enlargement of mammary glands in males; sometimes may secrete milk.

hyperesthesia   increased sensitivity to sensory stimuli such as touch or pain.

neurofibromatosis   a genetic disorder affecting neural tissue growth, presenting as multiple hyperpigmented areas with the appearance of multiple cutaneous and subcutaneous tumors in late childhood.

otitis media   infection of the middle ear.

pectus carinatum   abnormal prominence of the sternum, also known as pigeon chest.

pectus excavatum   congenital depression of the sternum, also known as funnel chest.

phimosis   stenosis of the prepuce, which prevents retraction of the foreskin over the glans penis.

resonance   quality of sound produced by percussion of the chest; absence of resonance is a flat percussion note, diminished resonance is a dull percussion note.

stridor   high-pitched blowing sound produced by obstruction of the upper airway.

witch's milk   whitish discharge from newborn infant's breast, stimulated by hormones from maternal circulation.

Bibliography

BARNESS, L. A. *Manual of Pediatric Physical Diagnosis*. Chicago: Mosby, 1991.

BATES, B. *Guide to Physical Examination and History Taking*. 6th ed. Philadelphia: J. B. Lippincott, 1995.

BERKOWITZ, C. D. *Pediatrics, a Primary Care Approach*. Philadelphia: W. B. Saunders, 1996.

BETZ, C., HUNSBERGER, M., AND WRIGHT, S. *Family-Centered Nursing Care of Children*. 2nd ed. Philadelphia: W. B. Saunders, 1994.

BURNS, C., BARBER, N., BRADY, M., AND DUNN, A. *Pediatric Primary Care: A Handbook for Nurse Practitioners*. Philadelphia: W. B. Saunders, 1996.

DAINS, J., BAUMANN, L., AND SCHEIBEL, P. *Advanced Health Assessment and Clinical Diagnosis in Primary Care*. St. Louis: Mosby, 1998.

ELLIOT, D., AND GOLDBERG, L. *The History and Physical Examination Casebook*. Philadelphia: Lippincott-Raven, 1997.

ENGEL, J. *Pocket Guide to Pediatric Assessment*. 2nd ed. St. Louis: Mosby, 1993.

JACKSON, P., AND VESSEY, J. *Primary Care of the Child with a Chronic Condition*. St. Louis: Mosby, 1996.

MARLOW, D., AND REDDING, B. *Textbook in Pediatric Nursing*. 6th ed. Philadelphia: W. B. Saunders, 1998.

OSKI, F., DEANGELIS, C., FEIGIN, R., McMILLAN, J., AND WARSAW, J. *Principles and Practice of Pediatrics*. Philadelphia: J. B. Lippincott, 1994.

SEIDEL, H., BALL, J., DAINS, J., AND BENEDICT, G. *Mosby's Guide to Physical Examination*. 4th ed. St. Louis: Mosby, 1999.

THOMAS, C., ED. *Taber's Encyclopedic Medical Dictionary*. Philadelphia: F. A. Davis, 1993.

WEBER, J., AND KELLEY, J. *Health Assessment in Nursing*. Philadelphia: J. B. Lippincott, 1998.

WONG, D. *Nursing Care of Infants and Children*. 5th ed. St. Louis: Mosby, 1995.

PEDIATRIC ASSESSMENT

follows a comprehensive history by then doing a → COMPREHENSIVE PHYSICAL

requires/relies upon effective → COMMUNICATION ABILITIES/SKILLS

begins with a → COMPREHENSIVE HISTORY

COMMUNICATION ABILITIES/SKILLS **aids in doing a** → COMPREHENSIVE PHYSICAL

COMMUNICATION ABILITIES/SKILLS **aids in doing a** → COMPREHENSIVE HISTORY

COMPREHENSIVE PHYSICAL

requires collection of →

DATA:
- General survey (age dependent)
- Mental and physical status
- Height and weight
- Head circumference
- Skin
- Head
- Eyes, ears, nose and throat (includes neck)
- Thorax and lungs
- Breasts
- Cardiovascular system
- Abdomen
- Male and female genitalia
- Musculoskeletal system
- Nervous system

COMMUNICATION ABILITIES/SKILLS

requires being →

aware of:
- Developmental cognitive stages/abilities of child
- Communication abilities of child/adolescent
- Observational ability of nurse
- Rapport with parent and child

using methods →

such as:
- Facilitation
- Reflection
- Clarification
- Empathic responses
- Asking about feelings
- Confrontation
- Interpretation

COMPREHENSIVE HISTORY

requires collection of →

DATA:
- Date of history
- Identification data—patient name, nickname, age, sex, place of birth, etc.
- Source of referral
- Source of information
- Reliability of historian/history
- Chief complaint
- History of present illness—concise chronology of illness
- Past history—includes birth history of prenatal, natal, and neonatal
- Development/growth history
- Current health status—medications, allergies, diet, screening tests, immunizations, etc.
- Sleep patterns
- Feeding patterns
- Family history
- Psychological history
- General review of systems

Concept Map 2-1

65

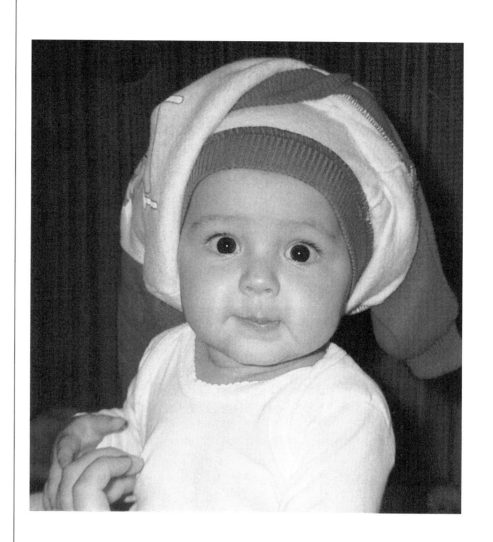

❧

$\mathcal{G}$ROWTH AND DEVELOPMENT

$\mathcal{I}$NTRODUCTION

Growth and development are ongoing processes that are multifaceted and interrelated, encompassing the vast changes that take place in the lifetime of an individual. Infants grow through childhood to adolescence needing parents or parent surrogates to survive, and eventually to assume the role of adults in society.

Growth and development derive from maturation and learning. *Growth* refers to an increase in physical size—the whole or parts—and can be measured. Growth charts include height, weight, and skin-fold diameters, and are established through cross-sectional studies for both sexes from infancy to adolescence. The genetic potential for growth differentiates one child from another and may be exceeded or hampered at any stage. Assessment of growth delays or abnormal acceleration indicates disorders requiring intervention. **Development** refers to an orderly and sequential increase in skill and capacity to function. Although used interchangeably with development, *maturation* refers to an increase in functionality of traits that are genetically transmitted. Both growth and development are influenced by heredity and environment. While heredity determines the extent of growth and development, environment determines the degree to which inherited potential is achieved.

The pediatric nurse needs to know about growth and development patterns in children to be able to **assess** each child's level, design interventions for deficits, and teach parents about facilitating the achievement of

Development. Increase in capability.

Assessment. Process of collecting information about the child and his/her family in order to make a nursing diagnosis.

Anticipatory guidance. Process of understanding developmental needs, and teaching parents and caretakers to meet the child's needs.

optimal growth and development according to norms appropriate for the child's age and sex.

Various tables for growth and development provide tools for the nurse to gauge the child's level. The Denver Development II instrument is commonly used for children from birth to 6 years to screen for otherwise unsuspected developmental problems, or to monitor children at risk for developmental delays. Beyond age 6 and through adolescence, physical, intellectual, and emotional and social competencies are evaluated via age-specific behaviors.

To achieve the goal of early identification of developmental delays, developmental screening needs to be a continuous process occurring at every well-child visit. The usual schedule is approximately 12 well-child visits by 3 years of age and yearly through adolescence. **Anticipatory guidance** can be provided as needed for parents and caregivers to optimize environmental factors supporting the development of the child's potential.

Chronologic divisions used in pediatric assessment for the development of physical, intellectual, and emotional and social competencies include:

Newborn or neonatal life: from childbirth to the first year of life
Toddlerhood: from ages 1 to 3
Preschool years: from ages 3 to 5
School-age years: from ages 6 to 11
Adolescence to young adulthood: from ages 12 to 21 years

NEWBORNS AND INFANTS (0 TO 1 YEAR)

Physical Growth

The average weight of a full-term newborn is 3000 grams at birth. A loss of 10% birth weight occurs in the first 3 to 4 days of life from extracellular losses, but is regained at the rate of 5 to 7 ounces per week. Weight doubles by 5 months and triples by 1 year. Height increases approximately 1 inch per month for the first 6 months and doubles by 1 year. The fontanels should be soft and flat. The head circumference at birth averages 13.5 to 14.5 inches and is generally .75 inches larger than the chest. The head and the chest circumferences, however, are equal at 1 year; thereafter, the chest circumference is larger than the head circumference. The posterior fontanel closes at 2 to 3 months; the anterior closes at 12 to 18 months.

The texture of the skin is smooth and velvety. Color is race-dependent, but can vary. At birth the skin may be covered with a grayish white cheesy substance called the vernix caseosa. It is composed of a mixture of sebum and desquamate cells, which can be removed easily with the first bath. The vernix caseosa acts as a barrier and moisturizer to the newborn. Lanugo, which is a fine, downy hair (peach fuzz), can be observed after the removal of the vernix caseosa. The presence of milia, minute profuse white or yellow papules around the face, is normal. Mongolian spots are also common in Asian, black, and East Indian infants. The umbilical cord remains should be dry and usually fall off during the first or second week of life.

At 6 to 7 months, the primary teeth erupt, with the central incisors erupting first. Six teeth can usually be counted at age 1.

The normal temperature of an infant taken via a tympanic thermometer ranges from 97 to 99 degrees. An apical pulse of 140 to 160 at birth is normal, and varies with activity or disease process. Infants are obligatory nose breathers from 3 to 4 months and respirations average 30 to 60 per minute.

Motor Development

Motor development tends to parallel central nervous system maturation, progressing from the **cephalocaudal** (head to toe) for gross motor skills and proximodistal (central to the periphery) for fine motor skills (Table 3-1).

The disappearance of primitive reflexes precedes the appearance of purposeful behavior in response to specific stimuli. Controlled use of the upper extremities precedes that of the lower extremities, and truncal mastery occurs prior to mastery of the lower extremities. There is greater variation in the timing of gross motor development and the acquisition of fine motor skills. Assessment of alertness, responsiveness, and concentration is

Cephalocaudal development. Process by which development proceeds from head to feet.

◙

TABLE 3-1
MOTOR SKILLS DURING INFANCY

Age	Gross Motor Skills	Fine Motor Skills
1 month	Rounded back when pulled to sitting position, turns head to side	Involuntary hand movements
2 months	Raises head and chest, and can hold in position	
3 months	Raises head to 45 degrees, slight head lag when pulled to sitting position	Holds hand in front of face
4 months	Lifts head and looks around, rolls from prone to supine position	Voluntary movements with ulnar surface of hand
5 months	Rolls over from supine to prone and back, sits with back upright	Grasps rattle with hands held together
6 months	Sits with shaky posture, raises abdomen off chest when prone	Drops object in hand to reach for another object offered
7 months	Sits alone, uses hands for support	Transfers objects between hands
8 months	Sits unsupported	Start of thumb and finger grasping
9 months	Creeping begins, abdomen off floor	Bangs held objects together
10 months	Pulls self to standing position	Picks up small objects
11 months	Stands securely holding on to objects	Offers toy and releases
12 months	Sits from standing position	Feeds self with cup and spoon

a more reliable indicator of the progression of development. Gross motor skills are poor indicators of the child's mental capacity.

Psychosocial Development

Infants can easily differentiate faces and objects during their first month. At 2 months, they begin smiling. Infants' cries are strong when they are hungry or uncomfortable. At 3 months, they explore and stare at the environment. The primary caregiver, usually the mother, is easily distinguished at 4 months. At 6 months, infants play. Stranger anxiety occurs at 7 to 8 months, and from 10 to 12 months separation anxiety occurs.

Erik Erikson (1963) uses biologic markers as critical periods in the development of a person, in which specific problems arise and must be solved satisfactorily in order to advance to the next stage. Psychosocial development occurs within the context of the social and cultural environment.

Erikson's psychosocial crisis of trust versus mistrust is resolved during the first year of life. The mother or primary caregiver is the significant person for the infant and determines, to a great extent, the development of the infant's sense of trust, which is a foundation for other psychosocial tasks. Trust is developed when the caregiver is prompt and consistent in meeting the needs of the infant. Mistrust, on the other hand, develops when the infant does not obtain security in immediate gratification of his/her needs because of lack of concern and constancy by the mother or primary caregiver.

Feeding time during the first 3 months of life is the most important social activity for the infant. Comfort time is also important. During the first 2 months of life, crying is the only way the infant knows how to convey his/her desires to the caretaker. As soon as vision, vocalization, and motor development progress, the infant learns to communicate what he/she wants by using hand and foot movements as well as facial expressions. Tactile stimulation from the caregiver is important at this stage. The infant and the caregiver must develop a symbiotic relationship in which both are satisfied. When this synchrony occurs, the infant develops a strong sense of trust in himself/herself and in the world around him/her.

During this stage of development, maturation of the nervous system allows the infant to distinguish himself/herself as separate from the mother and others. At this stage also, the infant learns to tolerate small doses of frustration, and learns to trust that gratification of needs can be delayed but will eventually be provided by the mother or caregiver.

Psychosexual Development

Sigmund Freud focuses on a single motive governing behavior: the desire to satisfy biologic needs, which is governed by sexual instinct. According to his theory, certain regions of the body assume a prominent psychological significance, with each stage building on previous ones as sources of new pleasures and conflicts. Freud believed that children who encounter severe conflicts at any stage of their development might be reluctant to move on to the next stage, causing impairment and psychosis.

Freud's first stage of psychosexual development is the oral stage. Factors affecting attitude development during infancy include touch, tone of voice, and the mother's or caregiver's acceptance. Sexual gratification centers around sucking, biting, chewing, and vocalizing. Behaviors during the later part of the first year of life move to random self-discovery and pelvic rocking. According to Freud, infants with unresolved conflicts at this stage have problems in later life with pessimism, envy, submission, and self-belittlement.

Cognitive Development

Cognitive development, according to Jean Piaget, takes place in several stages through the processes of assimilation and accommodation. Children assimilate new knowledge, skills, and ideas to existing schema familiar to them. New situations that do not fit the existing schema are accommodated into the present one in order to solve more difficult tasks and complex problems. These two processes allow children to achieve an accurate understanding of the world around them, have a firm grasp of reality, and solve their problems accurately and effectively.

The first stage of cognitive development, the sensorimotor stage, occurs during infancy through the early part of toddlerhood. During this phase, the infant progresses from reflexive behavior to imitation, repetition, and ability to anticipate events. Table 3-2 gives the four phases of the sensorimotor stage during infancy, and expected behaviors during each phase.

☒

TABLE 3-2

PIAGET'S PHASES OF SENSORIMOTOR STAGE OF COGNITIVE DEVELOPMENT IN INFANCY

Age	Phase	Behaviors
1 month	Reflexive	Reflexes in response to environmental stimulus
1–4 months	Primary circular reactions	Repetitive and voluntary actions
		Beginning stimulus response
		Recognition of familiar objects, sounds, odors
4–8 months	Secondary circular reactions	Imitation begins
		Object permanence
		Play brings pleasure
		Shows affect
8–12 months	Coordination of secondary schemata	Searches for hidden objects
		Anticipates events

The three most important events that take place during the sensori-motor phase are separation, achievement of object permanence, and use of symbols. First, separation of the infant from the environment and from other objects evokes anxiety. This coincides with the development of trust described in Erikson's psychosocial stage of infant development. The second important event is the achievement of object permanence, or the realization that out of sight does not mean permanent disappearance. The third most important intellectual achievement is the ability to use symbols, which allows the infant to think of an object without actually experiencing it. The recognition of symbols is the beginning of the understanding of time and space.

During the primary circular reaction phase, the infant shows evidence of accommodation as he/she starts to incorporate and adapt to the reactions of caregivers and the environment. In the secondary circular reaction phase, the infant repeats behaviors in the primary circular reaction phase and awaits responses to his/her actions. The new process empowers the infant, bringing into his/her behavior three new phenomena: (1) imitation, which needs to be reinforced; (2) play, which brings pleasure to both infant and caregiver; and (3) affect, which is a manifestation of the infant's feelings.

The fourth phase is very transitional. The infant uses previous knowledge as a foundation for adding new intellectual skills. This phase marks the beginning of intellectual reasoning.

Language Development

Language development is closely linked with cognitive development. Landmarks of language development in the infant are given in Table 3-3.

⊠

TABLE 3-3
LANGUAGE DEVELOPMENT IN THE INFANT

Age	Language Development
Neonate	Crying
1 month	Cries when uncomfortable, throaty sounds
1–3 months	Coos, vocalizes, differentiated crying
4–5 months	Simple vowel sounds, laughs, vocalizes to other voices
6 months	Babbling sounds, addition of some consonants to vowels
7–8 months	Chains syllables ("mama, dada"), no meaning attached Responds to simple commands
9–12 months	Patterned speech, meaning to "mama" and "dada" Imitates speech sounds
12 months	Two to three words with meaning Recognizes objects by name, imitates animal sounds

Moral Development

Lawrence Kohlberg (1968) theorized that children develop moral reasoning at the same rate that they develop cognitively. Because of limited cognitive development in the infant, Kohlberg's theory of moral development does not start until the next stage of development, toddlerhood. However, parents' responses to crying with stern discipline and withholding of love may affect the child's development of trust. This may have adverse effects on the child's moral development.

Health Maintenance

Nutrition The infant's total caloric intake should equal 100 to 115 calories per kilogram per day. For the first year, a child is either breast-fed or bottle-fed with an iron-fortified formula. Iron is necessary to decrease the risk of anemia. At 2 months there is a hypoactive erythropoietin production, and from 6 to 9 months the maternal iron stores are depleted. Fluoride and vitamin supplements should be given to nursing mothers. Solid foods are introduced at 4 to 6 months of age.

Foods should be introduced one at a time in small quantities and in the following order: rice cereal, strained fruits, vegetables, and meats, then finger foods when the infant starts teething. At 6 months, begin introducing the cup and finger foods, and help increase self-feeding at 10 to 12 months by introducing the spoon. The most common food allergy sources in infants are egg whites, milk, oranges, tomatoes, nuts, chocolate, and wheat or corn cereals. Symptoms may include urticaria, nausea and vomiting, respiratory symptoms, and abdominal pains. Singular addition of foods is necessary to enable the parents to determine the source of the allergic reaction.

Play One of the most important concepts that children learn is how to play. It is through play that they learn about the world and their place in it. It is also through play that children learn what they can do, and therefore develop qualities such as likes and dislikes that will affect their entire life.

Through socialization, children learn to get along in the world around them and to obtain the necessary social tools that will allow them to live in society. During the first 5 years of life, children pass through 4 phases in developing social competence in play. Infants up to 1 year old investigate other infants as objects in their environment. Children between 2 and 3 years of age play pretend roles, imitating a mother, father, etc. Children in their preschool years become increasingly aware of their peer group and can point out characteristics of their playmates, and they will acquire 2 or 3 playmates whom they like best. In play, children learn the sex role that society imposes on them, as well as norms of behavior, moral ethics, and values.

The specific functions of play include enhancement of sensorimotor skills, creativity, and intellectual and social development. Content play begins with social affective play, in which the infant takes pleasure in the relationship with others. For example, the infant learns to smile in order to elicit his/her parents' positive attention.

During the first 3 months of life, play for the infant is dependent on the caregiver. Cuddling and cooing sounds from the caregiver elicit cooing sounds and the social smile.

By age 3 to 6 months, interaction with the caregiver increases. Using rattles, soft toys, and mirrors to stimulate vocalization is suitable at this time. By 8 months, the infant is selective of parents as the focus of his/her attention and enjoys playing peek-a-boo, pattycake, and repetitive games.

By 12 months old, increased sensorimotor skills allow the infant to enjoy push-pull toys, large balls, activity boxes, blocks, and books.

Safety Considerations The key to preventing accidents is keen observation of infants, and remembering that they are explorers of the environment. Thinking abstractly is not an acquired skill as yet. The parents or the caregivers are the responsible thinkers for them. Total attention should be focused on the child, with the eyes as well as the mind.

Management of airway obstruction is taught to parents in basic CPR (cardiopulmonary resuscitation) classes. Prevention of aspiration and suffocation includes teaching parents to keep the following items out of the purview of the infant: plastic bags, small toys, and other small objects. Parents should also avoid tying strings and ribbons around the neck of the child to accommodate pacifiers or for bottle propping.

To prevent the child from falling, parents should use high chairs, car seats, bed rails, and gates for stairways, and should never leave the infant unattended. All sharp or pointed objects, toxic substances, and medications should be out of reach of the child, locked in a cabinet. The telephone number for poison control should be posted prominently on the telephone, with syrup of ipecac nearby. Parents should know how to properly use syrup of ipecac.

Parents should be educated about controlling burn accidents, including keeping the child away from the kitchen, avoiding flames, and keeping electric wires out of the child's reach. Checking the temperature of bathwater prior to baths is a simple precaution against scalding.

Immunizations Scheduled immunizations during infancy, toddlerhood, preschool, school, and adolescence, as recommended by the American Academy of Pediatrics, are presented in Table 3-4.

Immunizations are recommended for infants and older children to protect them from common communicable diseases. The most common reactions to immunizations include redness, swelling and soreness at the injection site, mild fever, fussiness, and malaise. MMR (measles-mumps-rubella) immunization produces mild rash or joint stiffness 1 to 2 weeks after the injection. Immunizations are usually delayed when a child has any serious illnesses or if an allergic response is noted. The most common allergic component of the vaccine is the egg for the MMR injection. DPT (diphtheria-pertussis-tetanus) injection is contraindicated when a child experiences inconsolable crying and irritability lasting 3 hours or more after the immunization, a fever of or greater than 105, or a high-pitched

◙

TABLE 3-4

IMMUNIZATION SCHEDULE RECOMMENDED BY THE AMERICAN ACADEMY OF PEDIATRICS

Age	Immunization
Birth	Hepatitis B-1
1–2 months	Hepatitis B-2
2 months	DPT-1 (diphtheria-tetanus-pertussis)
	OPV-1 (oral polio vaccine), HbCV-1 (hemophilus influenza, type B conjugate vaccine)
4 months	DPT-2, OPV-2, HbCV-2
6 months	DPT-3, HbCV-3
6–18 months	Hepatitis B-3
15 months	MMR (measles-mumps-rubella), HbCV-4
18 months	DPT-4, OPV-3
4–6 years	DPT-5, OPV-4, MMR-2 (optional)
11–12 years	MMR-2 if not given earlier
14–16 years	TD (tetanus and diphtheria), repeat every 10 years

cry. OPV (oral polio vaccine) is contraindicated in children with altered immune systems or possible contact with a person with HIV, malignancy, leukemia, or on chemotherapy. Inactivated polio vaccine can be substituted.

TODDLERS (1 TO 3 YEARS)

Physical Growth

Height and weight become more proportioned during this phase of growth, except that boys are slightly taller than girls. The estimated adult height can be predicted by multiplying the height at age 2 by 2. BMR (basic metabolic rate) is decreased from what it was in infancy, hence the rate of weight gain declines because of decreased appetite. The child grows 2 to 2.5 inches and 4 to 6 pounds yearly. The chest circumference is equal to the head circumference, and the transverse is greater than the anterioposterior diameter. The abdomen protrudes and the abdominal girth is greater after 2 years. With the increasing age and size, pulse and respirations also decrease. The normal pulse at this age is 80 to 120 and respirations are from 20 to 40. Temporary teeth or deciduous teeth all erupt by 2.5 to 3 years of age. Visual acuity is 20/40 and depth perception is increasing. The physiologic systems mature, and at 18 months bowel control is usually accomplished. At 2 to 3 years, children are usually pottytrained, and bladder control is established.

Motor Development

This is the stage in which the child learns to walk independently, progressing to running, jumping, and then climbing. Table 3-5 presents the development of gross and fine motor skills during toddlerhood.

Psychosocial Development

Based on Erikson's stages, this is the stage of autonomy versus shame and doubt. At approximately 15 months, the child learns to move independently, and anxiety toward strangers decreases. In exerting their autonomy and sense of will, children in this stage say "no" frequently and experience temper tantrums when frustrated or angry. The significant persons are the parents. Toddlers give hugs and kisses to familiar people and at 18 months imitate housework tasks they have observed being done. Temper tantrums peak at age 2. At this age, the child may cooperate with toilet training.

◙

TABLE 3-5
MOTOR SKILLS DURING TODDLERHOOD

Age	Gross Motor Skills	Fine Motor Skills
13–18 months	Walks alone, jumps in place, falls Creeps up stairs, comes down backwards Runs but falls	Holds and drinks from cup Takes shoes and socks off Helps take off shirt Helps unzip clothes
24 months	Walks steadily Kicks ball forward Jumps in place Walks up stairs, both feet on step Goes down stairs holding on Picks up objects without falling	Uses one hand to hold cup Uses spoon without spilling Undresses self Puts on shirt Turns doorknobs Builds tower of 6–7 cubes
30 months	Walks on tiptoes, climbs stairs with one foot on step, throws ball 3–4 feet	Holds crayons in fingers, imitates lines and circles, pours with spills
36 months	Rides a tricycle, balances on one foot but falls after 2 seconds	Draws recognizable figures Puts small objects in bottle

Parallel play may also occur. The child may learn to play simple games or play alone. At 30 months, the child begins to cope with separations for approximately 3 to 4 hours. At 3 years of age, daytime toilet training is usually completed, temper tantrums decrease, and role playing, or imitating adult behavior, is observed.

Psychosexual Development (Anal Stage)

According to Freud, during toddlerhood children center their interest in the anal region. As cephalocaudal growth progresses, the anal region and the sphincter muscles develop. Children are able to withhold or expel their feces at their own will. The nurse needs to reinforce to the parents that toilet training should develop in a climate of understanding and warmth, since this process has a lasting effect on the formation of the child's adult personality. Children who develop an anal personality become stingy or overgenerous, rigid or tardy, orderly or messy. Parents need to know that what the child can do physically has a great influence on his/her perception of self, which in turn greatly influences social development and independence. A warm, positive experience in toilet training gives the child confidence and success, which is very important for the accomplishment of future developmental milestones.

Cognitive Development

According to Piaget, this is the stage when the child is active and loves to experiment to achieve goals. Relationships between shapes and similar concepts are established and early signs of memory development are seen. Between 18 months and 2 years of age, children have a sense of time and are very egocentric. They see things only from their own point of view. They are able to infer from observing and experiencing, and predict causes and effects from those experiences. From ages 2 to 4, children go through what Piaget calls the preoperational stage. This is the stage when they "make believe." Increased use of language is noted, and they are able to construct 3- to 4-word sentences. There is also an increased sense of time and space. The child begins to realize that situations are interrelated and important.

Language Development

At 15 months, toddlers' favorite word is "no." At 18 to 20 months, they understand simple requests and gestures. By age 2, the child has a 275- to 300-word vocabulary, uses his/her own first name, and knows "I," "me," and "you." This is also the stage when they seem to talk continually. By 3 years of age, vocabulary increases to 900 words, first and last names are mentioned, plurals are formed, and the child can name one color and use complete sentences.

Moral Development

According to Kohlberg, toddlers are at the preconventional or premoral levels. The issues are based on their egocentric, cognitively biased, and limited considerations. Children at age 3 behave according to the punishment-obedience orientation.

Health Maintenance

Nutrition The required caloric intake for this age is 100 calories per kilogram per day. Toddlers can be finicky eaters. They may have a voracious appetite one day and want next to nothing the next day. Parents should not force children to eat when they are not hungry and should instead give children food choices in small portions. Finger foods are especially helpful at this age.

The child should have regular dental care during the developmental period when teeth are erupting, and should be taught correct teeth-brushing techniques with a soft-bristled toothbrush at least twice a day. Dental caries caused by going to bed with a bottle of milk or juice may occur. To prevent "bottle mouth" dental caries, avoid bottles with milk or juice at nap or bedtimes. Avoid "sweet" snacks as well.

The major task during toddlerhood is to master toilet training. The child should be physiologically ready and walking well. The child should have the ability to communicate the need to use the bathroom for urinating or defecation, and the caregiver should be keen and observant as to the child's nonverbal behavior.

Play At the toddler stage, the child obtains pleasure from parallel play, meaning he/she plays independently, but also enjoys the company of other children. Toddlers are possessive of their toys and have difficulty sharing them. As the toddler grows older, increased socialization is encouraged and he/she learns to share toys and engage in more **cooperative play**.

Sensorimotor activity is the major component for muscle development and also serves as a release of energy in children. Through sensorimotor activity, toddlers explore the world in which they live. Appropriate choices of toys for this age group include push-pull toys, balls, blocks, musical and talking toys, thick crayons, and tricycles.

Safety Considerations The leading cause of death for children ages 1 to 5 is the accident. As with infants, precautions against aspiration and suffocation should also be practiced. Keeping an eye on the child is of first priority. Teaching the child to avoid hazards is also important, including not putting small items in their mouths or asking a caregiver before doing so, not playing on or near stairs, staying in a safety restraint seat in the car, staying away from stoves and open flames, never touching matches, never swimming without an adult, never touching weapons or sharp objects—

Cooperative play. Play that emerges during school years. Children learn to play together.

including scissors, knives, and power tools—or pointing them at other people, and never going anywhere with someone they do not know.

Hemoglobin and hematocrit should be checked yearly, and a lead screen performed.

Preschool Children (3 to 6 Years)

Physical Growth

During this stage, the child gains height in proportion to weight. The child grows 2 to 2.5 inches a year, has an erect posture, and appears thinner and taller. The average weight gain is 5 pounds per year.

Motor Development

Children at this age skip and hop, roller-skate, and jump rope. They are able to play throw and catch games and walk backward heel to toe at age 5, and are able to dress and undress themselves. Fine motor skills for preschoolers allow them to wash their hands and feet, button and unbutton clothes, and tie shoelaces.

Cognitive and motor development allow the toddler to progress from copying a circle or square to copying diamonds and triangles. By age 5, the child can use simple tools.

Psychosocial Development

According to Erikson's stages, this is the stage of initiative versus guilt. Children investigate and initiate new skills to accomplish tasks, and feel satisfied when a task is accomplished. Also, they are aware of punishment and discipline when they misbehave. The preschool child is able to identify gender roles. Parents need to encourage the child to explore different things, praise acceptable behavior, support creativity, and avoid corporal punishment or taking food away for discipline. It is also of utmost importance for parents to instruct the child to use caution when he/she is approached by strangers; however, that cautious behavior should not instill a fear of all other people in the child.

Psychosexual Development (Phallic Stage)

According to Freud, during the late preschool years the child becomes preoccupied with his/her genitalia as a body area from which pleasure is received through self-stimulation. This self-stimulation is different from the sexual drive that adolescents and adults experience. Freud stresses that at this period, boys and girls experience a period of intense attachment with the parent of the opposite sex, and demonstrate hostility with the parent of the same sex. This phenomenon is called the Oedipus complex. Before the phallic stage the mother becomes the primary love object for boys and girls. The conflict resolution starts when the child begins the identification process with the parent of the same sex, which includes incorporating the qualities of the parent of the same sex into his/her own personality. The completion of this stage is what Freud has termed super-ego formation or the development of a conscience. What this means is that the child can see the difference between right and wrong based on the instruction and the modeling of the parent.

The most important nursing intervention at this stage is to explain to the parent that this is a normal process that all children go through. More important, in relation to the masturbation that the child exhibits, is for the nurse to reinforce to the parents that the child's behavior is innocent, and that it will go away. Parents also need to hear that the child should be told that this behavior is all right if done in his/her own room, but it should not be done in public.

Cognitive Development

Piaget describes this stage as the intuitive stage. The child plays a tug-of-war between perceptions and logic. He/she is also able to draw a person with six major parts—head, two arms, two legs, and a body. When liquid is poured in a tall glass and the same amount is poured in a smaller glass, the child perceives the tall glass to be greater than the smaller glass. Objects are fixed in quality. Children understand "before nap" and "after dinner," the concept of time in correlation to events. Magical and fantasy thinking is also at peak for this age. They are able to construct sentences and frequently use the word "why" in their attempt to understand concepts and situations.

Language Development

A 3-year-old has a vocabulary of 900 words: 3 to 4 words are formed in sentences; plurals, pronouns, and past tense of verbs are used; and numbers may be repeated. By 4 years, vocabulary is increased to 1500 words; speech is more concrete, and frequent questions are asked; verbs, adjectives, and prepositions are added to sentences. By age 5 the child has 2100 words in his/her vocabulary, 6 to 8-word sentences are used, including opposites and similarities, 4 or more colors, coin denominations, definitions of shapes or color, and counting to 10. At age 6, objects are described by compositions. Vocabulary increases 600 words per year from then on.

Moral Development

This stage is described by Kohlberg as the stage of naive instrumental orientation. The actions of children in this stage are geared to satisfying their own needs rather than the needs of others. At this age, children are able to have a concrete sense of justice. Their idea of reciprocity and fairness is "I'll hold your toys if you'll hold my toys." But they still lack the concepts of loyalty and gratitude. At this stage children adopt the moral values of their parents as standards for evaluating their own behaviors and the behaviors of others. This adaptation strengthens the child's sense of identification.

Health Maintenance

Nutrition The caloric intake should be 90 calories per kilogram per day. The child is now a self-feeder, but may be finicky with the quality or the taste of food.

Play As children begin preschool, they engage in **associative play**. In this form of play, they begin to borrow toys or materials from other children. Preschool children learn to refine their movements and master their dexterity. During this period of development, play becomes more differentiated and involved, and sometimes more complex. Children also learn to be creative by experimenting with raw materials and by exercising their imagination. In dealing with preschool children, the nurse must be aware that creativity is fostered by solitary activity, and should reinforce this activity.

Associative play. Play that emerges in preschool years as the child learns to interact with another child.

Intellectual development is facilitated through play using puzzles, books, games, films, etc. The most important aspect in the area of intellectual development is assimilating new experiences on top of previous ones, and understanding the difference between reality and fantasy. Imaginary playmates are normal at this age and disappear as the child gets more involved with friends at play.

Toys appropriate for this age include tricycles, skates, puzzles, coloring books, paints, and crayons. Dolls, puppets, and miniature communities are effective for role play. Books and electronic games stimulate cognitive development.

Safety Considerations The preschool child is less prone to falls because of the increased development of fine and gross motor skills. Seat belts to prevent injury during motor vehicle accidents, safety training about crossing the street, and why to avoid strangers are primary issues to be addressed. Parents should educate the child on safety procedures and should be good role models by setting examples for their children.

At 3 years old, children are aware of the anatomical differences between the sexes. This is the time when they imitate the roles of mommy and daddy and play "doctor" to explore their curiosity. Masturbation is normal and healthy at this age if it is not excessive. Parents should not punish their children and should explain that this should be done in private. Sexuality questions and birth process questions should be answered honestly and openly by the parents in understandable words to the child.

Children at this age also go to preschool and nursery school. This can increase the child's self-esteem and at the same time provide group learning experiences of various types, increasing the child's interactions with peers. This is excellent preparation for attending regular school, and stimulates the child in social, physical, and language development. The parents should encourage and prepare the child, and be interested in school activities.

School-Age Children (6 to 12 Years)

Physical Growth

Growth at this stage is regular and slow. This is the start of pubescent changes. Growth averages 2 inches per year and weight gain is 5 to 7 pounds per year. The face of the school-age child is growing faster than the skull and facial changes may be noted. Permanent teeth are acquired and the eyes acquire a 20/20 vision. Physiologically, the body systems are stabilizing and assuming the capacity of an adult. Secondary sex characteristics occur, including hair under arms and in the pubic areas, and girls' breasts may begin to enlarge. The leg length is also increasing and the child may experience growing pains from the stretching of muscles and the growth of the long bones.

Motor Development

Muscle strength doubles and coordination and refinements of motor skills are evident in the school-age child. For the child to develop new muscles, it is important that the nurse encourage regular exercise. Activities could include jumping rope, skating, bicycling, running games, swimming, and playing outdoor games like baseball, soccer, or football. A growth spurt may begin and as a consequence the child may seem clumsy.

The child also learns to refine drawing, painting, and writing skills. Left- or right-hand dominance is also predicted at this time. The child is able to make useful articles and to utilize knives, tools, and common utensils. Creativity also predominates and is expressed in stories, poems, and writings.

Psychosocial Development

Erikson describes this stage as the crisis of industry versus inferiority. It is important to emphasize interactions with friends and encourage group activities with same-sex peers. Peer pressure peaks at this time and children also become sensitive to social norms. They view the parent as an adult, not a peer, and a teacher's approval will aid in their development of industry. Children are able to play games with rules, explore the neighborhood in which they live, and use the phone frequently for communication with peers.

Psychosexual Development

Freud called the period between toddlerhood and adolescence latency. In this period Freud describes children as constructing their personality based on the previous stages. Children channel their energy into acquiring more independence from home. Teachers become very important in their life, and they help children to refine the skills they previously learned. The acquisition of new skills plays an important part in the development of their emergent personality. The nurse needs to reinforce to the parents that at this stage it is very important for them to support any activity that the child chooses and not to force any sport or activity at which the child is not going to be successful. The nurse also needs to educate the parents on the reality that the child who cannot do well in sports and in school becomes a candidate for problem behavior in school and later on in life.

Cognitive Development

Piaget describes this stage as the concrete operations stage. The child is able to think in a logical manner, comprehend and tell time, and understand days and seasons. The child is able to think abstractly and reason, to handle and classify problems, and is independent in making and testing a hypothesis. At this stage the child functions in the present and is able to view things from different perspectives, but is bound to rules. The cognitive skills and attention spans are increased.

Language Development

The child's vocabulary is rapidly expanding and objects are described with shape, color, and size. This age group likes to read and is eager to learn new words and their meanings. They know how to use the calendar and are able to tell time.

Moral Development

From egocentrism to logical patterns of thought, the child then moves through the stages of conscience and moral standards. This growth in judgment and moral thought progresses between ages 6 and 12. Rules are first perceived as covering limited situations, definite with no reason or explanation. From this, the children learn the standards for acceptable behavior. Children ages 6 to 7 know the rules and what they are supposed to do, but are unaware of the reasons. Judgment is based on the consequences, and rewards and punishment serve as their guides. When a conflict arises between a child and an adult, the adult is right, and the child is wrong. At this age, children also interpret accidents and bad luck as punishment.

Older schoolchildren judge an act by intentions and cause, rather than by consequences. They become more empathetic to the needs of others. Rules of conduct are based on cooperation and respect for others, and are considered in terms of mutual agreement. Young children judge an act as either wrong or right; older children take a different point of view and will take this into account to make a judgment. They understand the Golden Rule: "Do unto others as you would have others do unto you."

Health Maintenance

Nutrition Preferences for junk food prevail at this stage, resulting in a higher incidence of malnutrition. Caloric need increases to 2500 calories per day, with an increased need for snacking. Parents and schools should educate children on the fundamentals of proper nutrition. Food advertised in the mass media has a large, sometimes negative influence on their choices of food.

Permanent teeth are acquired at this time and it is the best time to build on the oral hygiene taught to the child as a toddler. Biyearly checkups, proper teeth-brushing and flossing, and balanced nutrition, including avoiding large intakes of sweets, are some of the major preventive measures for maintaining healthy teeth.

Play According to Piaget, children move through the stages of mental activity in an orderly and sequential manner. School-age children's thought process changes from preoperational thought (preoperational thought is "egocentric"; in this sense egocentric does not mean selfish but the inability to put oneself in the place of another) to concrete operational (thought becomes increasingly logical and coherent). Early in this stage, children play collaboratively with other groups of children, maintain mutual respect, and also create detailed rules to ensure equality among them. School-age children engage in symbolic play. This play is useful because the child is aware that many wishes and feelings are not socially acceptable. Children engage in play discussions and create drawings and paintings, which give them the necessary means for coping with their own feelings.

The school-age child reflects through play a new level of development, along with increased physical and intellectual skills. The child continues to refine gross and motor movements and eye-hand coordination. To perfect these skills children need to be given the opportunity to participate in sports or games in which they feel good about themselves. School-age children need to learn the concept of interdependence, that is, to function in a group. It is not unusual to see the child preoccupied with rules and regulations involving the play.

At this age, the child also enters the stage of "industry vs. inferiority." The sense of industry is explored by creating crafts. Collecting stamps, dolls, stones, etc., enables the child to collect information about the world. Also at this stage, children develop an interest in pets, which contributes to a sense of industry.

Safety remains a very important component of play. At this stage of development, children cannot realistically judge their physical abilities; therefore they need to be told what the dangers are of engaging in certain sports and in the use of firearms.

Safety Considerations The most common cause of injury and death at this age is motor vehicle accidents. Wearing and using seat belts in the car, and street and bicycle safety, including wearing of safety helmets, should be mandated. Water safety should be stressed to prevent drowning. Guns, matches, and any fire-producing materials should be kept away from the child. Children are very curious at this time and should be taught the importance of safety rules to avoid potentially fatal hazards.

The child should continue to have health screenings every 2 years, with laboratory values of hemoglobin and hematocrit, baseline cholesterol, urine analysis, and inspection for scoliosis all included.

Formal sex education should start with the parents and be reinforced at school. Misconceptions and myths about sex should be discussed in an open and honest manner, with every attempt made to answer all the child's questions at his/her level of understanding. The parents should also be aware of any negative or positive impact the mass media produces on the child's view of intimate relationships. Drug and alcohol abuse are also important issues to be addressed by parents and teachers, who should serve as role models for the child.

𝒜DOLESCENTS (12–16 YEARS)

Physical Growth

During adolescence, a growth spurt occurs in girls earlier than in boys. Boys have an increase in muscle mass with a normal weight gain of between 15 and 65 pounds. Girls also gain between 15 and 55 pounds, and their body fat proportion increases in relation to their muscle mass.

Secondary characteristics also develop at this stage, with the female maturing with menarche at 11 to 14 years. Increased breast tissue develops, hips widen, and there is an increase in vaginal secretions. Pubic and axillary hair also increases.

Males have an increase in pubic, facial, chest, and axillary hair, with an increase in penis size. Spermatozoa are also produced and nocturnal emissions sometimes occur at this stage of development. Males experience a broadening of their shoulders and chest and their voice deepens. Acne may develop and an increase in perspiration is common. The functioning of the physiological systems is approaching that of the adult.

Psychosocial Development

Erikson describes this stage as identity versus role confusion. With this stage of maturation, the adolescent is integrating present with past social skills. Various roles are tried, searching for an appropriate and comfortable state of being that Erikson refers to as "fit." Career choices and questions of "What do I want to be?" play a tug-of-war within their psyches. Peer relationships and being the same as their peers—fitting in—play an internal role in their development. Intimate sexual relationships may begin to develop and adolescents may become sexually active. Body image is of utmost importance. Physical appearance is a reflection of this image and efforts are continually made to adapt to changes that are occurring in the body.

Relationships become increasingly detached from parents as adolescents search for ways to interact with their peers and with other adults. This is one of the steps toward the independence the adolescent seeks. This search for independence is sometimes hard for both the child and the parents because the child wants to act like an adult and the parent must monitor what level is appropriate for the child.

Psychosexual Development

Freud describes this period as the period of development when the aggressive drives of the Oedipal stage become reality. According to Freud, a truce between the id and the ego results, until the emergence of the true sexual drive. At the beginning of the latency period, the superego becomes internalized. The child learns from the values of the parents. The outlook of latency is black and white: Family rules are clear in the child's mind and he/she bases principles on the ones that he/she has learned.

Following this period, the last significant phase in psychosexual development is the genital stage. The stage begins with puberty, with the maturation of the reproductive sex hormones. The sexual organs become the major source of anxiety or pleasure. Also at this time, the adolescent starts forming lasting relationships with friends. This is the time that he/she starts looking for a spouse with whom to spend the rest of his/her life.

Cognitive Development

Piaget describes the adolescent stage as the formal operations stage, where adolescents are able to think abstractly, deductively, and inductively, and to deduce conclusions from their own hypotheses. Egocentrism is exhibited, and the ability to use introspection develops.

Health Maintenance

With the rapid growth of the adolescent, adequate calcium and iron should be monitored. Girls need about 2200 calories per day; boys need 2700 calories. Snacking and fast food options predominate in the appetites of the adolescent. Outdoor sports are popular and adolescents who participate in athletics have increased nutritional requirements. Body image is of primary concern to the adolescent. It is at this age when adolescent obesity, anorexia nervosa, and bulimia in females may occur. Positive self-image should be fostered, and education about their developing bodies and the importance of good nutrition is imperative.

The major cause of death for adolescents is accidental injury. Motor vehicle accidents are prevalent at this time because at age 15 or 16 the adolescent can obtain a driver's license. Education about traffic laws should be stressed. Drinking alcohol and driving should never be allowed. Education on alcohol and drug abuse should also be emphasized by the school and the parents.

Adolescents experience many emotional events, including dealing with their changing bodies, changing expectations from others, and involvement with opposite or same-sex partners in intimate relationships. One solution adolescents appear to be taking more often is suicide. It is a permanent solution to a temporary problem. Parents, clergy, and educators should be observant as to any signs of withdrawal, moodiness (extreme swings of mood), and depression. Getting adolescents to talk about their emotions or feelings is difficult sometimes, but it is one way to reassure them that the way they are feeling is only part of growing up and will go away as they get older. Open expression of feelings without physical violence should be fostered in the home and at school.

With clinical screenings, a breast and testicular examination should be included. Gynecological exams, a regular physical, eye examination, and proper posture to prevent scoliosis should also be emphasized. In school, sex education classes should discuss the anatomy and physiology of males and females, sexually transmitted diseases, pregnancy, birth control, and alternative life-styles.

Critical Points in Growth and Development Issues

Pediatrics has changed from focusing on the child alone to including the entire family. The ultimate goal of pediatrics is to involve the family in the care of the child and to empower the parents, so that total care of the child comes from home and not from medical personnel. To attain this goal, the main issue remains the preparation of nurses as teachers for families, to guide them and empower them with knowledge in the care of their child.

Among the many issues involved in empowering parents is teaching. Beginning with the first physical examination of the child, the nurse should teach not only routine feeding, bathing, and clothing of the baby, but also incorporate issues of child safety, moral behavior, and what it means in terms of development. Carol Gilligan (1992) states that babies have the capacity for empathy as early as 2 months of age. She gives the example that children start to cry when other people or babies cry. Introduction of discipline and appropriate ways of setting limits will avoid behavior problems as the child grows. Instructing the parents on the cognitive development of the child will allow parents to begin thinking of their child as an individual. While doing the physical exam and plotting charts, the nurse can also project to the parents the ways to care for the infant to prevent future problems, especially related to physical growth with regard to racial and ethnic characteristics. For example, if the projection for the child is to have a short stature, parents can be helpful to the child by directing him/her to excel in areas where height is not a factor.

New parents are especially nervous and apprehensive with their first baby, and all their attention is focused on the area of physical care of their infant. Issues about the baby as an individual, his/her temperament, likes, and dislikes, are seldom taken into consideration unless there is a problem. This issue has a serious impact on how the baby is cared for and the effects that the baby's temperament has on his/her relationship with the other members of the family.

Temper tantrums, bed wetting, thumb sucking, sleeping at an appropriate time, toilet training all should be discussed based on research rather than opinion. In keeping such issues before the parents, the nurse has the opportunity to show alternatives to parenting in these areas while maintaining respect for the parents' own cultures and backgrounds.

Close attention to general, physical, and developmental examinations often suggests the correct diagnosis and the appropriate care for children. The evaluation of growth and development at each visit is most important to nurses, to enable them to teach the parents and minimize future problems.

$\mathcal{Q}$UESTIONS

History: Sara, a black newborn, is 4 hours old and weighs 7 pounds. Normal newborn; 40 weeks' gestation; uncomplicated labor and birth. Apgar scores 9-9; first child of a 28-year-old mother.
Plan: Child to go home with parents in 48 hours.
Nursing problems: Transition to extrauterine life.
Family integration: Support, help, risk of anxiety-altered role performance.

1. Mrs. Brown has not decided if she is going to breast-feed or use formula. She seems to be anxious and somewhat hesitant to make the decision. Which statement related to breast-feeding is important when talking to Mrs. Brown?

   A. Breast milk is digested better than formula.
   B. Babies like breast milk more than formula.
   C. Breast milk has higher protein content than formula.
   D. Breast milk never causes allergies.

2. The nurse touches Sara's cheek. Sara turns toward the stimulus and opens her mouth This reflex is called:

    A. Moro
    B. Rooting
    C. Babinsky
    D. Sucking

3. At 3 months of age, Sara has a cold. Sara's mom is complaining that she is worried Sara might stop breathing. The nurse explains that:

    A. Babies breathe through their mouth and the cold will pass.
    B. It is normal for babies to hold their breath for up to 1 minute.
    C. Babies at this age are obligatory nose breathers.
    D. It is normal for babies to turn red and then blue.

4. Sara is due for her shots. OPV is contraindicated if:

    A. Sara has a cold.
    B. Sara has a brother at home with leukemia, on chemotherapy.
    C. The family is negative for AIDS.
    D. Sara does not like sugar and has a positive history of diabetes.

5. At 6 months Sara should sit with support, be able to roll back to her stomach and vice versa, and to reach and grasp at objects. Her parents should be taught that:

    A. The child requires full-time protection.
    B. The child requires only limited supervision.
    C. Accidents are not frequent for this age group.
    D. Babies do not choke easily.

6. Mrs. Brown is told that from 12–35 months of age, Sara will continually explore her environment, start to imitate household tasks, and insist on doing everything by herself. Mrs. Brown is told that this developmental period is critical because the parents need to:

    A. Continue with complete protection.
    B. Begin to teach the toddler about safety.
    C. Have more patience with the inquisitive child.
    D. Begin firm discipline.

7. Mrs. Brown complains to the nurse that Sara, at 3 years of age, is frequently having temper tantrums. The nurse explains that:

    A. This is abnormal behavior and the child needs a psych consult.
    B. It is okay to isolate Sara when she starts acting up and to leave her alone.
    C. This is normal for this age because Sara is trying to establish her autonomy.
    D. It's important to reason with the child that this is a negative behavior.

8. Mrs. Brown is told that from 3–5 years of age, Sara will be able to understand 90% of speech. She will become more autonomous and will want more freedom. Mrs. Brown should also know that at this stage, children need close supervision and lessons regarding:

   A. Poisons
   B. Walking
   C. Playing
   D. Running

9. Mrs. Brown is told that from 6–11 years of age, most children have acquired all basic motor skills, physical growth slows down, and they are involved outside of the home with friends and going to school. At this stage, the most important knowledge that the child requires is:

   A. A sense of confidence and responsibility.
   B. A sense of security and caution.
   C. A sense of alertness.
   D. A sense of realism about danger.

10. Parents of 6- –11-year-old children have a poor knowledge of many developmental issues and erroneous beliefs about caution. This occurs because parents:

   A. Have a low level of perceived vulnerability.
   B. Have different beliefs about development.
   C. Find safety to be an obstacle.
   D. Find caution to be offensive.

11. Children from 13–19 years old are very vulnerable because of their age and their lack of experience. Adolescent behaviors result in actions that can be potentially stressful to the family system. What is the most important parenting skill that parents must have at this stage?

   A. Communication
   B. Alertness
   C. Guidance
   D. Firmness

12. To adolescents, one of the most important things is:

   A. School grades
   B. Having good and popular friends
   C. Body image
   D. Parents

13. What principles and characteristics of growth and development need to be explained to every teenager?

   A. Physiological changes that cause anxiety
   B. Physiological changes that do not cause anxiety
   C. All physiological changes
   D. Physiological changes related to their own gender

ANSWERS

1. *A.* Breast milk is digested better than formula.

2. *B.* The *rooting* reflex is elicited whenever the infant's cheek and lips are touched and the infant is hungry.

3. *C.* Babies are obligatory nose breathers at this age; all the other answers are false.

4. *B.* OPV is a live virus.

5. *A.* A child who is able to reach out and turn by himself/herself needs full-time protection.

6. *B.* The child still needs to be protected and supervision needs to be reinforced. Teaching and protecting the child become pivotal during this developmental stage.

7. *C.* Temper tantrums are actions to establish autonomy, according to Erikson.

8. *A.* Poisoning is one of the most prevalent injuries at this time.

9. *A.* Confidence is the basic trait children need in order to succeed in life. Their future is assured if they have confidence in themselves and have learned responsibility for their actions at an early age.

10. *B.* Parents think that the child at this age is more mature than he/she really is, and therefore, parents do not perceive the child's high level of vulnerability.

11. *A.* The most often voiced complaint from adolescents is that they are not understood. The most difficult task the parents face is listening without interrupting. Communication is the most important parenting skill at this age.

12. *C.* Body image is very important to teenagers. (See answer for question 13.)

13. *C.* Teenagers need to learn about physical and mental changes, and that others in their age group are going through the same things. An understanding of how everyone's body and feelings change gives the teenager a sense that he/she is not alone in this world.

$\mathcal{G}$LOSSARY

anticipatory guidance   process of understanding developmental needs, and teaching parents and caretakers to meet the child's needs.

assessment   process of collecting information about the child and his/her family in order to make a nursing diagnosis.

associative play   play that emerges in preschool years as the child learns to interact with another child.

cephalocaudal development   process by which development proceeds from head to feet.

cooperative play   play that emerges during school years. Children learn to play together.

development   increase in capability.

$\mathcal{B}$IBLIOGRAPHY

ALTSCHULER, S. M., AND LUDWIG, S. *Pediatrics at à Glance*. Philadelphia: Appleton and Lange, 1997.

BETZ, C. L., et al. *Family Centered Nursing Care of Children*. 2nd ed. Philadelphia: W. B. Saunders, 1994.

BOYTON, R. W., et al. *Manual of Ambulatory Pediatrics*. 3rd ed. Hagerstown, MD: Lippincott, 1994.

BURNS, E. C., et al. *Pediatric Primary Care*. Philadelphia: W. B. Saunders, 1996.

EISENBAUER, L. A., AND MURPHY, M. A. *Pharmachotherapeutics and Advanced Nursing Practice*. New York: McGraw-Hill, 1998.

FITZPATRICK, T. B., et al. *Color Atlas and Synopsis of Clinical Dermatology*. 3rd ed. New York: McGraw-Hill, 1997.

FOX, J. A. *Primary Health Care of Children*. St. Louis: Mosby, 1997.

GILLIGAN, C. Mapping the moral domain. In Terkel, S.: *Ethics*. New York: Lodestar, 1992.

GRODZIN, C. J., et al. *Diagnostic Strategies for Internal Medicine*. St. Louis: Mosby-Year Book, 1995.

HARRISON, T. R., et al. *Principles of Internal Medicine*. 14th ed. New York: McGraw-Hill, 1998.

HAY, W. W., et al. *Current Pediatric Diagnosis and Treatment*. Stamford, CT: Appleton and Lange, 1997.

JACKSON, P. L., AND VESSEY, J. A. *Primary Care of the Child with a Chronic Condition*. 2nd ed. St. Louis: Mosby, 1996.

KHER, K. K., AND MAKKER, S. P. *Clinical Pediatric Nephrology*. New York: McGraw-Hill, 1992.

KNOOP, K. J., et al. *Atlas of Emergency Medicine*. New York: McGraw-Hill, 1997.

KOHLBERG, L. Moral development. In D. I. Sill, (ed.), *International Encyclopedia of Social Sciences.* New York: Macmillan, 1968.

LAGERQUIST, S. L. *Critical Thinking Exercises.* Boston: Little, Brown, 1996.

LORIN, M. I. *Review of Pediatrics.* Stamford, CT: Appleton and Lange, 1993.

OSKI, F. A., et al. *Principles and Practices of Pediatrics.* Hagerstown, MD: Lippincott, 1994.

PANSKY, B. *Review of Gross Anatomy.* 6th ed. New York: McGraw-Hill, 1996.

PIZZUTILLO, P. D. *Pediatric Orthopedics in Primary Practice.* New York: McGraw-Hill, 1997.

WEINBERG, S., et al. *Color Atlas of Pediatric Dermatology.* 3rd ed. New York: McGraw-Hill, 1998.

WHALEY, L. F., AND WONG, D. L. *Nursing Care of Infants and Children.* 5th ed. St. Louis: Mosby, 1994.

*H*ELPFUL INTERNET SITES

PEDINFO: An Index of the Pediatric Internet at http://www. pedinfo.org An excellent site that covers nearly all topics within this review. It has a wealth of information and is worth a visit. It is written for health care professionals but others could also use the information.

Bright Futures at http://www.brightfutures.org/ A site dedicated to growth and development health care issues and problems. An excellent resource for health care professionals concerning particular issues and problems at various development stages.

The Cochrane Neonatal Collaborative Review Group at http://silk. nih.gov/silk/cochrane/Cochrane.htm This site is dedicated to providing systematic reviews of importance in informing providers and consumers about the effect of treatments and in identifying priorities for new research. This site has a wealth of current research in many areas for neonatal health care professionals. The materials are written at a high level and are comprehensive.

Paediapaedia™ An Imaging Encyclopedia of Pediatric Disease at http://www.vh.org/Providers/TeachingFiles/PAP/PAPHome.html For those who need an online encyclopedia of pediatric diseases that includes images. This site is part of the "Virtual Hospital" Web site and is an excellent resource.

University of Michigan Center for Human Growth and Development at hyperlink http://www.umich.edu/~chgdwww/home.html This is an excellent site concerning various issues and research surrounding human growth and development.

University of Minnesota, Kansas, and Oregon at hyperlink http://ici2.coled.umn.edu/ecri/default.html This site supports research conducted in October, 1996, by the Early Childhood Research

Institute on Measuring Growth and Development (ECRI-MGD) to produce a comprehensive, individualized measurement system for children with disabilities from birth to 8 years of age, and their families. This site contains links to many other sites that provide a wealth of information on childhood growth and development.

Zero to Three at hyperlink http://www.zerotothree.org A site dedicated to the child from 0 to 3 years of age that contains a wealth of information for parents and professionals alike.

International Society on Early Intervention at hyperlink http://weber.u.washington.edu/~isei This site is dedicated to providing effective early intervention programs for vulnerable children and their families. It has an excellent set of resources for forging families.

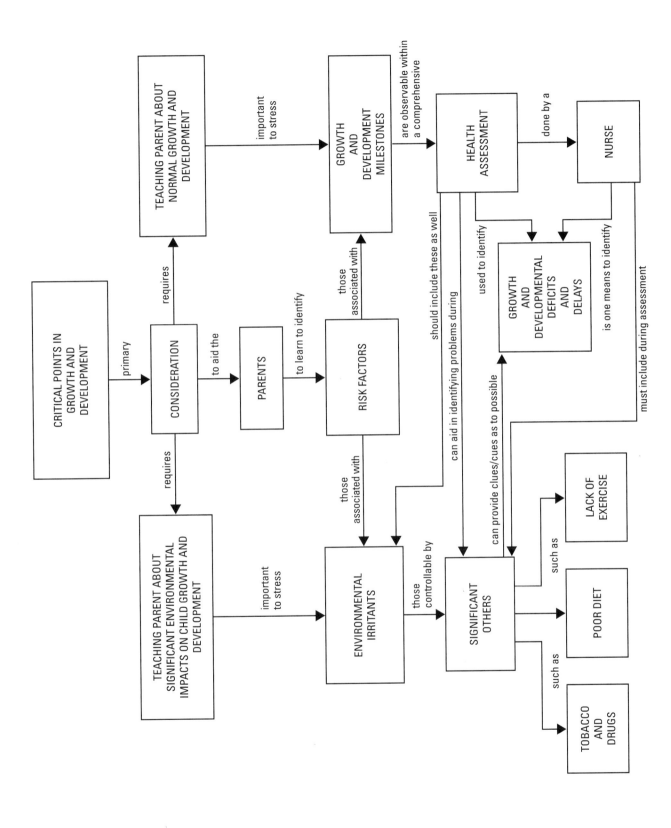

Concept Map 3-1

95

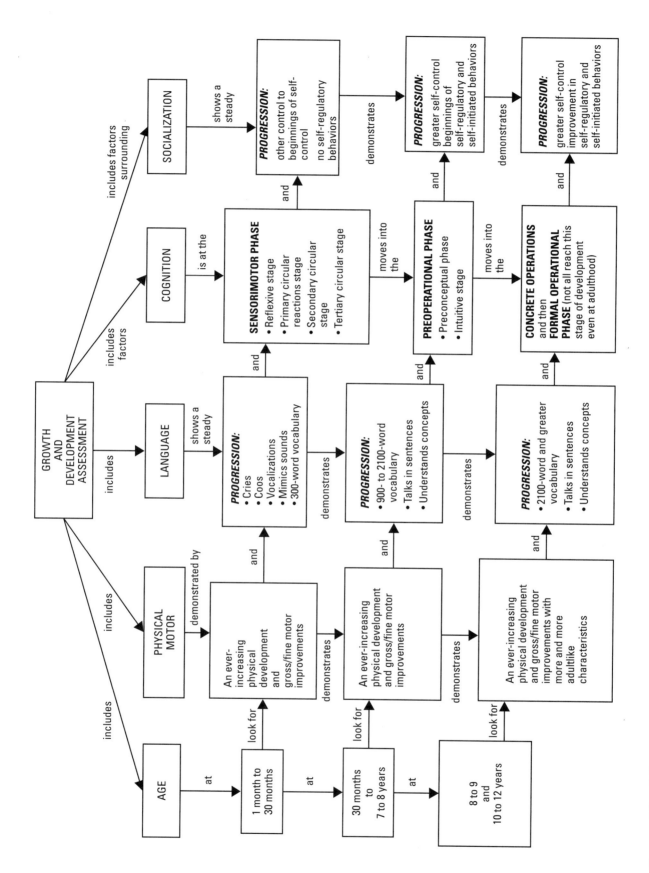

Concept Map 3-2

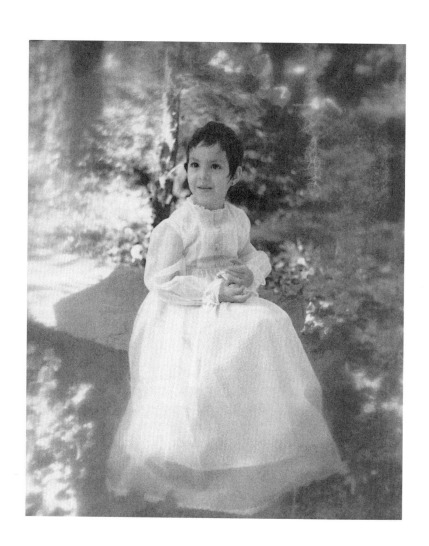

ℋEALTH PROMOTION

ℐNTRODUCTION

Health promotion is a process that emphasizes teaching attitudes and skills in order to help individuals to choose a life-style that will maximize their health potential. Wellness is a way of life. Pediatric health promotion is based on the belief that if children learn the value of wellness early, it will become their way of life.

Health care providers need to instruct parents to teach their children self-responsibility for wellness. Programs such as PACT (Participative and Assertive Consumer Training), designed by the University of Colorado School Nurse Practitioner Program, are great resources for nurses helping children become more actively aware of wellness. Another program that promotes self-responsibility for wellness in children is the Health Activities Project (HAP) of the University of California Lawrence Hall of Science, Berkeley. These two programs are examples of many others in the United States available to nurses and to other health care professionals as sources for promoting wellness.

Nurses play an important role in the development of realistic attitudes toward health in parents and children. Nurses have the advantage of seeing parents and children together in well-care clinics, hospital units, or rehabilitation centers. Nurses must promote wellness by involving children and their parents in the implementation of an individual plan for each family to maximize the wellness of each child.

Physical fitness in children contributes to the wellness of our society. It is well known that regular exercise lowers cardiovascular risk, improves attention span and self-reliance, and lessens anxiety and depression (Bailey, 1973). It is also well documented that one of the most important variables in children's participation in exercise is parental participation. Parents are important role models (Cooper, 1975).

Physical fitness guidelines for children younger than 10 have been developed only recently. It was not until 1979 that Samuels and Samuels suggested the first set of guidelines for young children.

1. Begin a new activity slowly.
2. Do warm-up exercises.
3. Avoid fatigue or overtraining.
4. Do cool-down exercises to stop the session.
5. Maintain a regular exercise pattern 3 to 5 times a week.

Samuels and Samuels also emphasized that young children should focus on activities that help them perfect the gross and fine motor skills (hand-eye coordination, balance, and agility). For older children, Samuels and Samuels suggested, team **sports** are useful for developing physical skills and confidence, rather than causing stress through competition (Samuels & Samuels, 1979).

As the treatment of professional athletes evolved, new medical techniques were developed. Sports medicine developed as a subspecialty of orthopedic surgery. The same treatment and prevention techniques used to treat professional athletes were eventually applied to college athletes and finally to children who suffered sports injuries. As changes in medical treatment evolved, the nurse's role in the care of children with sports injuries also changed. Nurses became more sensitive to the importance of sports in children's lives, to the impact that an injury has on a young athlete, and to the reality that an injury can be felt throughout life, physically and emotionally.

In 1990, *Healthy People 2000: National Health Promotion and Disease Prevention Objectives* for the year 2000 (U.S. Departments of Health and Human Services, 1990) were published. They include the following objectives for physical activities and fitness for children:

1. To increase to at least 30% the proportion of children age 6 and older who participate in light to moderate physical activity for at least 30 minutes per day.
2. To increase to at least 20% the proportion of teenagers 18 years old and older, and to increase to at least 75% the proportion of children between the ages of 6 and 17 who engage in vigorous physical activity for 20 minutes or more, 3 or more days a week.
3. To reduce to no more than 15% the proportion of children age 6 and older who engage in no leisure-time activity.
4. To increase to at least 40% the proportion of children age 6 and older who regularly engage in physical activities.
5. To increase to 50% the proportion of children who are involved in physical activities.
6. To increase to at least 50% the proportion of school education class time that students spend being physically active.

Sport. An individual or group athletic or competitive form of amusement/entertainment normally done for enjoyment.

Healthy People 2000 is the blueprint for what is envisioned for health promotion and maintenance for the nation for the next century. Physical activity is seen not only as a basic health need, but, more importantly, its preventive nature is seen as the main component of health care in the United States. The change from focusing on curing disease to focusing on prevention has come about because it has been reported that American youth are not involved in physical activity sufficient for healthy cardiovascular development. The health care of the nation depends on the preventive measures that people assimilate into their life-styles, including healthy habits like physical activities and optimal nutritional choices. These are essential components in growth and development. Healthy children become healthy adults. Thus, the nurse involved in the care of children needs to stress both to parents and to children the importance of making appropriate nutritional choices and maintaining physical activity levels to ensure optimal cardiovascular endurance.

Assessment

Often, the first time a child has a complete physical examination is when it is required before participation in a sports activity at school or in Little League baseball, football, soccer, and so on. The examination is geared to identify conditions that could be aggravated while participating in the sport, which would make it dangerous for the child to participate. This examination can also identify medical conditions that have gone undiagnosed. Dayment (1991) states that sometimes this examination is the only one that a child has during the year. Although this may seem inconceivable, it is further evidence that well visits to health care practitioners by children are not a priority of the health care industry.

The American Academy of Pediatrics recommends that sports examinations should be done every 2 years, at least 6 weeks before the child engages in a sport, in order to allow time for a follow-up if the child has any problems. Ideally, the examination should be done by the pediatrician that knows the child; however, more often, it is the practice to have mass physical examinations in the school districts or centers where the children will be participating.

When assessing a child for participation in any type of sport, the nurse needs to pay special attention to the following: previous trauma, cardiovascular disease, asthma, seizure disorder, infectious mononucleosis, skin infections, and anatomical abnormalities. The nurse needs to be familiar with the child before making any kind of recommendation. If problems arise, the first step that the nurse must take in problem solving is to identify the family's strengths and weaknesses regarding wellness. To solve the problem, the child must have a positive self-concept and cognitive ability, and the child and his/her family must have the proper attitude regarding health. Most children undergoing this type of examination fear that any condition that is discovered will disqualify them from sports participation.

Nurses need to be sensitive to the anxiety that this examination produces in children and take steps to minimize that anxiety.

Nurses should use the form from the AAP, because its questions are geared to uncover risk factors. The physical examination is a simple 12-step examination, which focuses on musculoskeletal alignment, flexibility, precondition, effective measures of abnormalities, and injury sequelae. One vital part of the examination is the assessment of Tanner stages, because this allows for the evaluation of skeletal and sexual maturity.

GUIDELINES FOR INJURY PREVENTION

The percentage of children who are injured during sports participation is between 25 and 28% a year, according to McClain and Reynolds (1989). Rates of **injuries** are higher in boys than in girls, and injuries increase as children get older. Injuries to high school athletes are most prevalent. Sprains and **strains** are the most common injuries, followed by **contusions** and **fractures** (Overvaugh & Allen, 1994).

Injury **prevention** encompasses not only the physical examination, but also the psychological and psychosocial needs of young athletes and their families. Nurses involved in sports medicine should be aware that the most important treatment of young athletes is the rehabilitation process, which should be geared toward maximizing the safety of the child before he/she returns to the sport after an injury.

MANAGEMENT OF ATHLETIC AND OTHER INJURIES

Emergencies

The role of the nurse in the care of children with an athletic injury is to prevent a catastrophic injury, such as spinal cord injury or cessation of breathing. The first nursing intervention is to apply first aid and then to secure help from the medical team. Once the injury has been identified and the extent of the damage has been assessed, the nurse stabilizes the child and the injury. A variety of nursing interventions are used immediately after an emergency has occurred, based on the location of the injury. For example, if the child has suffered a fracture, the nurse immobilizes the limb and makes sure that the child will not faint because of the pain and will remain stable until reaching the hospital. In the case of an eye injury, the nurse covers the eye and helps with transporting the child to the hospital.

Nurses in pediatric emergency departments take care of children with a broad range of illnesses, from simple colds to grave emergencies. The care of these emergencies has become more complex as demands on health care professionals have increased. In addition, the nurse has to face his/her own emotions when treating the new kinds of emergencies that surface every day.

Injury. A physical hurt. Can be described as a harm, sprain, damage, mutilation, impairment, blemish, cut, gash, scratch, stab, lesion, bite, fracture, hemorrhage, sting, bruise, sore, cramp, twinge, trauma, abrasion, burn, swelling, wound, scar, distress, or laceration.

Strain. A musculoskeletal injury involving muscles, joints, and connecting tissues. Injury can occur from unusual twists or movements on a joint or muscle group.

Contusion. Structural damage to bones.

Fracture. The rupture, breakage, or dysfunction or displacement of one or more bones. Can be classified by degree of injury to tissue and bone, i.e., simple to compound, etc.

Prevention. Anticipation of potential harm because of various factors such as being at risk because of age, sex, heredity, genetics, environment, and the like, and the introduction of interventions to reduce or eliminate the potential harm.

Scope of the Problem Injury is the leading cause of death in children age 1 to 15 years. Motor vehicle-related injuries account for 47% (division of injury control); homicide, 14%; drowning, 10%; fire burns, 8%; and other injuries, 14%. In view of these statistics, Betz (1994) states that childhood injuries ought to be seen not as imminent events, but as events that can be controlled and prevented. The child's age and cognitive development are the main determinants of the occurrence of an injury. Toddlers and preschool children are at high risk for injuries because of their lack of judgment and high level of curiosity. Preschool- and school-age children are also at high risk for injury because they like to play with firearms and are also more trusted to play by themselves and to play outside the home without close supervision from their parents. Environmental and sociocultural factors also play an important role in the occurrence of injuries.

The main role of the nurse in the management of injuries is in education in order to prevent them. Most injuries occur as the result of the child's interaction with his/her environment, and no one intervention is more effective than another. The nurse needs to assess not only the child and his/her environment, but also the strengths and weaknesses of the family, in order to educate the family about injury prevention. Family-centered teaching is required, where the family is the center of attention, not a specific child.

Bites Human and nonhuman bites are common among children; most of the bites are not serious. Dog bites account for 90% of the bites requiring medical attention; cat and rodent bites account for the other 10%. After assessment, the seriousness of the bite determines treatment. Most children are treated as outpatients. Wounds are cleansed and debrided, which minimizes the possibility of infection. If the child has not had a tetanus toxoid vaccine, it is given immediately, and if the wound is large, rabies prophylaxis should be considered, depending on the animal and the area where the animal lives. If the animal is a raccoon, bat, or skunk, the child is given the prophylactic treatment, which consists of passive and active immunoprophylaxis. Human rabies immune globulin is given as soon as possible to cover insufficient active antibody production. Prophylactic antibiotic is useful for wounds at high risk for infection. The patient is asked to come back to the clinic for follow-up care. At the same time that the nurse treats the child for the bite, he/she needs to make an environmental assessment of the home and the family's surroundings. The main nursing goal for this assessment is not only to remove the hazard from the child's life, but also to help improve his/her environment. Children need to learn about the hazards posed by animals, and parents need to learn to anticipate potentially hazardous conditions for their children.

Burns The treatment of **burns** starts immediately after the child is admitted to the hospital. A physical examination includes laboratory studies to determine treatment. Hospital treatment is based on fluid management, supportive care, wound care, and pain medications. Burns are treated according to their extent, seriousness, and cause. Decreasing mortality from burn injuries depends solely on prevention.

Burn. Injury to tissue that can be caused by chemicals, friction, or flame.

In addition to medical care, the nurse must use counseling modalities of clarification to deal with any guilt that the parents are feeling. With counseling, parents often develop the capacity to make the right choices and create a climate in which their children's health is a major priority. Children also benefit from counseling in that they develop a strong sense that they know how to make the right choices for their own health.

Aspiration. Introduction of a foreign object or liquid into the airway canal.

Foreign Body Aspiration Foreign body **aspiration** is a significant health hazard to young children, particularly those between the ages of 6 months and 3 years. Most foreign bodies are small objects that lodge in the trachea, causing acute obstruction, which can result in death by obstructing the stem of the bronchus. The nurse taking care of a child with suspected foreign body aspiration must be alert to the subtle signs and symptoms, since the diagnosis is often missed. If diagnosis is not made immediately the child may present symptoms of wheezing, which could be misdiagnosed as asthma or pneumonia. The diagnosis is based on the child's history and the report of a pulmonary condition that developed suddenly. The most helpful supporting tests are inspiratory and expiratory bilateral decubitus chest radiographs. Treatment consists of removing the foreign body by bronchoscopy. The degree of urgency depends on the location where the foreign body is lodged. Nurses taking care of infants or toddlers with suspected foreign body aspiration need to gear their teaching toward the parents, because these young children do not understand what is going on. Based on health promotion knowledge, the nurse must do a risk assessment for the child and teach the parents strategies that will protect the child's health, such as the rationale for keeping all small items away from the child's reach.

Poisoning. The accidental or intentional ingestion of a substance that is considered harmful or toxic to a system. Toxic substances from such agents as bacteria are also classified as a poison since such substances can potentially harm a system's ability to survive.

Poisoning The incidence of **poisoning** has declined in the United States because of intensive educational efforts by health care providers and the implementation of childproof medication containers since the 1970s. Despite these efforts, however, estimates of annual poisonings among children age 1 to 5 years old exceed millions, and of those, it is reported that 100 children die from accidental poisoning each year. The diagnosis is not obvious, and it is difficult to obtain because often the parents cannot give a clear account as to when the accident occurred. Routine laboratory tests play an important role in the diagnosis and management of the poisoned child. The three goals of treatment are preventing further drug absorption, providing antidotal therapy, and hastening the elimination of the absorbed poison. Treatments vary according to the poison. The nurse's main role in the treatment of the child who has ingested poisons is to support the child and the parents during a very crucial time, and to reinforce safety consciousness by teaching preventive measures to be used in the house and in the environment.

Health Teaching

Preventing problems before they arise by educating and counseling parents and children is the key for the nurse in health teaching. Lack of knowledge as to why problems occur while participating in sports, for example, is the main cause of most injuries. One area of prevention, in which parents and children can both participate, is learning about proper nutrition. Adolescents need to compensate for growth and activity with their nutritional intake. There is an erroneous idea that ingesting sugar prior to participating in a sport enhances performance. Parents need to know that carbohydrate consumption just prior to playing can be detrimental. Parents and children also need to be taught that protein supplements are not needed. Although protein is needed for growth and development, over-the-counter supplements may contain incomplete proteins, which are useless. Muscles come from exercise and a consistently healthy intake of appropriate nutrients. An overall healthy diet should be encouraged, including plenty of fruits and vegetables, especially dark green leafy vegetables; carbohydrates in the form of pasta, bread, or crackers; and protein from lean meat, fish, and chicken. Milk and calcium products are vital for strong bone development and healthy teeth.

During competition, muscle cramps and dehydration can be avoided by simply wearing lightweight, loose-fitting clothing. In addition, children sweat less than adults, so they should be encouraged to consume cool drinks while playing, at least 100 to 150 cc every 15 to 30 minutes. The best fluid for young athletes to drink during competition is plain, cool water. Children should rest in the shade for at least 10 minutes before rejoining the team, and they should be acclimatized for at least 7 to 10 days prior to playing in an unfamiliar climate. All children should use sunscreen products. During the summer, insect repellent is important if mosquitoes are prevalent, especially in the early evening.

Physical activity should be encouraged from infancy. Team sports participation can begin as early as 6 years of age. The child should be given a balance of guidance and encouragement. Handicapped children also should be encouraged to participate in sports, and children with academic problems should not be discouraged from participating. Boys and girls should be encouraged to compete and play together.

In addition to encouraging team sports, parents should teach children to swim. For the most part, drowning is a preventable accident, especially if the child knows how to swim and fully understands the buddy system. Bicycle safety training for children should include the importance of wearing a helmet and knowing hand signals and bicycling road etiquette.

Nutrition

Food always has been more than what we eat. People celebrate with food and mourn with food. How, when, and where we eat are just as important as what we eat. Our learning about food begins right after birth. Formula or breast milk is sufficient nutrition for an infant to about 6 months of age. But getting the correct amount of nutrients is not the sole reason for feeding a baby. Breast-feeding or bottle-feeding is a necessary bonding time for parents and infants.

During the first 6 months of life, it is not advisable to substitute cow's milk because when breast milk or formula mixes with the acid in the infant's stomach, it turns into a soft curd or custard texture, which is easy for the baby to digest. However, when pasteurized or raw milk is introduced into the baby's stomach and mixes with the acid there, a tough, clumpy curd forms, which is very difficult for the baby to digest.

Water is acceptable after 2 months and should be encouraged between feedings. The ideal water for infants is clean, fluoridated, and low in nitrate and sodium. Boiling water only concentrates chemicals, so if tap water has a high nitrate concentration, another water source should be used until the baby is on a mixed diet. Nitrate is dangerous for the baby because his/her body will change it to nitrite, which can interfere with the amount of oxygen his/her blood can carry. Sodium in excess can cause blood pressure to rise, just as in adults.

Also at 6 months, the baby develops an eating pattern of 5 to 6 times per day. Because his/her stomach is maturing and becoming more efficient, the baby is able to consume sufficient quantities of nutrients during the day, allowing him/her to sleep through the night.

Between 4 and 6 months of age, formula or breast milk is still sufficient. Solid food is not needed for proper nutrition; however, rice cereal with iron is acceptable. Parents should be advised not to begin feeding their infant cereal until the baby can sit upright without assistance. Infants should never be given cereal diluted in a bottle, because of the danger of choking. The addition of cereal to the diet is more social than nutritional, so sitting in a highchair with the rest of the family is the most important part of adding the cereal to the baby's diet. In addition, the baby gets used to the feel of solid food in the mouth and the way it feels in the stomach.

By 6 months, the feeding pattern should be stabilized, and the baby should sleep through the night and be ingesting larger quantities of formula during the day. A consistent growth pattern is the best indicator of the state of the baby's nutrient intake.

Adding solid foods to the baby's diet should be predicated on developmental achievements in hand-to-mouth coordination and the maturity of the digestive system. For instance, one reason for adding food at 4 to 6 months is because, developmentally, at this time the baby has the beginnings of a swallowing pattern. The baby can transfer food from the front of the tongue to the back. The baby also begins hand-to-mouth movement. He/she sits with support and intestinal amylase begins to increase, allowing for starch digestion, so cereal with iron is an acceptable addition. Also, at this time the infant's iron stores are becoming depleted and need to be replenished.

Asking the nurse will help parents understand the developmental stages at which foods are added and the approximate age at which the addition is appropriate. Keep in mind that infant development varies and so should the timing of adding different foods to the baby's diet.

By 12 months, the baby should have formula supplemented with diluted regular milk. He/she should have 4 servings a day of fortified cereals and breads; 4 servings a day of table food including soft pieces of fruits and vegetables and juices; and protein intake—ground beef, eggs, fish, peanut butter, legumes, and cheese—of 2 1-ounce servings of meat or the equivalent.

Finicky eaters cause stress to parents. If a child is taught from the start that eating is a social function and that everyone eats a variety of foods, there will be fewer problems. Too much emphasis on food consumption— whether the child eats too little or too much—may confuse the child into thinking that the way to the parent's heart is through what he/she eats. This pressure will stunt the growth of the child's own regulatory process with regard to food. Help parents to understand that the best way to influence their child's eating habits is to set a good example.

What about the child who eats too much? Children go through growing spurts when they seem to eat everything that isn't nailed down, often followed by a period when they aren't hungry and don't seem to eat enough. These are normal behaviors that result from increased or decreased need.

Children who complain about being hungry all the time, or children who don't eat enough and whose growth pattern appears to be interrupted or slowed, should be checked for underlying medical causes or eating disorders. Boredom or understimulation is a contributing factor to overeating and sometimes undereating. Although boredom is not considered a medical problem, it should be addressed with just as much caution. Parents should understand that they can remedy their child's boredom by giving more attention to the child and not making food an issue. Parents need to be given the information they can use to understand the apparent whims of their child's appetite.

An extremely fragile age is the preteen and teenage years. Girls want to diet while boys want to "bulk up." This is the time when bones are strengthening for adulthood and appropriate nutrition is of vital importance. Parents should be made aware that arguing with a teenage girl about dieting will only strengthen her resolve. Parents should, instead, help their daughter with her self-image.

Teenage boys who want to train with weights should be encouraged in healthful pursuits. However, setting appropriate weight limits is important to prevent injury. Parents should also be warned about the possible problem of drugs used to enhance physical appearance. They should watch for unbridled aggression, severe mood swings, and puffy face and hands. Again, a healthy self-image is the key to healthy teenage years.

Nutrition is what we eat, but it is more than that. Nutrition has ties to our childhood, our parents, and our self-image. The nurse's job is to help parents understand how to bring all those ties together to help their healthy child grow to be a healthy teenager and finally a healthy adult.

$\mathcal{S}$UMMARY

This chapter gives a comprehensive foundation of aspects of health care as it relates to managing common injuries and teaching how to prevent them.

Included are the basic aspects of nutrition and common parenting concerns about injuries and accidents. The family is the most vital support that the child has. It is imperative that the nurse see the family as a unit when caring for the child or when giving instructions for his/her care. By treating the family as a unit, the nurse ensures that the child will be taken care of. Family units are an extremely important resource for the health care team. By seeing the family as a unit, the nurse acknowledges the impact that the illness of any one of the members has on the functioning of the rest of the unit.

CRITICAL POINTS IN HEALTH PROMOTION AND ILLNESS PREVENTION

In teaching and counseling parents about health promotion and what to do in case of emergencies, it is very important that the nurse make developmental, environmental, and risk assessments of the family as well as the child. Families, like children, differ greatly according to the age of the marriage and the ages of the children. The most important information that the nurse can obtain is the family's understanding of where they believe they are in their cycle of development.

Families are not only shaped by their own convictions regarding religion and culture, they are also greatly influenced by unpredictable events that often have a tremendous impact on the way that they function. Young families with young children not only have the pressure of having to take care of the children, but also have the pressures of undergoing adjustment to marriage, to the financial world, and to the complexities of a new family. Families with adolescents undergo a great transformation involving the evolution of a new generation. Teenagers are testing the extent of their potential, and parents have the responsibility of monitoring the teens for safety while still encouraging them to develop as individuals. As parents shift their relationship with their sons or daughters, parents have to cope with feelings of fear and uncertainty as their children declare their independence. This is the time that families should be refocusing their goals to accommodate the growing independence of the children and the parents' realization that they are aging. Sometimes parents have the added responsibility of caring for their own aging parents. Nurses need to be keenly aware that the family's functioning only comes from within and that the family's biggest treasure is the reciprocal relationships that they developed along the way.

The nurse caring for a child with a medical emergency first must try to identify the cause of the emergency in order to optimize care, and to restore or preserve vital signs. The nurse must be able to assess the child rapidly, remembering that the primary nursing intervention is to establish a patent airway. After that, the nurse quickly assesses vital signs and level of consciousness, and then proceeds with subsequent treatment as the condition warrants. Once the immediate care has been given to the child, the nurse's next step is to obtain important historical and physical information that may indicate how the emergency developed. This includes information on the child's status prior to the accident, growth and development details, and routine. At the same time the nurse observes the parents and obtains a family history. In assessing the child and observing the parents, the nurse needs to be aware that there is always the possibility of child abuse or neglect. It is important to remember, however, that when parents have a child with an emergency, they are panic-stricken and deserve all the support and care that the nurse can give. Parents should be informed of what is going on as soon as possible, and should be allowed to stay with the child if possible. The nurse also needs to remember that the goal of health promotion is to reduce the risk of disease and maintain optimum functioning.

As American society changes, people are living in a more migratory society where grandparents and other close relatives often are not available to help with the care of the children. Many children live with one parent and that parent usually has to work outside the home. The worst reality is that not all the children of this country have access to medical care; in many instances the first time that the child is seen by the medical team is when he/she comes to the emergency room. Therefore, the nurse should also educate parents on how to access medical care, making them aware of the resources available within the community. Although many efforts are used to promote better care for children, the sad truth is still that the real needs of the families and children of America often are not met and that parents should be educated and counseled as to how to improve their own access to medical care.

$\mathcal{Q}$UESTIONS

Sports Injuries

History: Johnson is 12 years old, 5 feet 7 in., 200 lbs. He plays on the junior varsity football team at his junior high school. While on the field, he tackles the opponent and falls to the ground. Fire rescue is called to the scene and he is routed to the nearest emergency room.

Plan: Management and evaluation of extent of injury. Prevention of injury.

Nursing problems: Assessment of extent of damage.

Intervention: Teaching.

1. Johnson is on a backboard. Immobilization is essential because:
   A. Johnson might have a spinal cord injury.
   B. It is definite that he has broken bones.
   C. To teach him a lesson not to play football again.
   D. It's easier to transport him on the backboard.

2. Johnson is cleared for a spinal cord injury and is taken out of the backboard. However, he complains of right upper leg pain. No swelling or gross deformities are noted and circulation, movement, and sensation in the right distal extremities are within normal limits. An x-ray is obtained and no fractures are noted. He is diagnosed with soft tissue injury. Management includes:

A. Nothing.
B. Ice, rest, and ibuprofen for pain.
C. Ben-Gay and an ace bandage.
D. Warm compresses.

3. It is noted that Johnson is obese. Upon discharge the nurse should teach his parents:

A. Proper nutrition and the health hazards of obesity.
B. Nothing; it is none of the nurse's business.
C. To let him continue with his eating habits; "more is better," so he can play football in college.
D. Nothing; his eating habits are cultural and the nurse has no control over the situation.

4. The *National Health Promotion and Disease Prevention Objectives for the Year 2000* include increasing children's physical activities and fitness. With this in mind, during physical examinations the nurse could:

A. Encourage children to participate in appropriate sports.
B. Have everyone try out for the football team.
C. Encourage children to play video games to prevent them from getting injured.
D. Encourage children to eat whatever suits them.

5. In teaching Johnson and his parents about injury prevention while on the football field, the nurse should tell them:

A. About the importance of protective gear, a helmet, hydration, and sunscreen.
B. Eating a lot of pasta or carbohydrates will increase Johnson's performance.
C. Resting while at practice is not important.
D. To rub the body with alcohol after each game.

Nutrition

History: Susan is a 5-month-old whose mother brings her to the clinic for her immunizations. She is a normal, healthy baby with no significant illness. Her mother asks questions about Susan's formula.
Plan: Educate.
Nursing problems: Compliance.

1. Susan is on Enfamil with iron, and is taking 3–4 ounces every 2–3 hours. Her mother asks if Susan can drink regular milk. The nurse answers:

   A. At this age, regular cow's milk is okay.
   B. Nonfat milk would be better, so the baby won't be so chubby.
   C. Regular milk is not recommended because the child's stomach is immature and the acids make it difficult to digest the milk.
   D. Regular milk causes diarrhea.

2. Susan's mother asks the nurse about the right time to feed the baby solid food. The nurse replies:

   A. 4 months is okay.
   B. Cereal first, in a diluted bottle.
   C. When the child can sit upright.
   D. At 6 months solid food is not needed.

3. During the teenage years, the nutrition focus emphasizes:

   A. Fat intake.
   B. Self- and body image.
   C. Prevention of obesity.
   D. Prevention of drug abuse.

Fracture of the Leg

History: Doug is a healthy 7-year-old. His father is an accountant and his mother stays home and is very protective of Doug. Doug started to play soccer a month ago and his mother states that the children are too rough and not polite. This morning while Doug was playing, his mother yelled at him to be careful, but he fell down and hurt his right leg.

Plan: Doug will go home with his parents and his leg will be checked during regular visits to the orthopedic doctor. The nurse decides that she needs to teach Doug's mother parenting skills and assess the cause of her overprotectiveness. She will also teach her about cast care and follow-up treatment for Doug.

Nursing problem: Altered parenting. Close monitoring of pain. Close monitoring of edema due to fracture. Teaching of cast care.

Chief concerns of the nurse: For Doug, the chief concern is to relieve his immediate pain and edema, and deal with decreased mobility of his leg. For his mother, to learn parenting skills along with how to care for Doug.

1. During the admission assessment, the nurse realizes that Doug's mother answers all the questions and that Doug clings to his mother. The nurse's plan of care should include:

   A. Encouraging Doug to take care of his cast.
   B. Not allowing his mother to talk while the nurse is giving instructions.
   C. Encouraging Doug, his mother, and his father to take care of the cast.
   D. Clarifying that accidents happen only when children are not alert.

2. In trying to teach Doug's parents appropriate parenting skills, the nurse should provide opportunities for the family to:

   A. Express their fears and concerns.
   B. Read a manual about parenting.
   C. Visit a support group for abused children.
   D. Talk to the doctor alone to express their concerns.

3. Doug's parents tell the nurse that Doug's father had a femur fracture 2 years ago and that it took a long time to heal. The nurse responds that Doug's fracture will heal differently because children's bones are more:

   A. Stable.
   B. Porous.
   C. Short.
   D. Complete.

4. Doug's mother asks the nurse what she must do to prevent edema in Doug's leg. The nurse answers:

   A. Limit movement.
   B. Give medication for pain every 4 hours.
   C. Elevate the leg above the heart.
   D. Elevate the leg on a small pillow.

5. Doug is being discharged after his leg is placed in a cast. The nurse is planning Doug's discharge teaching. What is the most important thing that the nurse must teach about Doug's care?

   A. The cast should be kept clean at all times.
   B. The pain should be assessed every 4 hours.
   C. The circulation must be watched closely.
   D. The cast should not be touched for at least 12 hours.

Burns

History: Alicia, a 3-year-old, is brought to the emergency room by her mother. Mrs. Castillo states that Alicia pulled the tablecloth down and hot water spilled all over her. Mrs. Castillo is very upset and does not understand the diagnosis.

1. Mrs. Castillo asks the nurse what the characteristics of second-degree burns are. The nurse answers:

   A. Blisters cover the entire burn.
   B. The tissue will turn bright red.
   C. The child will not feel pain.
   D. The tissues will be white in color.

2. The nurse knows that the major complication from burns is:

   A. Pain.
   B. Infection.
   C. Edema.
   D. Scarring.

3. What is the best treatment to prevent infections from burns?

    A. Prophylactic antibiotics.
    B. Extensive debridement.
    C. High-protein nutrition.
    D. IV antibiotics.

4. All children with burns should receive a tetanus booster immunization if they have not received a booster in the last:

    A. 2 years.
    B. 4 years.
    C. 5 years.
    D. 7 years.

5. Children that have not received prior immunization should receive:

    A. Tetanus immune globulin and primary immunization.
    B. Only tetanus immune globulin.
    C. Only tetanus booster immunization.
    D. Only primary immunization.

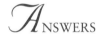

Answers

Sports Injuries

1. *A.* Immobilization is essential until spinal cord or neck injuries are ruled out and because of possible fractures.

2. *B.* For pain and for management of soft tissue injuries, Johnson can use ice, rest, and a nonsteroidal anti-inflammatory.

3. *A.* Proper nutrition should be emphasized to prevent cardiovascular problems.

4. *A.* Encouraging children to participate in physical activities and sports would help promote health.

5. *A.* All of the other answers are false.

Nutrition

1. *C.* Formula or breast milk, when mixed with acid in the child's stomach, makes a curdy substance that is easy to digest.

2. *C.* Eating solid foods is warranted when the child can physically sit upright to prevent choking. All the other answers are false.

3. *B.* For teenagers, self-image is key.

Fracture of the Leg

1. *C.* Family participation helps develop an individual's self-concept and responsibility.

2. *A.* Overprotectiveness can be caused by excessive fear.

3. *B.* The pliable bones of growing children are more porous than those of adults.

4. *C.* During the first hours after a fracture, the chief concern is that the extremity may continue to swell. A measure for reducing this potential problem is to elevate the body part, which increases venous return.

5. *C.* During the first hours after a cast is applied swelling may continue, and the cast may become a tourniquet, shutting off circulation and producing neurovascular complications.

Burns

1. *A.* Second-degree burns involve the epidermis. These wounds are painful, moist, red, and blistered.

2. *B.* Infection, both local and systemic sepsis, is the primary complication.

3. *A.* For minor burns, it is advised to apply topical antimicrobials and dressings to the burn wound.

4. *C.* When more than 5 years have passed since the last immunization, tetanus prophylaxis is instituted.

5. *B.* Only tetanus immunization.

$\mathcal{G}$LOSSARY

aspiration   introduction of a foreign object or liquid into the airway canal.

burn   injury to tissue that can be caused by chemicals, friction, or flame.

contusion   structural damage to bones.

fracture   the rupture, breakage, or dysfunction or displacement of one or more bones. Can be classified by degree of injury to tissue and bone, i.e., simple to compound, etc.

injury   a physical hurt. Can be described as a harm, sprain, damage, mutilation, impairment, blemish, cut, gash, scratch, stab, lesion, bite, fracture, hemorrhage, sting, bruise, sore, cramp, twinge, trauma, abrasion, burn, swelling, wound, scar, distress, or laceration.

poisoning the accidental or intentional ingestion of a substance that is considered harmful or toxic to a system. Toxic substances from such agents as bacteria are also classified as a poison since such substances can potentially harm a system's ability to survive.

prevention anticipation of potential harm because of various factors such as being at risk because of age, sex, heredity, genetics, environment, and the like, and the introduction of interventions to reduce or eliminate the potential harm.

sport an individual or group athletic or competitive form of amusement/entertainment normally done for enjoyment.

strain a musculoskeletal injury involving muscles, joints, and connecting tissues. Injury can occur from unusual twists or movements on a joint or muscle group.

$\mathcal{B}$IBLIOGRAPHY

ALTSCHULER, S. M., AND LUDWIG, S. *Pediatrics at Glance*. Philadelphia: Appleton and Lange, 1997.

BAILEY, D. A. Exercise, fitness and physical education for the growing child—A concern. *Canadian Journal of Public Health* 64:423, 1973.

BETZ, C. L., et al. *Family-Centered Nursing Care of Children*. 2nd ed. Philadelphia: W. B. Saunders, 1994.

BOYTON, R.W., et al. *Manual of Ambulatory Pediatrics*. 3rd ed. Hagerstown, MD: Lippincott, 1994.

BURNS, E. C., et al. *Pediatric Primary Care*. Philadelphia: W. B. Saunders, 1996.

COOPER, K. *The New Aerobics*. New York: Bantam Books, 1975.

DAYMENT, P. How to make team sports physically exciting. *Contemporary Pediatrics*, 8(A):93–106, 1991.

EDELSTEIN, S. F. *The Healthy Young Child*. Minneapolis/St. Paul: West, 1995.

EISENBAUER, L. A., AND MURPHY, M. A. (1998) *Pharmacotherapeutics and Advanced Nursing Practice*. 3rd ed. New York: McGraw-Hill, 1998.

FITZPATRICK, T. B., et al. *Color Atlas and Synopsis of Clinical Dermatology*. 3rd ed. New York: McGraw-Hill, 1997.

FOX, J. A. *Primary Health Care of Children*. St. Louis: Mosby, 1997.

GRODZIN, C. J., et al. *Diagnostic Strategies for Internal Medicine*. St Louis: Mosby, 1995.

HARRISON, T. R., et al. *Principles of Internal Medicine*. New York: McGraw-Hill.

HAY, W. W., et al. *Current Pediatric Diagnosis and Treatment*. Stamford, CT: Appleton and Lange, 1997.

JACKSON, P. L., AND VESSEY, J. A. *Primary Care of the Child with a Chronic Condition*. St Louis: Mosby, 1996.

KHER, K. K., AND MAKKER, S. P. *Clinical Pediatric Nephrology*. New York: McGraw-Hill, 1992.

KNOOP, K. J., et al. *Atlas of Emergency Medicine*. New York: McGraw-Hill, 1997.

LAGERQUIST, S. L. *Critical Thinking Exercises*. Boston: Little, Brown, 1996.

LORIN, M. I. *Review of Pediatrics*. Stamford, CT: Appleton and Lange, 1993.

MCLAIN, L. G., AND REYNOLDS, S. Sports injuries in high school. *Pediatrics* 84:446-450, 1989.

OSKI, F. A., et al. *Principles and Practices of Pediatrics*. Hagerstown, MD: Lippincott, 1994.

PANSKY, B. *Review of Gross Anatomy*. 6th ed. New York: McGraw-Hill, 1996.

PIZZUTILLO, P. D. *Pediatric Orthopaedics in Primary Practice*. New York: McGraw-Hill, 1997.

PROJECT HEALTH PACT. Denver: University of Colorado, School of Nursing, School of Nurse Practitioner Program, 1980.

SAMUELS, M., AND SAMUELS, N. *The Well Baby Book*. New York: Summit Books, 1979.

SATTER, E. *Child of Mine: Feeding with Love and Good Sense*. Emeryville, CA: Bull, 1991.

UNIVERSITY OF CALIFORNIA, BERKELEY WELLNESS LETTER EDITORS. *The Wellness Encyclopedia*. Boston: Houghton Mifflin, 1991.

U.S. DEPARTMENT OF HEALTH AND HUMAN SERVICES. *Healthy People 2000: National Health Promotion and Disease Prevention Objectives for the Year 2000*. Washington, D.C., 1990.

WEINBERG, S., et al. *Color Atlas of Pediatric Dermatology*. 3rd ed. New York: McGraw-Hill, 1998.

WEITEN, W. *Psychology, Themes and Variations*. 3rd ed. Pacific Grove, CA: Brooks/Cole, 1995.

WHALEY, L. F., AND WONG, D. L. *Nursing Care of Infants and Children*. 5th ed. St. Louis: Mosby, 1994.

WHITNEY, E. N., AND HAMILTON, E. M. *Understanding Nutrition*. 4th ed. Minneapolis/St. Paul: West, 1989. Chaps. 14 and 15.

WHITNEY, E. N., AND ROLFES, S. *Understanding Nutrition*. 7th ed. Minneapolis/St. Paul: West, 1996. Chap. 16.

WONG, D. L., AND WILSON, D. *Whaley & Wong's Nursing Care of Infants and Children*. 5th ed. New York: Mosby, 1995.

$\mathcal{H}$ELPFUL INTERNET SITES

PEDINFO: An Index of the Pediatric Internet at http://www.pedinfo.org An excellent site that covers nearly all topics within this review. It has a wealth of information and is worth a visit. It is written for health care professionals but others could also use the information.

University of Iowa Family Practice Handbook at http://www.org/Providers/Providers.html An excellent resource for health care professionals. This is an online 20-chapter resource that would be used by physicians in family practice. It is an excellent resource and worth a look.

U.S. Department of Health and Human Services at hyperlink http://www.healthfinder.gov   HealthFinder is a Web site that provides a wealth of information in many areas of child and adolescent health issues. There is information in Spanish as well as in English and the topics are well organized. The site is aimed at the lay public rather than strictly health care professionals.

Kids Health Organization at hyperlink http://www.kidshealth.org   A site created by the pediatric medical experts at the Alfred I. duPont Hospital for Children, the Nemours Children's Clinics, and other children's health facilities nationwide. The site is written for the lay public and has information on infections, behavior and emotions, food and fitness, and growing up healthy, as well as cool games and animations.

National Network for Health at hyperlink http://www.nnh.org   A site created for the promotion of healthy and safe individuals, families, and communities, created as part of a cooperative state research and education extension system. The site has numerous links to a wealth of information for both the lay public and professionals.

Institute for Family-Centered Care at hyperlink http://www. familycenteredcare.org   Family-centered care is an approach to health care that offers a new way of thinking about the relationships between families and health care providers. The Institute for Family-Centered Care, a nonprofit organization, provides essential leadership to advance the understanding and practice of family-centered care. The institute serves as a central resource for both family members and members of the health care field. This site shares information, facilitates problem solving, and promotes dialogue among individuals and organizations working toward family-centered care.

Collaborative Family Health Care Coalition at hyperlink http://www.cfhcc.org   The Collaborative Family Healthcare Coalition, founded in 1993, is a diverse group of physicians, nurses, psychologists, social workers, family therapists, and other health care workers, in both primary and tertiary care settings, who study, implement, and advocate for the collaborative family health care paradigm. It also includes researchers, educators, health care policy workers, and consumer group representatives. The Coalition functions as a communication network and information clearinghouse by holding an annual conference and maintaining Web site database listings and a list sever. A subscription to *Families, Systems & Health* is included with membership. It publishes a quarterly newsletter, *Working Together*.

Institute of Child Health Care Policy at hyperlink http://www.ichp.edu This site has a wealth of information concerning child health care policy issues.

The Cochrane Neonatal Collaborative Review Group at http://silk.nih.gov/silk/cochrane/cochrane.htm   This site is dedicated to providing systematic reviews of importance in informing providers and consumers about the effect of treatments and in identifying priorities for new research. This site has a wealth of current research in many areas for neonatal health care professionals. The materials are written at a high level and are comprehensive.

Virtual Naval Hospital Information for Providers at http://www.vnh.org/providers.html   This site is part of the University of Iowa's health care site and is linked to a very large set of databases on health care issues and problems that can be used by health care providers. This is an excellent starting place to discover information on various common diseases and their treatments.

Vanderbilt Pediatric Interactive Digital Library at http://www.mc.vanderbilt.edu/peds/pidl/index.htm   This site is dedicated to health care providers. It is a learning resource intended for all who are interested in the health and welfare of children. Topics include development; nutrition; acute illness; genetics/metabolism; neonatology; adolescent medicine; allergy/immunology; rheumatology; infectious diseases; gastroenterology; pulmonology; cardiology; heme-onc; nephrology; endocrinology; neurology; orthopedics/sports medicine; preventive medicine; psychosocial studies.

COMMON HEALTH DISORDERS AND DISEASES

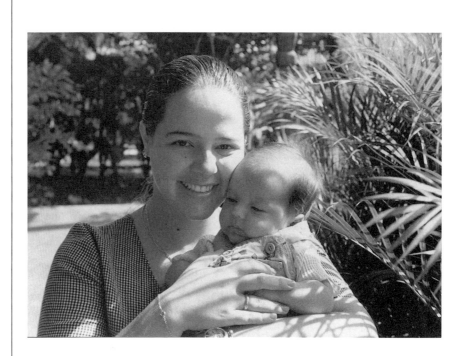

ℱEAR, ANXIETY, AND FEVER

ℐNTRODUCTION

For a child the world is both a magical and a menacing place. It is full of mysteries and dangers, real or imaginary, that are all but forgotten upon entering adulthood. A **survey** of 1000 children between 2 and 14 years of age found that 90% had some specific phobia. In another study of children between 6 and 12 years of age, more than 40% had many worries and fears. For these children, most of the anxieties and fears were not associated with a major psychiatric disorder or psychopathology. For the parent and for the nurse, deciding which anxiety or fear is serious enough to require treatment is difficult. The categories used for adult anxiety disorders are not adequate when applied to children, since children are constantly growing and changing, both physically and mentally. Fear can be normal at one age and become incapacitating a few years later. **Chronological** age is not the deciding factor as to what is normal or abnormal, physically or mentally, because children develop at different rates in both areas.

𝒲HAT IS FEAR?

The clue to understanding and judging whether a fear is normal or abnormal requires knowledge of the **psychodynamics** or roots of fear and anxiety.

Survey. A comprehensive appraisal of an area of study.

Chronological. Occurring in a natural sequence according to time.

Psychodynamics. The scientific study of mental action forces.

Startle response. The uncontrollable startle reaction that follows any stimulus for which there is usually no adaptation, such as a sudden noise.

Stranger anxiety. An anxiety or fear caused by the presence of a strange person. Children develop this at about age 6 to 8 months.

Mild transient. Temporary interference, usually with abrupt onset. Specific symptoms depend on the cause.

Fluid. A continuous process.

Disabling. An action that restricts the ability to perform an activity in the manner that is considered normal.

Boundaries. Limits set in accordance with development.

Newborns fear loud noises and the loss of physical support. Newborns and infants appear to have 3 innate fears: sudden motion, loud or abrupt noises, and being approached suddenly. Their **startle response** or crying is normal and expected. At 6 months of age, the child develops **stranger anxiety**, and this fear can persist until the age of 2 or 3. The fear of separation from significant others, such as caretakers, begins about the age of 1 and may last until 7 or 8 years of age. Preschoolers often fear animals, large objects, dark places, changes in their environment, masks, "bad" people, supernatural creatures, and sleeping alone. As the child matures mentally and physically, he/she may develop worries about death, examinations, and events such as wars or killings. Adolescents may develop many social and sexual anxieties and fears.

As the above examples indicate, normal fears and anxieties are **mild, transient,** and **fluid.** Fear and anxiety become a problem only if they interfere with activities normal for a given age. Fear and anxiety represent a mental health problem only if the fearful state lasts at least a month and becomes fixed. The National Institute of Mental Health estimates that 8% of boys and 11% of girls have clinically significant anxiety of some kind before the age of 18. One study estimated that 6% of all children aged 4 to 6 and 2.5% of all children aged 12 to 15 could be in need of treatment for abnormal fears and/or anxieties.

What factors contribute to children's fears? Researchers have identified 2 key factors that should be considered: maturity level and emotional susceptibility. Research on childhood fears shows that 25% of fears in 2-year-olds were related to loud noises, while only 3% of 12-year-olds had such fears. Children clearly outgrow some fears but appear to become more emotionally susceptible to others. An example of this is that fear of strangers may decline as fear of monsters under the bed rises.

Researchers have agreed upon no single classification of childhood fears. Generalized anxiety or specific phobias may be symptoms of many severe childhood psychiatric disorders, such as autism, major depression, and schizophrenia. Such symptoms can also be associated with organic reasons, such as brain damage.

Anxiety disorders, on the other hand, fall into several distinctive patterns and are more easily classified than fears. Most anxiety disorders have symptoms of exaggerated, prolonged, or **disabling** versions of normal childhood fears. Some are similar to adult anxiety disorders. The **boundaries** between the various anxiety disorders are disputed, and researchers are continuously attempting to redefine such boundaries and classifications.

Common Childhood Fears

All human beings feel fear at times. It is an innate reaction to potential danger and the need for self-protection and survival. A threatened sense of security appears to underlie many childhood fears. Fears, big and small, are a universal fact of childhood.

Infants' fears usually stem from real objects and events, while those of preschoolers can be born of an active imagination. Dependent on others for even basic needs, young children appear to be prone to more fears and anxieties than are adults. Basic fears can be expressed even before the child can talk. The startle response or crying by infants exposed to loud noises or who feel they are falling clearly demonstrates such basic responses. As children grow older, they develop more complex fears and anxieties that arise from the rapid changes in their emotional makeup and their expanding perceptions of the world.

By their second year, children's interest encompasses the world around them. More mobile, they explore their environment; their sense of security is easily shaken by new or unusual experiences. Sudden, unfamiliar sounds, such as a barking dog or a vacuum cleaner, can startle them and cause them to be fearful and anxious. Throughout the toddler stage of development, the child's fears seem to be more and more ill founded rather than less so. The reason for the ill-founded nature of their fears comes from children's immature sense of spatial relationships and their **distorted** sense of their own size in relation to size of the things around them. A child may show fear of the toilet or a bathtub, based on a concern that he/she will be sucked down the drain.

A 2-year-old is better organized and more secure than an infant or newborn. The 2-year-old may fear the dark, a bath, thunder and lightning, toilet training, loud noises, animals, doctors and nurses, strangers, or separation. The 3-year-old adds to this list and even adds a fear of people or animals that have an unusual appearance. Four-year-olds may add the fear of the loss of a parent or even loss of control (emotional control).

The main reason for an increase in irrational fears after 18 months of age is because of the child's awakening sense of imagination. This sense of imagination begins to become intermingled with various emotions such as anger and jealousy. Often these strong feelings find expression in fears of imaginary enemies, such as robbers, monsters under the bed, and bogeymen. Fears arising from this emerging ability to use imagination reach a peak between the ages of 3 and 5. Struggling to distinguish between fantasy and reality, children can invent fantastic explanations for things they do understand, and often, in the process, assign human feelings, abilities, and motives to inanimate objects.

Children also acquire fears through experiences. A child once bitten by a dog may acquire a fear of all dogs. A painful inoculation in the past may cause the child to cry and cringe at the mere idea of going to the doctor's office. Divorce, separation, and other abrupt changes in a child's environment may be the trigger for the development of fears.

Since each child is an individual, what will cause a fear reaction within a child is difficult to predict. Realistic scenes of violence on television in contrast to cartoon characters getting shot are a case in point. The child may react to the real scenes as self-threatening, whereas the cartoon characters' violence simply gets a laugh. Another case is the use of words and expressions in casual adult conversation, which may trigger fears in the child. Such statements as, "My boss is going to kill me," may be taken as a fact and start the child worrying that the parent's life is really in danger.

Children between 4 and 5 years of age are often unpredictable in their behavior. For the most part, the child of 5 is not fear-filled. The change

Distorted. The process of modifying unconscious mental elements so that they can enter consciousness without being censored.

Ritual. A routine that the individual feels is essential and should not fail to be carried out.

that one sees in the 5-year-old is that the fears become more concrete or real and less imagined. These fears include bodily harm, falling, dogs, the dark, death, and mom or dad not returning home.

By this age and beyond, the child may have developed a surprising array of psychological strategies for dealing with his/her own anxieties. Through pretend play, normally around ages 3 to 5, the child may take on the role of superhero so that imagined fears can be played out. Although small and less powerful, the child is able to become the all-powerful hero who can fend off those who would do harm. Another strategy is to confront the fear by experimenting with its source. Often, a child who is fearful of a flushing toilet or bathtub drain will attempt to flush a toy down the toilet or place a toy near the drain while it is emptying. When the parent is able to retrieve the toy from the bath or toilet, the child is relieved, being reassured that if it cannot happen to the toy it cannot happen to him/her. At times a child becomes strongly attracted to an object or event that once caused them great fear. A child fearful of dogs may suddenly become interested in every dog he/she sees, going up to the animal or admiring it. Others may develop **rituals** around fears. Children fearful of bedtime may be comforted by a familiar routine such as having a bath, brushing their teeth, having a story read, and then a kiss goodnight. The routine is comforting and reinforces their sense of security.

Death

For the child younger than 5, death is equal to separation. At 5 and older, the child develops a personal sense about death. Death becomes someone who carries you off. The child develops a sense of vulnerability and requires honest and direct answers to be reassured. Often the death of a pet is the child's first experience with death. Such experiences can set the tone for an honest discussion in which the child can express his/her feelings about the sense of loss. Euphemisms at this age should be avoided, such as "Grandma is in a deep sleep" or "was laid to rest." The explanation "Grandma died because her heart stopped working" is more concrete and something the child can understand. Often children ask if they will die, and such questions need to be answered in an honest and direct manner.

Beyond Childhood and into Adolescence

The child at 5 and beyond is using his/her concrete intellectual capacity. Formal operations or the ability to conceptualize and use abstract logic does not appear until much later (logical and formal reasoning begins in middle adolescence or even later). Using abstract reasoning or lengthened bits of reasoning falls on deaf ears with this age group. Being a concrete thinker, the child's thinking process is mostly black and white, and therefore makes him/her unable to see gray areas in logic. Being concrete in their thinking means that children can begin to determine for themselves what is real and what is not. For the 5-year-old and even for the older child, it becomes important for the nurse to start laying the groundwork for abstract reasoning and formal logic by responding to a child's fears in a positive, supporting manner. Such a positive and supportive approach should continue to help the child learn to face many situations throughout his/her development.

School-aged children are developmentally beginning to realize that they can work through their fears or to learn to cope in positive ways. The school-aged child and adolescent are able to recognize that they will outgrow fears and that fears do not have to immobilize them. The 5-year-old, the school-aged child, and adolescents may learn to call upon their own inner strengths to deal with their fears. Developing a sense of mastery, they are able to call upon such successes for assistance in mastering new territories.

The number one fear of adults, teens, and older school-aged children is the fear of public speaking. This fear develops for a number of basic reasons and may be difficult to eliminate. One factor is the need to appear socially competent while also needing social affiliation and a sense of belonging (fear of rejection and social disapproval). These can be strong motivators not to "appear foolish." A list of people's most common fears is as follows:

Public speaking	Injections
Making mistakes	Hospitals
Failure	Taking tests
Disapproval	Open wounds, blood
Rejection	Police
Angry people	Dogs
Being alone	Spiders
Darkness	Deformed people
Dentists	

Management of Fears

There are several key points that the nurse needs to consider when attempting to deal effectively with children's fears. These key points should also be reinforced with the child's parents or significant others. Since most fears are informally learned, parents and others reinforce what is considered normative for the child and what is not. The following are guidelines for parents and caregivers:

Respect the child's fears—they are very real to him/her.
Understand that the child will normally outgrow most fears.
Allow the child to gradually work through a fear.
A particular fear is related to the child's personality.
A variety of fears are experienced by children at different ages.
Become familiar and informed about children's fears and learn to gently guide a child through such fears.
Provide a safe and supportive environment in which the child can learn and grow.

Cause for Concern

Obsessive. A neurotic mental state of having an uncontrollable desire to dwell on an idea or an emotion.

When a fear becomes so intense that it interferes with a child's daily activities, then it is a cause for concern. An **obsessive** fear of dogs, for example, may cause a child to fear going outside, and can make life difficult both for the child and for the family. If a nurse sees that a child's particular fear is unusually severe or long-lived, it is time to suggest professional help for this particular problem.

For the most part, however, the nurse realizes that a fear is at best short-lived, and will vary from child to child. One means of reducing fears is to support the child's sense of security and sense of independence that is both age- and ability-appropriate. Another means is to provide the child with the opportunity to explore and learn about his/her fears in a supportive environment. The child requires opportunities to develop a sense of competence and self-reliance. Meeting fears head-on provides that opportunity. Time and experience are the child's greatest weapons in learning to cope with fear.

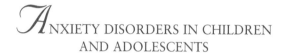

ANXIETY DISORDERS IN CHILDREN AND ADOLESCENTS

Anxiety disorders. Ongoing exaggerated worry and tension, even when there is no reason for it.

Anxiety disorders cause people to feel excessively frightened, distressed, and uneasy during situations in which most others would not experience such symptoms. Left untreated, these disorders may dramatically reduce the child's or adolescent's productivity, and can significantly diminish the individual's quality of life. Research shows that anxiety disorders in children and adolescents lead to poor school attendance, low self-esteem, deficient interpersonal skills, alcohol and drug abuse, and adjustment difficulties.

Anxiety disorders affect 1 in 10 young people and are the most common mental illnesses in America. Unfortunately, these disorders are difficult to recognize since the child is constantly growing and changing physically and mentally. Often, those suffering from anxiety disorders are too ashamed to seek help. They fail to recognize that these disorders can be treated effectively.

The Difference Between Fear and Anxiety

Stimuli. Factors that increase functional activity.

Panic. Acute anxiety, terror, or fright that is usually of sudden onset.

Fear is associated with a strong, unpleasant attitude or emotion in response to painful, dangerous, or unexpected **stimuli**. Fear is viewed as an attempt to gain control over a specific threatening situation (Wolman, 1979). On the other hand, anxiety is an extended emotional response, characterized by extreme apprehensiveness, resulting in **panic** and crisis in its extreme. Anxiety is considered more pervasive in one's personality, and it lacks the clear and concise focus on a specific object or event that fear connotes (Theodorson & Theodorson, 1970; Beck, 1976).

Fear is recognized as a functional, learned response by a child to painful, dangerous, or unexpected stimuli, real or imagined. As such, normal, age-appropriate fears should be accepted as part of the child's internal map of personal and social reality. Recognizing fears' functional nature and that they are learned, a nurse may use fear-producing situations as a constructive force in supporting the child's psychological growth and development.

Anxiety, on the other hand, has a set of distinctive features and in its extreme forms is considered dysfunctional and even life-threatening. Feeling nervous is a normal and even beneficial response to a varied set of challenging situations. When faced with having an IV inserted for the first time, going for a job interview, or taking a critical test, for example, it is not abnormal to experience uneasiness and apprehension, have sweaty palms, or even have butterflies in the stomach. Such responses serve a useful purpose in alerting one to prepare to handle an upcoming event.

Anxiety disorders, however, differ greatly from the above normal feelings of apprehension and nervousness, which can be associated with a specific situation. Anxiety disorders are mental health illnesses and as such are not normal or useful. Psychological symptoms include overwhelming feelings of panic, fear, and apprehension that are associated with uncontrollable obsessive thoughts and painful and intrusive memories and nightmares. There are a variety of physical symptoms that include heart palpitations, numbness, and muscular tension.

Anxiety disorders can be distinguished from normal feelings of apprehension and nervousness by several features. Symptoms of anxiety disorders often occur for no apparent reason, and these symptoms persist. The continuous anxiety or panic that is being experienced serves no functional purposes because the feelings are often unrelated to any actual or impending experience. Rather than working as a call to action (functional fear or anxiety), these overwhelming emotions have a devastating effect, damaging relations with friends, family, and fellow students, reducing one's school or work productivity, and making everyday experiences potentially terrifying. If left untreated, anxiety disorders can immobilize the child or adolescent, propelling them to take extreme measures such as refusing to go to school or to leave their home, to avoid the situations that they see inducing or aggravating their anxiety.

Classification of Anxiety Disorders

Anxiety disorders are a group of mental illnesses that include panic disorder, phobias, obsessive-compulsive disorder, posttraumatic stress disorder, and generalized anxiety disorder. These illnesses arise from biochemical changes in the brain, genetic vulnerability, psychological makeup, and life experiences. Each of the anxiety disorders is characterized by particular symptoms, and, as is the case with physical illnesses, the severity and duration of symptoms vary among individuals. The characteristics of anxiety disorders are both emotional and physical.

Panic Disorder Panic disorder is characterized by repeated and unexpected panic attacks. Panic attacks are bouts of overwhelming fear of being in danger that are accompanied by at least 4 of the following symptoms:

Pounding heart
Chest pain
Sweating
Trembling or shaking
Shortness of breath
Sensation of choking
Nausea or abdominal pain
Dizziness or lightheadedness
Feeling unreal or disconnected from oneself
Fear of losing control, "going crazy," or dying
Numbness
Chills or hot flashes

Panic attacks can accompany several types of anxiety disorders, not just panic disorder. Because of the symptom of heart pain, those with panic disorder often mistakenly think that they are having a heart attack.

Panic disorder typically first occurs in late adolescence or early adulthood but can also begin in childhood. Women are twice as likely as men to experience it. Research shows that there is a strong family relationship, suggesting that some people may be genetically predisposed to the disorder.

Phobia. Uncontrollable, irrational, and persistent fear of a specific object.

Phobias A **phobia** is an uncontrollable, irrational, and persistent fear of a specific object, event, situation, or activity. Approximately 5 to 9% of all Americans will experience one or more phobias that will be from mild to severe to disabling. Phobias are normally first evidenced between the ages of 15 and 20 years, but also occur in early childhood. Phobias affect people of both genders and all ages and races. The fear associated with the phobia can cause individuals to go to great lengths to avoid the source of their dread. An extreme response to a phobia is panic anxiety.

There are three types of phobias:

1. *Specific phobia* is characterized by extreme fear of an object or event that is not harmful under general conditions (e.g., fear of flying since the plane will crash; fear of dogs since they will bite; fear of storms since one will be hit by lightning). Those with specific phobias realize that their fears are excessive, but cannot overcome the emotion associated with the phobia. Children may have fears of certain objects or events, but this is not a phobia until it interferes with daily activities of school, work, and home life.

2. Significant anxiety and discomfort that are related to fear of being embarrassed or scorned by others in social or performance situations mark *social phobia*. There are many situations that can trigger social phobia, including public speaking, meeting people, dealing with authority figures, eating in public, or using a public restroom. Those with social phobia will avoid situations that trigger the pho-

bia. Diagnosis is based on when the phobia is severe enough to interfere with normal, expected routines or is excessively upsetting to the individual.

3. *Agoraphobia* is fear of experiencing a panic attack in a place or situation from which escape may be difficult or embarrassing. Anxiety associated with agoraphobia is so severe that individuals seek to avoid the cause of their terror. Different from social phobia, agoraphobia involves fear of situations such as being alone outside one's home, being home alone, being in a crowd, traveling in a vehicle, or being in an elevator, tunnel, or on a bridge. Agoraphobia can be so debilitating that it causes the person to be housebound.

Obsessive-Compulsive Disorder Obsessions are irrational thoughts that frequently recur and cause great anxiety, but cannot be controlled through rational reasoning. Common **obsessions** include preoccupations with dirt or germs, repeated doubts (Did I turn off the stove? Did I lock the door?), thoughts about violence or hurting someone, and a need to have things in a very particular order. The individual realizes that the thoughts are unreasonable and are not related to real-life problems, but this knowledge is not sufficient to make the unwanted thoughts go away. In an attempt to get rid of the unwanted thoughts, people with obsessions use compulsions, or repetitive ritualized behaviors, to reduce the anxiety associated with the obsessions. Repeated hand washing, turning the stove off and on, and following rigid rules of order (for example, putting on clothes in the same sequence every day) are but a few examples of rituals used to reduce the anxiety. Compulsive behaviors can become excessive, disruptive, and time consuming, often taking up to more than an hour a day to complete, and can interfere with daily activities and social activities.

Obsessions. Irrational thoughts that frequently recur and cause great anxiety.

Obsessive-compulsive disorder (OCD) often begins in adolescence, but can be seen in early childhood. The disorder appears equally in men and women, and appears to run in families. It is not uncommon for other disorders such as depression, eating disorders, or substance abuse to accompany obsessive-compulsive disorder. This disorder affects about 2% of the American population annually.

Posttraumatic Stress Disorder Posttraumatic stress disorder (PTSD) occurs in children and others who have survived a severe or terrifying physical or emotional event. Normally the person who has posttraumatic stress disorder reexperiences the ordeal through recurrent nightmares or memories of the event, a feeling that the trauma is recurring, and extreme emotional, mental, and physical distress when exposed to situations that may remind him/her of the traumatic event. In addition to the painful memories, nightmares, and flashbacks, other symptoms include the feeling of numbness or being detached, having trouble sleeping, feeling jittery or on guard, and depression.

Many events can trigger posttraumatic stress disorder, including war, natural disasters, childhood physical or sexual abuse, and witnessing abuse or injury to another person. Symptoms normally occur with 3 months of the event, but can surface many months or years later. The severity and duration of the event and the individual's nearness to the event appear to affect the development of posttraumatic stress disorder. People with the disorder are susceptible to drug and alcohol abuse, other anxiety disorders, and depression.

Generalized Anxiety Disorder (GAD) Ongoing and exaggerated worry and tension characterize generalized anxiety disorder. GAD sufferers worry constantly, even when there is no apparent reason for doing so. The focus of such exaggerated concerns can be health, family, work, or money. In addition to experiencing distorted anxiety that interferes with daily functions, they are also unable to relax; are easily tired and irritable; have difficulty concentrating; and may experience insomnia, muscle tension, trembling, fatigue, and headaches.

Those suffering from generalized anxiety disorder differ from those suffering from other anxiety disorders in that GAD individuals usually do not avoid specific situations. As found in other anxiety disorders, those suffering from generalized anxiety disorder sometimes may have accompanying depression, substance abuse, and another anxiety disorder.

The illness typically begins in childhood or adolescence. It occurs more often in women than men, and appears to run in families. Each year between 2 and 4% of all Americans experience generalized anxiety disorder.

What Is the Cause of Anxiety Disorder?

Strong evidence suggests that heredity, brain chemistry, personality, and life experience all play important roles in the development of anxiety disorder. There is clear evidence that anxiety disorders run in families. Research studies have found that if one twin has an anxiety disorder, the other will more than likely have an anxiety disorder. This is not true for fraternal twins, only for identical twins. But these findings strongly suggest a heredity linkage that may be activated in combination with life experiences that predispose some people to these illnesses.

Brain chemistry appears to play a major role in the onset of anxiety disorders. Research studies demonstrate that anxiety disorders are often relieved by medications that alter levels of brain chemicals. Brain functioning likewise may play a part as well. Research currently being conducted is attempting to determine whether specific areas of the brain are unusually active in those patients with anxiety disorders.

Personality also plays a significant role. Studies have found that those individuals with low self-esteem and poor coping skills may be prone to anxiety disorders. It is not certain whether anxiety disorder in childhood may itself contribute to low self-esteem later on. Along with personality, life experiences may affect the individual's susceptibility to the development of an anxiety disorder. Researchers think that the relationship between anxiety disorders and long-term exposure to abuse, violence, or poverty is an important area for further investigation.

Treatment for Anxiety Disorder

Before treatment can begin a proper diagnosis must be made. A complete history and physical examination and a psychiatric evaluation need to be done. Evaluation serves to identify physical and/or mental conditions that may be contributing to, or mimicking, the anxiety disorder. Once evaluation has been done and a diagnosis has been made, treatments are prescribed. Treatments are aimed at reducing the symptoms, allowing the individual to pursue a more normal and healthy life.

Each anxiety disorder has its own unique set of characteristics. Most anxiety disorders respond well to two types of treatments: medication and psychotherapy. Such treatments can be prescribed alone or in combination. Antidepressants, benzodiazepines, and other antianxiety drugs are used to treat anxiety disorders. Selective serotonin reuptake inhibitors have been found to be effective in treating obsessive-compulsive disorder, whereas other anxiety-reducing drugs have been found useful in relieving the symptoms of posttraumatic stress disorder. Medications can take weeks or a month to provide the full expected effect. Patients are often monitored by a mental health professional to determine if a change in dosage, another drug, or a combination of drugs is needed.

Three types of psychotherapy have been found to be useful in treating the symptoms of anxiety disorder: behavioral therapy, cognitive-behavioral therapy, and psychotherapy. Behavioral therapies seek to change responses to certain classes of stimuli thought to trigger the anxiety. Relaxation therapy techniques, such as deep breathing, gradual exposure to what is frightening, and other forms of biofeedback methods have been successful in reducing anxiety disorder symptoms. Cognitive-behavioral therapy seeks to have patients not only reduce their responses to certain classes of stimuli, but also to come to recognize that certain patterns of thinking can also be triggering their responses. Changes in those patterns of thinking can also reduce their responses to triggering events and/or objects. Lastly, psychotherapy is based on the concept that symptoms result from unconscious mental conflict, and that uncovering the meaning of symptoms is needed to relieve them.

FEVER

Nurses have recognized fever (pyrexia) as a sign of disease for a number of years. Physiologically, fever represents a disturbance in normal thermoregulation. The disturbance is demonstrated with an upward shift of the body's core temperature from its normal set point (37°C or 98.6°F or lower) to 1 or more degrees higher. Fever is considered a naturally occurring physiologic event in which the body actively seeks to elevate its temperature.

Fever Classifications

Several classification schemas are used to describe fever. Fevers can be classified as low (oral reading of 99°–100.4°F, or 37.2°–38°C), moderate (100.5°–104°F, or 38°–40°C), or high (above 104°F, or above 40°C). Fever over 108°F (42.2°C) causes unconsciousness and, if sustained, leads to permanent brain damage.

Along with low, moderate, and high, fevers have been further classified as remittent, intermittent, sustained, or relapsing. A remittent fever is the most common type and is characterized by daily temperature fluctuations above the normal set point range for the individual. Intermittent fevers are those that have a daily temperature drop into the normal range, and then have a rise back up above the normal set point for the individual. An intermittent fever that has wide fluctuations and typically produces chills and then sweating is called hectic or septic fever. Sustained fevers are those that have persistent temperature elevations with little or no fluctuation. Relapsing fevers are those that alternate between feverishness and afebrile periods.

Another classification includes the duration of the fever: brief or prolonged. A brief duration is less than 3 weeks. Prolonged fevers, e.g., fevers that last longer than 3 weeks, also include fever of unknown origin (FUO). FUO, as a diagnosis, can be used only when careful examination fails to detect an underlying cause for the fever.

Pathophysiology of Fever

An individual's normal temperature or baseline temperature varies with time of day (lowest in morning or baseline), physiologic events (ovulation, exercise, intense crying), and habits (smoking, excessive drinking of fluids) (see Concept Map 5-1: Pathogenesis of Fever). Elderly patients tend to have lower baseline temperatures and often produce less impressive fever response to pyrogenic stimuli than younger patients. Elderly patients and young children and infants often lack the resources to mount a prolonged physiologic effort (fever) against various infections. Often elderly patients with infections fail to mount a febrile response and instead present with confusion, loss of appetite, or even hypotension without fever.

Fever can be explained pathophysiologically with three basic reasons. The first and most prominent pathophysiological reason involves the raising of the body's normal set point. The second type of fever is one that is a result of heat production exceeding heat loss. With this type of fever, the set point is normal, and heat loss mechanisms are active; however, fever occurs either because the body raises its metabolic heat production or the environmental heat load exceeds normal heat loss mechanisms. Fever of this origin can be found in such mechanisms as aspirin overdose, malignant hyperthermia, hyperthyroidism, or hypernatremia. The third type of fever is caused by a defective heat loss mechanism that cannot cope with normal heat load, as found in heat stroke, anticholinergic drug poisoning, and burns. As with the second type of fever, the third type involves no change in the set point.

Fever of physiologic origins is considered a result of a normal defense mechanism caused by phagocytic leukocytes. Fever is then a bodily response to pyrogenic substances such as infectious agents, immunologic mediators, or toxic agents which stimulate phagocytic leukocytes into action as part of the body's normal defense mechanism. Phagocytic leukocytes, especially in response to a bacterial infection, release a protein known as endogenous pyrogen into the bloodstream. This protein circulates in the bloodstream and interacts with specialized receptors in the thermoregulatory center of the anterior hypothalamus. The response of the hypothalamus is to move the set point up 1 or more degrees.

Fever, an increase in the core temperature set point of 1 to several degrees, can be found during both infectious and noninfectious illnesses. Fever has become highly associated with infections. This is in part because fever is considered a naturally occurring event with infectious agents, which are often the reason that a patient has a fever. As a naturally occurring event, it is seen as a response of the body's immune system against an invasion. When the body's defense mechanisms attempt to destroy the invading agents, toxins are liberated. In response to the toxins the body's white blood cells (leukocytes) release interleukin-1 (a pyrogen) into the bloodstream. Pyrogen substances act on the hyperthalamic thermostatic neurons, increasing the body's normal set point. To reach this new set point, the patient shivers, increasing heat production, and also becomes pale from skin vasoconstriction. This pattern of events of increased heat production, shivers, and vasoconstriction continues until the new set point is reached. Because it is a reaction to infectious agents, fever is considered a natural defensive response, and the higher set point may be detrimental for the bacteria or their toxin. For the patient, extremely high set points (42°C or greater) cause heat shock and may be fatal if not treated. Many fevers are self-limiting because the body's defenses are able to reduce the effects of the offending agent, whereas other fevers can be life-threatening and require aggressive and immediate interventions to aid the body's defenses. The antifever influences of such medications as aspirin prevent the effects of pyrogen on the hypothalamus. For self-limiting fevers, this may be the treatment of choice. Often, additional interventions such as antibiotics and IV therapies are required in order to reduce the effects of the infectious agents until the body's defensive mechanisms are able to do so on their own. If the infection is treated with antibiotics or other agents, the body is better able to mount a defense. The results are a decrease in pyrogen secretions to a point that they no longer influence the hypothalamus, and the body's thermostat returns to its normal set point. In response to decreased pyrogen secretions, the body attempts to cool down by skin vasodilatation and sweating.

Fever and Hyperthermia

Fever is an elevation in the body's core temperature that is mediated by an increase in the hypothalamic heat-regulating set point. Although exogenous substances may precipitate fevers, the increase in the body's core temperature is achieved through physiological mechanisms. In contrast, hyperthermia is an increase in body temperature that overrides or bypasses the normal homeostatic mechanisms. A general rule of thumb is that body temperatures that exceed 41°C are rarely physiologically mediated and strongly suggest hyperthermia. Hyperthermia may be seen after vigorous exercise, in patients with heatstroke, as a heritable reaction to anesthetics, as a response to phenothiazines, and in some patients with central nervous system disorders such as paraplegia. Some patients who suffer from severe dermatoses may also be unable to dissipate heat and experience hyperthermia.

Heatstroke (as hyperthermia) is normally associated with some form of prolonged exposure to high environmental temperatures, humidity, and strenuous exercise. A body temperature greater than 40.6°C characterizes heatstroke. Concurrently the patient presents with altered sensorium or coma, and the cessation of sweating. Treatment for heatstroke is to immerse the patient in cool water until the core temperature reaches 39°C and get the patient to a hospital for possible intravenous infusion of fluids necessary to correct fluid and electrolyte losses.

Etiology of Fever

Infections are generally considered the most likely causes of febrile reactions (see Concept Map 5-1). Yet it is important to remember that fever can frequently occur in many noninfectious illnesses. Many noninfectious illnesses, such as collagen vascular disease (e.g., systemic lupus erythematosus, rheumatoid arthritis, Reiter's syndrome, vasculitis), hypersensitivity reactions (e.g., to medications and various blood products), neoplastic diseases (especially the lymphomas, primary and secondary tumors of the liver, and renal cell carcinoma), hemorrhage (especially retroperitoneal, subarachnoid, and intraarticular), and thromboembolic disease (e.g., thrombophlebitis, pulmonary embolism), can present with fever as one of the clinical presentations. Even with such a variety of causes, the nurse will first wisely assume that a presentation of a fever in an ill child is due to an infectious agent until other diagnostic efforts fail to identify and document an infectious etiology.

Since most diseases have the capability of producing fever, the characteristics of the fever curve are of little or no help in suggesting the etiology of the fever. Patients who present with fever often can be grouped as having (1) fever without localizing symptoms and signs, (2) fever and a rash, or (3) fever and lymphadenopathy. The majority of healthy patients who present with fever alone will defervesce spontaneously or within 2 or 3 weeks present with localizing clinical or laboratory findings. Some infectious agents that produce such patterns can be from viral agents such as influenza; from bacterial agents such as *Salmonella typhi* or *S. paratyphi*; from postanimal exposure agents such as *Coxiella burnetti* (Q fever), *Leptospira* (water contaminated by urine of dogs, cats, rodents, or small animals); or from granulomatous agents such as *Mycobacterium tuberculosis*. Those patients who present with both fever and a rash need to be evaluated for bacterial diseases, viral infections, rickettsial diseases, and Lyme disease, all of which have as clinical presentation both fever and a rash. Patients who present with both fever and generalized lymphadenopathy need to be evaluated for mononucleosis syndromes such as Epstein-Barr virus (EBV), cytomegalovirus (CMV), toxoplasmosis, and granulomatous disease. And those who present with fever and regional lymphadenopathy need to be evaluated for pyrogenic infection from such agents as *Staphylococcus aureus*, for tuberculosis, cat-scratch disease, ulceroglandular fever, and oculoglandular fever. Some sexually transmitted diseases also produce inguinal lymphadenopathy, such as syphilis. Bubonic plague presents with fever, headache, and a large mat of inguinal or axillary lymph nodes. Plague is an especially important consideration with patients who have had possible exposure to fleas and rodents in the western United States.

Although frank rigors are strongly suggestive of bacterial infection, such chills can also be seen in patients with nonbacterial diseases, including viral illnesses (AIDS), protozoa infections (such as malaria), drug reactions, and inflammatory diseases. The first priority in assessing a patient with fever should be to determine the degree of urgency that is suggested by the clinical presentation (signs and symptoms).

Diagnostic Approach to Fever

Urgency of the clinical presentation (e.g., the clinical signs and symptoms) determines the priority of evaluation and treatment of febrile patients. Febrile patients who present with a short or brief history of a rapidly evolving illness and who appear toxic and acutely ill require urgent diagnostic assessment and treatment. Evaluation should lead to a prompt therapeutic intervention. When the reason for an aggressive intervention is warranted, it is to prevent a morbid or even fatal outcome from an acute, fulminating disease. In contrast, a clinical presentation from a chronically ill patient, one with a known, nonthreatening condition that presents with fever, or one with a prolonged, lingering illness with either unremitting fever or recurrent episodes of fever, more than likely will not exhibit a sudden and precipitous deterioration requiring urgent treatment.

Clearly, urgency depends on the clinical presentation and the nurse's clinical judgment. The diagnostic approach for those patients who present with subacute-to-chronic signs and symptoms of fever should be a more prolonged and meditative one. Therapy in the subacute-to-chronic presenting patients should be delayed until a diagnosis is certain. The reason for the delay is that one does not want to obscure the clinical picture by providing an inappropriate administration of medication such as an antibiotic when another agent might be more effective. Since the clinical picture is not one of an acutely ill person, it is important to be more deliberate in assessment, diagnosis, and treatment. However, although acute and subacute-to-chronic febrile patients have different clinical presentations, they both have a presentation of fever and, therefore, the nurse should clearly include similar areas of investigation in gathering and interpreting data during the history and physical examination.

It is important to remember, during the history and physical assessment, that infants and young children experience higher and more prolonged fevers, more rapid temperature increases, and greater temperature fluctuations than older children and adults. In infants and young children, extremely high fevers can cause seizures, so appropriate precautions must be taken in such cases. It is important to instruct parents not to give infants and young children aspirin when the child has varicella or flulike symptoms because of the risk of precipitating Reye's syndrome. It is important also to ask whether they have attempted to treat an infant or younger child who has had fevers with aspirin in order to assess for Reye's syndrome.

Common pediatric causes of fever include varicella, croup syndrome, dehydration (from excessive exercise, diarrhea), meningitis, mumps, otitis media, pertussis, rubella, rubeola, and tonsillitis. Fever can also occur as a reaction to immunizations and drug treatments such as antibiotics. Any evaluation should include exposure to ill family members and others in the community (day care, school, etc.).

History and Physical Assessment in the Febrile Patient

Diagnostic Reasoning: Focus on History Assessment Clues Fever as a chief complaint is often reported as a subjective fever, i.e., flushing, chills, shaking chills, headache, malaise, or muscle aches, which are considered a fever by the patient or the parent but have not been validated by actually taking the temperature with a thermometer. Simply because the patient does not present with a fever does not mean that he/she does not have a febrile illness. Similarly, often a parent will report that the infant or child feels "hot." This is also not a precise indicator since during fever perfusion to the skin (vasoconstriction) is decreased and skin temperature can actually fall. Accurate temperature should be measured by using a thermometer. Because of diurnal variation in normal body temperature, frequent monitoring should be done to establish if in fact a fever does exist.

There are a number of factors to be evaluated by the nurse while assessing a febrile patient. Consider the following questions when assessing a patient presenting with fever as the chief complaint:

How do you know you have a fever? (How do you know your child has a fever?)
Has the temperature been measured? How?
Has there been any recent head trauma?
Has the patient had recurrent ear infections?
Has the patient been in contact with anyone who has had meningococcal disease?
Has the patient had any headache, lethargy, confusion, or stiff neck?
If the patient is an infant, how old is he/she?

Head trauma may provide access for infection, especially at the base of the skull. Children with recurrent ear infections or otitis media may have developed mastoiditis spreading to the meninges. Contact with anyone with meningococcal disease or *Haemophilus influenzae* puts that person at risk for contracting the disease. A typical clinical picture of meningitis is one of headache, fever, lethargy, confusion, vomiting, and stiff neck. Any patient with minimal neurological signs and symptoms should be evaluated for meningitis.

Infants Fever in children younger than 2 months of age is considered uncommon and must be viewed as serious. Neonates, infants, and young children are less able to mount a febrile response, and when they do, it is therefore a significant finding. Such fevers can be viral or bacterial in nature. Fevers in neonates may be traced to an underlying anatomical defect; urinary tract infection and bacteremia are often the first indications of a structural abnormality of the urinary tract itself. Infants with galactosemia may present in the first week to 1 month of age with gram-negative sepsis. Some infants can present with sepsis associated with delivery or acquired from instrumentation during delivery.

In infants and young children, behavior changes may be the only indicator that the child is ill. Mildly ill infants may act alert, active, smile, and feed well, whereas moderately ill infants may be fussy or even irritable, but continue to feed and can be consoled. Severely ill infants appear listless, cannot be soothed, and feed poorly or may not feed at all.

Questions being asked about the patient should include behavioral changes that the parent may have observed:

Is the child sleepier than normal?
Is the child more irritable?
How is the child acting?
How is the child eating?

Host Factors to Be Assessed One of the primary assessments that needs to be done is whether the child, as a febrile patient, is predisposed to infections that are likely to be fulminant or fatal. If so, these need to be detected and treated urgently since these patients can become acutely ill rapidly. Included in the history taking is looking for the possibility of gram-negative bacteremia, especially associated with patients with severe alcoholism, malignancy, or neutropenia. *S. aureus* bacteremia or endocarditis can be found in drug abusers, long-term hospitalized patients with indwelling plastic intravenous cannulas, or patients on hemodialysis. Fulminant bacteremia because of *Streptococcus pneumoniae, H. influenzae,* or *Neisseria meningitidis* is associated with fevers, especially in patients who have been splenectomized surgically or even spontaneously (due to hemoglobinopathy such as sickle cell disease). There are serious infections commonly associated with other conditions, such as bacterial peritonitis in cirrhotic patients and patients on chronic peritoneal dialysis. Another serious infection is pneumococcal peritonitis found in children with nephritic syndrome. Bacterial meningitis due primarily to *S. pneumoniae* is a serious infection associated with patients with cerebrospinal fluid rhinorrhea or otorrhea. Pyelonephritis is associated with patients with deranged urinary tract anatomy or dynamics that include neurogenic bladder, prostatic obstruction, indwelling Foley catheter, or nephrolithiasis.

Within the last 10 years, patients who are immunosuppressed as a result of HIV infection have raised additional concerns in the area of fever and febrile conditions. Such patients are highly susceptible to a variety of infections. These infections can present subacutely or fulminantly owing to the etiologic agents that can span all of microbiology, which include viruses, bacteria, fungi, and protozoa. Assessment and treatment require a comprehensive approach for such patients.

Questions that should be asked of the patient and/or the patient's family:

Do you have any chronic health problems? (Does your child have any chronic health problems?)

Have you (or your child) been treated recently for any health problems?

Have you (or your child) had any recent surgery?

Have you (or your child) been diagnosed with an infectious disease recently?

Are you sexually active? How many partners?

Are your immunizations up to date?

Does anyone in your family have tuberculosis or hepatitis?

Mortality Factors While taking a febrile patient's history, the nurse needs to be aware that certain health and medical factors can strongly influence the patient's ability to mount a defense against a fever. What other medical and health conditions might the patient have that may lower his/her ability to tolerate various infections? Does the patient present with coronary artery disease, congestive heart failure, or a chronic obstructive pulmonary disease? Does the patient have known medical conditions that seriously influence his/her ability to tolerate infections, such as sickle cell disease, diabetes mellitus, or adrenal insufficiency? Positive answers should impart a sense of urgency to the nurse's evaluation and treatment of the patient.

Epidemiologic Factors Part of the history taking should include an inquiry into recent travel, living conditions, or past exposure to diseases in order to help discover the epidemiology of the fever-producing agent. Has the patient traveled to exotic lands or within temperate regions of the United States? Has the patient changed his/her dietary habits (including milk products)? Has the patient had recent exposure to farm animals? Has the patient had any exposure to illnesses in family members or in the local community?

Have you been out of the country recently?

Have you been in the woods or camping recently?

Have you been staying on a farm?

Has a cat scratched you recently?

Have you been around any animals?

What immunizations have you had recently?

Localization of Symptoms When assessing the patient by taking a history, the site of the infection may be highlighted by focal complaints and referred to as localized pain, organ dysfunction, or organ irritability. (See Table 5-1). Such leads should be pursued early in the evaluation of the febrile patient. Many febrile, systematic illnesses that include generalized viral illnesses and severe bacterial infections are marked by spuriously localizing complaints, such as low back pain, **arthralgia,** headache, and abdominal pain.

Arthralgia. Pain in a joint, usually due to arthritis or arthropathy.

Temporal Sequence During the history taking, the nurse should develop a careful history of the temporal evolution of the signs and symptoms of the

❧

TABLE 5-1

LOCALIZING SIGNS AND SYMPTOMS

Possible Diseases	Symptoms
Meningitis, brain abscess, encephalitis, central nervous system vasculitis, sinusitis, mycoplasma pneumonia, and rickettsial infections	Headache and stiff neck
Pneumonia, pulmonary embolism, tuberculosis, pain, and lung abscess	Cough, tachypnea, chest
Parapharyngeal or retropharyngeal abscess, streptococcal pharyngitis, infectious mononucleosis, epiglottitis	Sore throat
Hepatitis, cholecystitis, liver abscess, and right lower lobe pneumonia	Right upper quadrant pain
Pyogenic vertebral osteomyelitis, Potts' disease, epidural abscess, pyelonephritis, retroperitoneal abscess, and endocarditis	Back pain
Diverticulitis, appendicitis, and pelvic inflammatory disease	Lower abdominal pain
Cystitis, pyelonephritis, urethritis, and prostatitis	Dysuria/frequency
Pyelonephritis	Constipation pain
Bacterial or amebic dysentery, pericolonic abscess, mesenteric ischemia, pseudomembranous colitis (antibiotic associated), inflammatory bowel disease, diverticulitis, and gonococcal proctitis	Diarrhea

febrile patient. Consider the duration of the fever (brief or prolonged). Fevers of prolonged duration are given the diagnosis of "fever of unknown origin" only when no underlying cause can be given after a comprehensive evaluation. Part of the temporal sequence is looking for cause and effect, such as exposure to an ill family member and then the development of the signs and symptoms, or changes in dietary habits, exotic travel, and the like.

Diagnostic Reasoning: Focus on the Physical Assessment The physical examination of the febrile patient normally begins with the skin and the mucous membranes. Included in this examination should be the conjunctiva, oropharynx, and anogenital region. With visual inspection, primary infection of the skin (such as cellulitis) may be detected. Inspect the skin for any integumentary evidence of disseminated infection: the petechial rash of meningococcemia or Rocky Mountain spotted fever, the embolic lesions of endocarditis, and the palpable purpura or necrotic papules of systemic vasculitis. Exanthematous diseases of childhood often produce classic eruptions; in adults, these diseases often have an atypical presentation.

While taking the history the nurse should note what physical examinations should be done as a follow-up to the clues being provided. Careful examination of febrile children should include the chest, heart, and abdomen. Examination of the musculoskeletal system should include a search for local tenderness, warmth, swelling, or erythema. During manipulation of all accessible joints the nurse assesses the presence of effusions or restriction of motion. Of particular attention should be a comprehensive search for localized or generalized lymphadenopathy. In acutely ill febrile children, the nurse should include an examination of the tympanic membranes, teeth, genitalia, rectum, and pelvis, and a comprehensive neurologic assessment. It is possible that one could discover an unsuspected cause of the fever that includes periapical dental abscess, sinusitis, otitis media, epididymitis or prostatic abscess, or pelvic inflammatory disease.

In summary, the physical examination of patients presenting with a fever should focus on looking for and ruling out the common causes before investigating more unlikely causes. Following is a list of what the nurse should include while completing a physical examination of a patient presenting with fever as a chief complaint.

1. Observe the patient: Does the patient look ill, dehydrated, seem lethargic, and respond appropriately?
2. Take vital signs and note temperature: Incidence of bacteremia, as well as specific infections, increases with the magnitude of the fever. Not all patients with extremely high fevers have infections, but they may be suffering from hyperthermia.
3. Observe skin and mucous membranes: Macular/papular rash may indicate a viral exanthema, infectious disease, or a drug sensitivity reaction. Vesicular rashes occur with viral infection. A petechial skin rash indicates meningococcemia or Rocky Mountain spotted fever.
4. Examine the head and neck: Percuss the sinuses and transilluminate for evidence of sinusitis. Examine and palpate the teeth for abscesses. Palpate the salivary glands for tenderness. Examine the

throat and tonsils for signs of infection, specifically for enlargement or red tonsils, lymphadenopathy, or tonsil or pharyngeal exudate. Inspect the ears and tympanic membrane for effusion, erythema, fluid, or purulent secretion. In the infant feel for a tense or bulging anterior fontanel.

5. Palpate the lymph nodes: Palpate all lymph nodes for enlargement and tenderness.

6. Examine the lungs and chest: Percuss and auscultate the lungs. Note adventitious sounds, decreased breath sounds, or areas of consolidation that may indicate lower respiratory tract infection or pneumonia. Note sputum for color, consistency, and presence of blood or odor.

7. Palpate breasts if indicated: Palpate for signs of inflammation, masses, tenderness, and discharge. Palpate axillary lymph nodes for presence and tenderness.

8. Examine genitourinary system if indicated: Palpate for suprapubic tenderness that may indicate pelvic inflammatory disease (PID) or urinary tract infection (UTI), and for costovertebral angle (CVA) tenderness, which suggests pyelonephritis.

9. Examine musculoskeletal system if indicated: Examination may suggest inflammation or infection of bone or joints, especially if there is swelling, increased warmth, or tenderness.

10. Perform neurological/mental state examination: Evaluate for signs of meningeal irritation. Note the presence of focal deficits and assess for disturbances in mentation, irritability, lethargy, somnolence, or coma that may indicate increased intracranial pressure. Seizures occur in 20 to 30% of children with meningitis.

Laboratory Studies There are no routine laboratory studies in the evaluation of the febrile patient. Presenting signs and symptoms and other factors determine what laboratory tests should be considered, if any. One factor that would call for the use of laboratory tests is the severity and acuteness of the patient's condition. Another factor would be the presence of debilitating or compromising underlying diseases. The occurrence of symptoms such as dysuria and frank pain dictates at least a urinalysis and urine culture. A cough, sputum production, or pleurisy suggests the need for a chest x-ray. Certain physical findings that clearly establish a diagnosis suggest a conservative use of laboratory tests. A child who presents with classic measles is one such example. One factor that would reduce the use of certain laboratory tests is beginning antibiotic therapy before obtaining blood cultures, since antibiotics inhibit the growth of bacteria in any blood cultures drawn. Another is that the patient presents having been started on antibiotic therapy at home, perhaps by the parent.

The Acutely Ill, Recently Hospitalized Patient Infants, young children, and older children who were hospitalized recently but not evaluated for fever, and who subsequently develop fever, may merit an initial battery of laboratory tests, to be ordered by the physician. Such tests might include white blood cell count with differential count, urinalysis, and perhaps a chest x-ray. Depending on the severity of the fever and the acuteness of the patient's condition, the physician might also order two blood cultures and request a clean-catch midstream urine or a catheterized urine specimen to be cultured. Patients who develop a cough or dyspnea may additionally require orders for a deep sputum specimen for Gram stain and culture. Patients with abdominal complaints may require some form of abdominal imaging, such as ultrasound or computer tomography (CT) scanning.

Regular monitoring of the patient's temperature is clearly a priority for febrile children and adults. Providing an increase in fluids and nutritional intake should be encouraged if permitted by the patient's condition. When administering prescribed antipyretic drugs, the resulting chills and sweating should be minimized if the dosing schedule is maintained. It is important to promote the patient's comfort by maintaining a stable room temperature and by frequently changing bedding and clothing.

Fever Management

Fluids The child with fever should be encouraged to take plenty of fluids to prevent possible dehydration. However, fluids that increase fluid loss, such as drinks containing caffeine, should be avoided.

Antipyretics Drugs such as acetaminophen and anti-inflammatory drugs restore the hypothalamic set point by blocking substances like prostaglandin and interleukins, which increases thermoregulation. Aspirin, unless otherwise prescribed by the physician, is no longer given to children because of its connection to Reye's syndrome. Antipyretics should not be routinely administered for fever, except if the fever is 40.5°C (104.9°F). Otherwise, they should be used only if the associated symptoms of fever such as malaise, arthralgia, and headache bother the child.

Physical Remedies External cooling such as tepid water sponging allows for evaporation. It works best if the child is given an antipyretic one-half hour prior to the bath. Without an antipyretic, the temperature set point in the hypothalamus does not decrease and the cooling bath may stimulate shivering, which will cause the temperature to rise. The combination of antipyretic and sponging has been supported by research as more effective in reducing the fever than antipyretics alone (Friedman & Barton, 1990; Steele, Tanaka, Lara, & Bass, 1990). In addition, it has been demonstrated that sponging is effective only during the first 30 minutes after the procedure (Agbolosu et al., 1997; Aksoylar et al., 1997). The use of alcohol is not condoned because the fumes can be a danger to the child.

The child with fever may be covered with a light blanket, particularly when he/she complains of being cold and shivering occurs. However, when these signs are over, the child should be uncovered to allow for evaporation of heat.

Although physical activity in itself is not contraindicated in fever, vigorous exercise should be discouraged, since it raises body temperature.

$\mathcal{P}$ AIN

Introduction to Principles of Pain Management

To manage pain and relieve a patient's **suffering** are crucial elements of a health care professional's commitment. The importance of appropriate and adequate pain management is further increased when benefits for the patient are realized: earlier mobilization, shortened hospital stay, and reduced costs. Infants, children, and adolescents can and do experience pain. Research studies demonstrate that despite the availability of effective techniques for pain management in infants and children, their pain is less effectively managed than the pain in adults. Recognition of this inadequacy in terms of traditional pain management in adults, infants, and children has prompted action in a number of health care disciplines including surgery, pediatrics, anesthesiology, nursing, and pain management groups. Part of the action has resulted in the development and issuing of clinical guidelines to help assist clinicians with decisions about acute and chronic pain management in children.

Suffering. A state of emotional distress associated with events that threaten the biological and/or psychosocial integrity of the individual. Suffering often accompanies severe pain, but can occur in its absence; hence pain and suffering are phenomenologically distinct.

Eight Principles of Pain Management

From the pain clinical guidelines eight principles of pain management have emerged that influence assessment, treatment, and outcomes in pain management of infants, children, and adults. The first principle is that unrelieved pain has negative short- and long-term physical and psychological consequences. No patient should be allowed to suffer with unrelieved pain. Initiating aggressive pain prevention and control before, during, and after surgery and other medical procedures, therefore, will yield both short- and long-term physical and psychological benefits. The second principle is that prevention is better than treatment in pain management. Health care professionals must be proactive in assuring that postoperative and medical procedures that are known to produce pain must be accompanied by aggressive intervention strategies to ensure that the least amount of pain is suffered by the patient. Once pain is established and severe, it is more difficult to control. Principles one and two suggest that to manage effectively a patient's pain and its effects, one must continuously assess and reassess both the pain intensity and duration, and those interventions that provide pain relief must be proactive and aggressive. Such assessment and interventions should be done at regular intervals and when necessary in order to avoid the negative short- and long-term consequences of unrelieved pain.

The third principle from the guidelines is that successful assessment and control depend, in part, on a positive relationship having developed among the nurse, the child, and the child's family. Part of this relationship is to recognize that the child and the family need to be informed that pain relief is an important part of their health care. Another part of this relationship is the willingness to share information about options available to them to control pain. Last, the parents and the child should be welcome to discuss their concerns, fears, and preferences with the health care team. This leads us to the fourth principle, which is that the child (if able) and the family (if able) should be actively involved and continuously encouraged to be involved in pain assessment and its management. Clearly not all pain can be eliminated in postoperative situations or in all medical procedures, but the child and family should be able to voice their concerns, be involved in pain management, and let the health care professional know when the pain is beyond tolerance or that the interventions are inadequate. The fifth principle is that any and all techniques that reduce pain to acceptable levels as part of the patient's health care management should be a realistic goal, especially in the care of infants, children, and adolescents. The sixth principle is that health care professionals need to learn about and to develop a better knowledge of the children in their care through routine assessments. Knowing the patient can in turn optimize the assessment of pain and its management. The seventh principle is that children who cannot communicate, or have difficulty communicating, about their pain require particular attention. Children, especially those who are cognitively or emotionally impaired or psychotic, or who cannot speak English or have a level of education or cultural background that differs significantly from that of the health team, require close attention. Included in this group are fetuses and neonates. Current research and current definitions of pain propose that from the second trimester a fetus has the capacity to experience pain, and, when confronted with painful stimuli, does actively respond through nonverbal cues. The eighth principle is that any unexpected and intense pain, particularly if it is sudden or associated with altered vital signs such as hypotension, tachycardia, or fever, should be immediately evaluated.

Pain Assessment Procedures

Based on the above principles pain assessment strategies of a child (infant to adolescent) should be tailored to the child's development level and personality style, and to the context and situation. It is important to obtain a pain history from the child and/or the child's parents at the time of admission (Table 5-2). A pain history is especially important for any patient who will be undergoing painful medical or surgical procedures. Part of this assessment should be to learn what terms the child uses to describe pain such as a "booboo," "owie," or "hurt." Such information can be elicited by asking simple questions when you note a bruise or cut or by asking questions about falling down while on the playground or riding their bikes. Included in the pain assessment should be eliciting the family's and child's culturally determined beliefs about pain and medical care.

Often one can see such cultural beliefs in action in the reactions of the child and parent to the various manipulations of the child's body while completing physical assessment or in the very act of meeting with a health care professional. Verbal and nonverbal cues that come from the parent or the child should be openly interpreted by questioning the meaning from the child and/or parent. Such questioning should be done in a nonjudgmental and nonthreatening manner using the "I noticed . . ." or "I'm not sure what was meant by . . ." form of questioning, which is less threatening than using "you" statements. If the child is in pain at the time of the history taking, then one can measure the child's pain using self-report and/or behavioral observation tools that have known reliability, validity, and sensitivity (Table 5-2). Such tools should be practical for the nurse to

☒

TABLE 5-2
ASPECTS OF PAIN

Definition

An unpleasant sensory and emotional experience that is associated with either actual or potential tissue damage or that is described in terms of such damage (International Association for Study of Pain)

Temporal Characteristics

Acute: less than 6 months
Chronic: 6 months or more

Physiology

Somatic pain
- Results from activation of peripheral receptors and somatic efferent nerves, without injury to nerves
- Can be characterized as either sharp or dull but typically well localized and intermittent
- Managed by a wide variety of nonopioid and opioid analgesics, anesthetic blocks, and neurosurgical approaches

Visceral pain
- Results from activation of visceral nociceptive receptors and visceral efferent nerves, without injury to nerves
- Characterized as deep aching, cramping sensation, often referred to cutaneous sites
- Managed by a wide variety of nonopioid and opioid analgesics, anesthetic blocks, and neurosurgical approaches

Neural (causalgic pain) pain
- Results from injury to peripheral receptors, nerves, or central nervous system
- Characterized as burning and dysesthetic
- Often associated with sensory loss
- In contrast to somatic and visceral pain management, neural pain responds minimally to nonopioid and opioid analgesics, anesthetic and neurosurgical approaches

(continued on next page)

TABLE 5-2 (CONTINUED)

Pathogenesis

Structural:

- Chronic and associated with such diseases as rheumatoid arthritis, metastatic cancer, and sickle cell anemia
- Episodes of pain alternating with pain-free intervals as in sickle cell anemia
- Episodes of waxing and waning pain in varying degrees of severity as in metastatic cancer

Psychological:

- Where neither structural nor physiologic mechanisms can be found to produce the chronic pain being described
- May be related to a structural disease or physiologic mechanism that may have been present in past but psychological aspects engender chronic physiologic factors long after structural or physiologic mechanisms are healed

Delusional:

- Pain that has neither structural nor physiologic mechanisms
- Occurs often with patients who have profound psychiatric disorders, such as psychotic depression or schizophrenia
- History is often so vague and bizarre, with a nonanatomical pain distribution strongly suggestive of the psychological disorder

administer and interpret, and simple and age appropriate for the child to respond to. Self-reports tools are more appropriate for the child over 7 years of age who can understand the concepts of order and numbers. Behavioral observations need to be used with preverbal and nonverbal children, and can even be used with verbal children as adjunct to the self-report measures. Behavioral observations include vocalizations, verbalizations, facial expressions, motor responses, body postures, levels of activity, and appearance. Behavioral observations need to be interpreted with caution. Some behaviors such as watching television, playing, and sleeping may be used as strategies to cope with pain.

Continuous severe pain, depression, fatigue, extreme illness, and the use of sedatives or hypnotics can blunt behaviors. Very ill children with severe pain may simply whimper and lie still in their beds rather than cry. Parents can be extremely helpful in the nurse's assessment of the child's level of pain. Often the nurse can use the parent's self-report when the child is either unwilling or unable to provide a self-report. Use physiologic measures to assess levels of pain and its management (e.g., heart rate, respiration, and blood pressure) only as an adjunct to either self-reports or behavioral observations. Physiologic measures are neither that sensitive nor that specific as indicators of pain.

Postoperative Assessment

Based on the above principles of pain management, the nurse should be assessing pain at regular intervals and especially if opioids are used. Assessment after major surgery should occur at least every 2 hours for the first 24 hours, and every 4 hours thereafter. More frequent assessment is necessary if pain is being poorly controlled. The child as well as the parent should be interviewed about the pain, specifically as to its duration and intensity, as well as about pain relief following a pain reduction intervention. The assessment of pain should be included with other routine assessments such as vital signs. The pain assessment should be documented either at the bedside or where such information can be easily and quickly accessed. The documentation should include a description of the pain (site, duration, and intensity) and the patient's response to interventions. Part of the documentation and assessment is noting the child's behavior, appearance, activity level, and vital signs. Changes in any and all of these are the early warning signs that the pain is not being well controlled. Before discharge, the nurse should review with the child and parents what interventions were used and their effectiveness, and provide any additional instructions or information required for home management of pain.

Management of Pain Related to Medical Procedures

Both hospitalized children and those who visit ambulatory clinics will at one time or another undergo procedures that are either uncomfortable or painful. Procedures can range from venipunctures and the insertion of intravenous catheters to even more stressful procedures such as lumbar puncture, bone marrow aspirates and biopsies, chest tube insertions, cardiac catheterization, circumcisions, and dressing changes. Children often describe such procedures as the most distressing aspect of their disease, clinic visit, or their hospitalization. Aggressive efforts on the part of the health care team, and especially the nurse, to reduce the child's level of stress and pain during such procedures are, therefore, truly warranted. What can be done to reduce the stress and the pain associated with various procedures will vary according to the procedure and the situation and the context in which it is being done. Interventions may consist of pharmacologic modalities, nonpharmacologic modalities, or both (Table 5-2). Using the following set of questions should help the nurse select the appropriate level of intervention to minimize pain and stress.

Why is the procedure being performed?
How do the parents think the child will react?
Has the child had a similar experience and what was the reaction to the experience?
What are the expected intensity and duration of pain?
What are the expected intensity and duration of the anxiety?
How often will the procedure be repeated?

The Management of Procedures Related to Pain If the nurse has the time and opportunity, the child and the family should be adequately prepared for the procedure. Preparation should be developmentally appropriate. The timing of the preparation should be adjusted to meet the individual needs and preferences. The nurse should be aware of environmental comfort (that is, privacy, lighting, noise levels, and temperature). Unless it is absolutely necessary, the procedure should not be performed in the child's bed or room. The parents or parent should be allowed to be with the child before, during, and after the procedure (with the older child or the adolescent the same-sex parent may be more appropriate). The parents should be well prepared in advance as to what their expected roles should be. Pharmacologic and nonpharmacologic options should be combined whenever it is appropriate and possible. Pharmacologic options should be given well enough in advance that they have the desired effect on the child before the procedure is performed. If the procedure is to be repeated, the child should be provided maximum treatment for the pain and anxiety for the first procedure so that anticipatory anxiety is minimized for subsequent procedures.

Pharmacologic Agents for Procedure-Related Pain A number of pharmacologic agents are available for use in reducing the pain and anxiety associated with procedure-related pain. Injected and topical local anesthetics can reduce pain sensation. Opioids, given either intravenously, orally, or transmucosally, can be given in increments and titrated to produce an analgesic effect. Oral and intravenous benzodiazepines can produce anxiolysis and sedation, but remember that they do not provide an analgesic effect. Other agents, such as nitrous oxide and ketamine, can be used by trained personnel and when appropriate monitoring procedures are available. General anesthesia is appropriate in some situations.

Nonpharmacologic Management of Procedure-Related Pain For those procedures that are considered less painful, such as venipunctures, or as adjuncts to pharmacologic strategies for the more painful procedures, nonpharmacologic strategies can be used alone. Strategy and intervention selection should be tailored to the needs, preferences, and coping styles of the child. During the history taking, and especially under the pain assessment portion of the history taking, the nurse can elicit from either the child or the parents what strategies have been useful to reduce pain and anxiety during less painful situations. The family members then can be used to encourage the child during these more painful procedures to call upon those strategies.

For infants clearly sensorimotor strategies would include the use of pacifiers, swaddling, holding, and rocking. For the older child, cognitive and/or behavioral strategies include the use of hypnosis, relaxation techniques (deep breathing, visualization, and so on), distraction (number counting, for example), music, art and play therapy, preparatory information, and positive reinforcement. In some children rehearsal before the procedure may be helpful. Child-centered participation strategies focus on involving the child in age-appropriate decisions about the procedure and in activities related to its conduct. Physical strategies include the use of heat or cold, massage, exercise, rest, and immobilization. Older children and adolescents who find nonpharmacologic strategies helpful may even prefer them to pharmacologic agents for procedures that are not excessively painful.

Anatomy and Physiology of Pain

The measurement of pain in children is a major challenge to researchers and health care professionals who want to make medical procedures and postoperative care for children less painful or want to reduce the pain associated with certain diseases. In order to measure it, one first has to identify what pain is. Part of the problem in identifying what pain is that pain has multidimensional physiologic and psychological features. Pain has been primarily viewed as a response to noxious stimuli that results from potential or actual physical injury, damage, or disease. Such a definition of pain is unidimensional since it lacks the interpretative aspects or the cultural and behavioral, cognitive, and emotional responses associated with pain. While pain clearly does have sensory features and, therefore, lends itself primarily to sensory description, it is above all a very powerful and demanding feeling state that can be expressed in both verbal and nonverbal cues that include both psychological and physiologic dimensions and responses. Once learned, pain is associated as part of an emotional response, that is, as a multidimensional psychological and physiologic response. The question for researchers and health care professionals in both researching pain and in its management and control, then, is at what stage in human growth and development does such a physiologic and psychological response to pain occur. When is the human system capable of recognizing and responding to pain?

The Perception of Pain

Pain by definition is subjective. Until recently it was thought that individuals learn the application of the word by experiences related to injury early in life. Biologists have long recognized that stimuli that cause pain are also liable to damage tissue. Accordingly, what is experienced consciously as pain is often associated with actual or potential tissue damage. Being consciously associated with various noxious stimuli, it is unquestionably a sensation in one or more parts of the body, but since it is also always a conscious association with unpleasantness, it has an emotional component as well. Pain in the absence of actual or potential tissue damage, or any likely pathophysiological cause, more than likely has a psychological reason for its existence. Psychological pain cannot be distinguished easily from pain due to tissue damage, and, therefore, should be reported in the same way as tissue-related pain.

Because of the cultural, behavioral, cognitive, and emotional judgments about the nature and severity of pain that others may be experiencing, the observer's judgments are heavily influenced by their own subjective preconceptions (prejudices and biases) about the nature of that experience. Such preconceptions come from having a strong association to a conscious sense about such past experiences; hence the observer looks for similar patterns of conscious awareness in others that include such constructive memories and thoughts, images, and feelings linked or associated with pain. In other words, we only assume that others are in pain when it fits our own preconceptions that such experiences are truly painful. Preverbal and nonverbal individuals and those individuals who do not share similar patterns of experiences (especially cultural) are at risk of having other evidence of pain denied, minimized, or ignored. This is clearly indicated in substantial behavioral evidence of pain in neonates, infants, and children, and findings that indicate destructive immediate and long-term consequences if such pain is not controlled.

Pain in neonates, infants, and children continues to be discounted, and, therefore, poorly controlled. One reason for this is that our current definitions favor the conscious adult concept of pain—early life experiences dictate the emergence of pain recognition, and infants do not have the psychological mechanisms to remember pain or the physiologic maturity to respond to pain. New research argues for the inclusion of verbal and nonverbal cues in one's assessment of states of pain since second-trimester fetuses have been found to have the neurological capacity to physiologically recognize and respond to painful stimuli. The proposition for using both verbal and nonverbal cues is based on the need for an explicit recognition that the experience of pain is an inherent quality of life rather than solely a learned response from a physiologic event. It is an inherent quality present in all viable newborns that can be demonstrated in nonverbal pain clues. The nature of the pain experience and its expression change during the course of a human's maturation and as a result of exposure to life experiences related to tissue injury.

Purpose of Pain

Pain is a protective mechanism of the body. The definition of pain provides the clues to recognizing that tissue damage (potential or actual) is the primary cause of most pain. The body's defensive reaction is to withdraw from a painful stimulus. The simple act of sitting too long can cause tissue damage and destruction because of lack of blood flow to the compressed area. It is the reason that one consciously or unconsciously shifts one's weight or turns during sleep. Coma patients or those who have lost the ability to sense pain can rapidly develop ulceration of the area of pressure unless special measures are taken to move the person from time to time.

The pain system in humans develops during the second and third trimesters with additional maturation changes over the next 2 years of life. Perception of pain changes little after such maturity has occurred. Emotional aspects of painful experiences, the interpretation of painful experiences, and the behavioral and cognitive strategies and repertoires undergo often profound and major changes throughout life. Hence one can see a large variation in psychological and emotional reactions in an individual to similar types of painful experiences.

The traditional view of neuroanatomy and neurophysiology of the pain system in premature infants, neonates, and even nonverbal infants was that they were highly undeveloped and required months to years to mature. Since such children were unable to describe the subjective nature of the phenomenon of pain they were experiencing, it was concluded that they were not capable of holding perceptions of painful experiences. Holding this traditional view led to the widespread practice of providing either very little or no anesthesia during surgery and no analgesia for invasive procedures or after surgery for such neonates and infants. Such practices were common for newborns, especially for the premature; if full-term infants were thought not to have fully developed perceptions of pain, then premature infants were thought to be even less developmentally mature. For such children, recommendations for analgesia or sedation while in intensive care were made with little regard for the developmental neurobiology of their pain mechanisms or even for the behavioral and/or physiologic clues and responses to pain and stress observed in the neonates and premature infants.

The theoretical framework for understanding the pain system begins with understanding the development and maturation of pain-related pathways that may be traced from sensory receptors in the skin to the cerebral cortex. The development of each of these components provides the framework to study and understand the development and maturation of the pain system. Many, if not most, ailments of the body can cause pain. The ability to recognize and diagnose an ailment depends to a great extent on the nurse's knowledge of different qualities of pain. Included in this knowledge is how pain can be referred from one part of the body to another, how pain can spread from the painful site, and, last, what the different causes of pain are.

Pain Qualities

Pain has been classified into three different major types: pricking, burning, and aching pain. Pricking pain is felt when one is stuck by a needle into the skin or when cut by a knife. It can be in a local or widespread area of the skin and is described as diffuse and irritating. Burning pain is the type of pain felt when the skin is burned. It is described as excruciating and the type of pain most likely to cause suffering in the patient. Aching pain is a deep pain rather than a surface or skin-level pain. It is described with varying degrees of annoyance.

Describing pain in greater depth is not needed since most people are familiar with pain and are able to describe its qualities in great detail. The issue is what causes the varying types and qualities of pain. Pricking pain is seen as a result of the simulation of type-A delta pain fibers found in the skin, whereas burning and aching result from the simulation of more primitive type C fibers. Since there are two types of fibers and these two fibers are associated with different qualities of pain, recognizing which type of pain is associated with which fiber can help differentiate the cause of pain.

Pain Receptors and Their Stimulation

The sense of pain (a perception) is contributed by free nerve endings (pain receptors) located in the skin and certain visceral tissues. Pain is caused by stimuli (**noxious** or unpleasant) of different natures. Strong "mechanical" stimuli (intense pressure), very hot and very cold "thermal" stimuli, and certain "chemical" stimuli such as acidic substances can all cause pain. Pain receptors (free nerve endings) have a high **threshold** of stimulation so stimulus strength must be high in order to activate them.

Since such strong stimuli are considered noxious, pain sensation is also called nociception (noxious perception). The pain receptors (free nerve endings) associated with pain sensation are called **nociceptors**. It is felt that nociceptive stimuli (noxious stimuli) cause tissue damage that can be anything from a simple itch to serve consequences such as an electrical burn. Tissue damage causes the local release of certain internal nociceptive substances (noxious substances) such as serotonin, substance-P, histamine, and kinin peptides found in the injured tissue. It is these substances that in turn then act on the free nerve endings, thus activating the pain signals.

Studies demonstrate that there appear to be two systems of pain transmission to the central nervous system where the signals are interpreted and reacted to. The two systems are associated with two distinct types of pain experience. The two associated types of pain can be seen when you prick your finger with a rose thorn. At first the sensation is of a sharp localized pain, followed a while later by a more dull and generalized pain sensation. The sharp pain sensation is the pain signal to arrive at the central nervous system. It is the prickling, localized, and short lasting type of pain. The second pain sensation is then later felt as a dull sensation. As a sensation it is longer lasting, considered more diffuse, and it hurts and aches but the aching source cannot be pinpointed and normally it is ascribed to a larger body part, such as the whole finger.

Physiologists think that the sharp pain is conveyed by thin but myelinated, relatively fast-acting, nerve fibers called type A-delta, and the hurting and aching pain is conveyed by unmyelinated, relatively slow-acting type C fibers. Once stimulated, conduction velocity in type A-delta is thought to be 10 times faster than the type C fibers hence the difference in which pain perception is felt first. Type A-delta and C fibers terminate at the dorsal horn in the spinal column and ascend by the spinothalamic pathway. The slow aching pain signals are thought to make a major input into the brain stem reticular formation and essentially terminate in the thalamus. The sharp, fast pain signals, however, ascend more directly to the thalamus as well as up to the sensory cortex. The sharp, fast cortical component of pain gives the fine localization capacity to the sharp/fast pain system and the ability to respond to localized pain quickly. The

Noxious stimulus. Stimulus that is potentially or actually damaging to body tissue. In some instances there is no lasting tissue damage (e.g., muscle pain due to excessive exercise).

Pain threshold. The least experience of pain that a subject can recognize.

Nociceptor. A receptor preferentially sensitive to a noxious stimulus or to a stimulus that would become noxious if prolonged. Avoid use of terms like *pain receptor, pain pathway,* etc., because they reflect anachronistic concepts and can mislead. Pain is a complex perception that takes place only at higher levels of the central nervous system.

slower subcortical projection of the dull/aching/slow pain system is associated with the aching/hurting component. Sensory cortex damage allows patients to feel pain and hurt, but they are unable to localize the source.

Spinothalamic Pathway

With entry into the spinal horn, the various sensory fibers become segregated into two categories. One is the thin fibers carrying pain, temperature, and crude tactile sensations. These pain sensations are collectively referred to as nondiscriminative pain modalities. These thin fibers terminate in the dorsal horn of the spinal cord. It is then in the dorsal horn where they synapse with the secondary relay cells, and the sensory input travels up to the thalamus. The thin fibers decussate (cross over) and enter the white matter of the dorsal horn to ascend in the "spinothalamic pathways" toward the brain. The spinothalamic fibers of this pathway terminate in the thalamus. The thalamus is considered the most important subcortical sensory relay/integration center. The spinothalamic sensory relay/integration center and its related modalities are considered to represent a basic, primitive somatic (bodily) sensory system. This primitive somatic sensory system is seen in all vertebrates.

A more highly developed somatic sensory system has evolved in higher primates and humans. This more highly developed somatic sensory system's pathway is taken by the large myelinated fibers (type A fibers) in the dorsal horn and physiologically represents this somatic sensory system. These myelinated type A fibers carry the sensory modalities of fine touch and pressure and proprioception (discriminative tactile sensory inputs) and are, therefore, considered the fibers for discriminative sensory modalities, whereas the more primary spinothalamic pathway contains the fibers for nondiscriminative modalities. These discriminative fibers (type A) enter the spinal cord but do not terminate or synapse in the dorsal horn (as do type C fibers). The type A fibers instead ascend without crossing over, up the sensory pathways of the posterior (dorsal) columns (called the funiculi), to terminate in the medulla where they make their first synapse.

In summary, there are two sensory systems, one that is considered primitive and a sensory system for crude tactile, pain (nociceptive), and temperature (thermal) signals. These signals are conveyed by unmyelinated small-diameter fibers (type C) up the spinothalamic pathway via the dorsal horn to the thalamus. The fibers of these cell bodies are small. The central terminals (synapses) of these fibers are in the spinal horn. It is in the synapse area that they release peptide transmitters (substance P by pain fibers) which permit impulses to be relayed up the spinothalamic pathway to the thalamus where these signals are then integrated. Fine touch and pressure and proprioceptive modalities (signals from joints and muscles) are carried by fast-conducting, large, myelinated fibers (type A) via the dorsal horn to the central medulla where then they are integrated. Type A fibers can be differentiated by the fact that they have larger cell bodies than type C, synapses in the medulla, and are myelinated.

Pain Inhibition

Recent studies have shown that electrical stimulation of certain neuronal groups of the brain stem reticular formation makes the conscious animal completely oblivious to pain stimuli. It is thought that descending control fibers from the reticular formation project to the dorsal horn of the spinal cord where it is thought that this projection suppresses the relay of pain signals to the brain. This ability to suppress pain signals is thought to be a protective mechanism to aid animals to cope with the debilitating and hurtful consequences of high physical stress and fighting. Psychologists think that through active training some people, including athletes, Yogis, soldiers, and others, are able to activate this descending inhibition system at will and thus reduce incoming pain signals. How this occurs is just beginning to be understood and is associated with studies surrounding endorphins.

Endorphins One means used by the higher reticular centers to inhibit pain is just beginning to be understood. Descending fibers activate certain "inhibitory interneurons" in the dorsal horn of the spinal column. Activation of these inhibitory interneurons causes the release of a peptide neurotransmitter called "enkephalin" which is one of the endorphins. Enkephalin is thought to suppress the transmission of pain signals by binding with particular receptor molecules (opiate receptors) found in the synapses of cells in the dorsal horn. Binding is thought to either decrease the amount of the neurotransmitter substance-P released by the type C pain afferents or to induce postsynaptic inhibition of the relay cells (signal relay inhibition). Morphine and other opiate analgesics are thought to act in the same manner as naturally occurring endorphins to relieve pain.

Afferent Pain Inhibition Current research suggests that interneurons of the dorsal horn in the spinal column may be involved in a different type of pain inhibition from that just described. Skin rubbing relieves the dull/hurtful pain sensation that comes from the rub area or a nearby area. Rubbing activates the large, fast-conducting tactile fibers (type A-alpha nerve fibers) while the pain is being conveyed by C fibers. Within the dorsal horn, tactile or touch fibers are thought to activate inhibitory interneurons that in turn inhibit the synaptic transmission of pain signals. This inhibition is called the gate theory of afferent inhibition. The theory hypothesizes that the more powerful tactile or touch signals limit the transmission gates in the dorsal horn to their own, suppressing and excluding access for the weaker pain signal.

Referred Pain Afferent pain fibers that originate in the same area show extensive convergence onto the dorsal horn relay cells in the spinal column. In some cases the convergence may take place from fibers from different areas, causing the relay cell in the dorsal horn to be activated by pain originating from a different body part. Normally one part is a visceral area of the body or an organ. This is thought to be the mechanism for the phenomenon called "referred pain."

Assessment and Diagnosis of Painful Disorders

Pain can be either acute or chronic. Pain of more than 6 months in duration is considered chronic. When assessing pain, several clinical features (signs and symptoms) differentiate acute from chronic (see Table 5-2). Patients who have severe acute pain normally can either provide clues or clear descriptions of its location, character, and timing. Many autonomic nervous system hyperactivity signs are often present, such as rapid heart rate and breathing, hypertension, diaphoresis, mydriasis, and pallor. Acute pain normally responds well to analgesic agents, and psychological factors play a minor role in the pain's pathogenesis.

In contrast, patients who suffer from chronic pain often describe less precisely the localization, character, and timing of the pain. Because the autonomic nervous system adapts, signs of autonomic hyperactivity disappear. Chronic pain does not respond as well to nonopioid and opioid analgesic agents as does acute pain. Psychological aspects and features (cultural, behavioral, cognitive, and emotional) are usually more pertinent than those found in acute pain presentations. Taken collectively, these features often cause the health care professional to believe that the patient is exaggerating the complaints. Since there is no objective measurement for chronic pain, the health care professional must, having taken into consideration the patient's age, cultural background, psychological makeup, and history of pain, accept the patient's report.

$\mathcal{S}$UMMARY

This chapter addresses fears, real and imagined. A child's fears are a normal part of growing up and in most cases can be predicted by age. Fears become problematic only if they inhibit the child's growth intellectually or emotionally or debilitate him/her in some way. A symptomatic approach to overcoming fears is addressed and teaching techniques for the nurse are highlighted. This chapter presents the management of the symptoms of fear developmentally and has an overview of how to use fear constructively for the child's optimal development.

This chapter also addresses parents' concerns regarding their child's fever. Parents rarely present to the clinic with a medical diagnosis of their child; instead, they talk about the symptoms, which they want alleviated as soon as possible, especially if the symptom is fever.

$\mathcal{C}$RITICAL POINTS IN THE MANAGEMENT OF FEAR, ANXIETY, AND FEVER

In organizing care for children with fear, anxiety, or fever, the nurse needs to be careful to obtain a clear history. All facts should be clearly organized and considered. It is most important for the nurse to realize that fear is an individual experience. Special attention should be given to determining the child's cultural background and therefore determining whether the symptoms described are the product of fear or anxiety. Even though this experience is very hard to diagnose or to differentiate, the treatment should be based an objective collection of data and not on what the nurse thinks is the best treatment. Assessment of the parents' beliefs is important since values are internalized and transmitted to children by parents and by the society in which they live. A nurse's responsibility, above all, is to examine all the family behaviors and also to examine his/her own assumptions and cultural biases. People from different cultures often have traditional beliefs that have been handed from generation to generation. Nothing is harder for parents than to see their own child hurt and not be able to help him/her. The care of these children requires acceptance of multiple realities, a clear understanding of the differences, and an open, sensitive intervention.

$\mathcal{Q}$UESTIONS

Diagnosis: Fever, Unknown Origin

History: Baby Clare, 16 months old, is brought to the emergency room by her mother with the complaint of fever for the last 3 days. The mother is very worried. She states that she has called the doctor's office with the complaint, but no one has been able to help with Clare's fever.

Plan: Clare will go home with her mother after the doctor diagnoses her and the nurse teaches her mother how to manage fever.

Nursing problems: Prevention of seizures, parent teaching, parent support, instructions on medication management for parents.

Chief concerns for the nurse: Control the baby's fever and treat the underlying cause of the fever. Teach the parent how to manage the fever and how to treat the disease that is causing the fever. A reality in pediatrics is that parents get very upset when their child has fever. Often, they panic or do not know what to do, and overuse the medication.

1. Which statement related to fever is correct?

   A. Fever is a reaction to an infection.
   B. Fever is an infection and needs to be treated rapidly.
   C. Fever is an elevation of the body temperature.
   D. Fever is a reaction to a viral infection.

2. Clare's mother asks the nurse if fever is a good thing because it alerts one to an infection. The nurse responds:

   A. Fever usually alerts to infections.
   B. Fever never alerts to infections.
   C. Fever is good only when the fever is low.
   D. Fever is never bad.

3. The mother asks if all fevers of all diseases are treated equally. The nurse responds:

    A. Since all fevers are a response to infections, all are treated the same.

    B. Fever is treated more aggressively according to the underlying conditions.

    C. Fever is treated differently in cold climates.

    D. Fever is treated differently if it is viral or infectious.

4. The nurse needs to know that although acetaminophen is the drug of choice to treat fever, on the basis of age and weight, the most important consideration when treating children is:

    A. Age

    B. Sex and age

    C. Age, sex, and weight

    D. Weight

5. Clare's mother asks the nurse under what circumstances she should use external sponging.

    A. External sponging with tepid water is always recommended as an alternative treatment for fever.

    B. External sponging with ice water is recommended as an alternative treatment for fever.

    C. External sponging with alcohol is recommended as an alternative treatment for fever.

    D. External sponging with tepid water plus acetaminophen is a slightly more rapidly antipyretic.

Diagnosis: Fear

History: Six-year-old Virginia is going to the hospital to have her appendix removed. Mrs. Miranda, Virginia's mother, is upset because Virginia is very frightened and does not want to cooperate with the hospital staff.

Plan: Virginia will cooperate with staff while she is in the hospital, go home with her parents feeling well, and, most important, learn that she can manage her fears.

Nursing problems: Teach the child to manage her fears. Reassure the parents that the child will learn to control her fears. Help other hospital personnel deal with Virginia's behavior.

Chief concerns for the nurse: The nursing intervention for a child who is going to have surgery is help in management of fear. The nurse needs to evaluate whether the type of preparation that the child has had for surgery is enough to cope with anxiety and fear. Not only the child, but also the parents, have fear mixed with anxiety and guilt. (Parents believe that they can take care of everything when they cannot, a defense mechanism that surfaces in guilt.) For the child and for the parent alike the nurse's chief concerns are to help them cope with the present problem and to help them grow from the experience.

1. What is the most important information that the nurse must obtain from Virginia while he/she is taking the nursing history?

   A. Find out how much Virginia has been told about the surgery.
   B. Find out what is the worst fear that Virginia has.
   C. Find out if Virginia is scared of the dark.
   D. Find out if Virginia sleeps alone at home.

2. After the nurse talks with Virginia, Mrs. Miranda tells the nurse that this is not the first time that Virginia has been in the hospital. The nurse tells Mrs. Miranda:

   A. I am glad that you told me. This means that Virginia is just being difficult.
   B. Children like more attention when they are in the hospital.
   C. Children's fears may not subside with repeated hospitalizations.
   D. She will feel better when she realizes that we like her very much.

3. Mrs. Miranda asks the nurse who is the best person to help Virginia with her fears. The nurse answers:

   A. Nurses are trained to take care of children's fears.
   B. Since the nurses are in charge of the floor, they are the best.
   C. The doctors will talk to Virginia before surgery; they are the best.
   D. A collaborative effort by the health care team is the best.

4. Mrs. Miranda tells the nurse that her oldest son had an appendectomy and that the preparation was different from the preparation for Virginia. What is the best answer that the nurse can give?

   A. Children are prepared based on their age and how much they understand.
   B. This is the policy of the hospital and we have to obey the rules.
   C. Girls are prepared differently than boys.
   D. Preparation depends on the education that the nurse has.

5. Mrs. Miranda asks the nurse not to tell Virginia that she is going to have a shot. She is concerned that Virginia may get upset. The nurse tells Mrs. Miranda:

   A. All right, but I have to give her the shot later on.
   B. If we want Virginia to trust us we must tell her the truth.
   C. Why don't we tell her father to tell her about the shot?
   D. Do you want the doctor to tell Virginia about the shot?

Diagnosis: Pain

History: Charlie Thomas is a 1-year-old boy who is brought to the hospital for a hernia repair. Mrs. Thomas is very upset because her son is going to have surgery and she is terrified that little Charlie is going to be put to sleep. While talking to the nurse she tells the nurse that her main concern is that Charlie will wake up soon after the surgery is finished. At the same time, she tells the nurse that she has heard that children at that age never feel pain and that she does not want anyone to give Charlie anything for pain. Mrs. Thomas also tells the nurse that she knows how annoying it is for the nurses when children cry, and that she will stay with Charlie after his surgery so that he will not cry a lot.

Plan: Charlie will go home with his parents when he has recuperated from surgery. His mother will understand the fallacies and the facts about pain and pain management.

Nursing problems: Risk for infant—mismanagement of pain. Knowledge deficit of parents about pain management and about pain in children.

Chief concerns of the nurse: For the baby, the chief concern is to make sure that Charlie is going to be comfortable and that he is going to recuperate well. For the parents, to teach them about the facts and fallacies about pain in children and also to relieve their anxiety as it relates to the use of opiates and analgesics.

1. Mrs. Thomas tells the nurse all her friends and her mother-in-law have told her that children do not feel pain until they are 4 years old. The nurse responds:

   A. That is not true.
   B. That is true.
   C. Can you tell me all that you know about pain in children?
   D. Let me call Dr. Sanches. He will explain this to you much better.

2. After assessing how much the mother knows about pain in children, the nurse explains to the mother that infants demonstrate feeling pain by:

   A. Sleeping a lot
   B. Disengaging from the parents
   C. Screaming a lot
   D. Having an elevation in temperature

3. Mrs. Thomas asks the nurse if children can tolerate pain better than adults. The nurse responds:

   A. Since infants do not talk, we do not know much about that.
   B. No; because of the immaturity of their central nervous system infants do not tolerate pain better than adults.
   C. Children's tolerance of pain actually increases with age.
   D. That depends on how well behaved the child is.

4. The nurse knows that the major concern among nurses on the floor is the lack of knowledge about the management of opiates to relieve pain in children. The major concern of the nurses is fear that the child will develop:

   A. Addiction
   B. Behavioral problems
   C. Drug tolerance
   D. Respiratory depression

5. In evaluating pain in children the nurse knows that he/she needs to evaluate both behavioral and physiologic changes. In using pain scales the nurse needs to be aware that if there is a discrepancy between the child's behavior and the rating, he/she needs to give credence to:

A. The pain rating on the scale
B. The mother's report
C. The child's behavior
D. The child's vital signs

$\mathcal{A}$NSWERS

Fever

1. *C.* Fever is simply an elevation of temperature above normal; however, a more exact explanation is that an elevation of body temperature is part of a specific biological response mediated and controlled by the central nervous system.

2. *A.* Biologically, fever has some role in defending the host against the infection and possibly against other diseases as well.

3. *B.* Fever in children at risk for febrile convulsions and with underlying neurologic and cardiopulmonary disease needs to be treated with great care.

4. *D.* Although acetaminophen is often prescribed on the basis of age, 60 mg/day/year of age, a weight-based dosage is more accurate. In general, the dose of acetaminophen is 10–15 mg/kg every 4 hours.

5. *D.* A well child with non-life-threatening febrile illness may benefit from sponging with tepid water plus acetaminophen, because this may make him or her feel better; research shows that the temperature only goes down 0.2°F of a degree with tepid sponging.

Fear

1. *A.* Before the nurse starts to tell the child about surgery or any other procedure it is very important to find out how much the child knows, and what his or her understanding of what is going to happen is. This process facilitates the use of the right interventions and helps to dissipate unrealistic fears.

2. *C.* Fears and fantasies about hospitalization are not dissipated with previous hospitalizations. It is always necessary to assess the fear that children have.

3. *D.* A collaborative health team is ideal in treating fears in children.

4. *A.* The age and stage of development of the child are the most important piece of information before starting any intervention in order to dissipate fears.

5. *B.* Parents should be told that it is very important not to lie to a child; children will lose trust if they find out that you have lied to them. The trust that the child develops for medical personnel is pivotal in the management of the childhood illness.

Pain

1. *C.* The knowledge of pain in children is not only misunderstood by laypeople, but also by professionals; therefore, in order to answer the question it is very important that the nurse must find out how much the parents know and what fallacies about pain need to be clarified for the parents.

2. *C.* Infants demonstrate behavioral, especially facial and physiological, indicators of pain. Facial changes are common indicators of pain and are especially valuable in assessing pain in nonverbal children.

3. *C.* Children's tolerance for pain increases with age.

4. *A.* A major concern that prevents nurses from giving pain medication to children is the fear of addiction. The Acute Pain Management Guideline Panel (1992) states that there is no known aspect of childhood development or physiology that indicates any increase of physiologic or psychological dependence from the brief use of opiates for acute management.

5. *A.* The difference in culture and in psychological development among children influences their responses and the exhibiting behaviors of pain. Therefore, if children's behavior appears to differ from their rating of the scales, the nurse should give more validity to the scale than to the child.

$\mathcal{G}$LOSSARY

anxiety disorders   ongoing exaggerated worry and tension, even when there is no reason for it.

arthralgia   pain in a joint, usually due to arthritis or arthropathy.

boundaries   limits set in accordance with development.

chronological   occurring in a natural sequence according to time.

disabling   an action that restricts the ability to perform an activity in the manner that is considered normal.

distorted   the process of modifying unconscious mental elements so that they can enter consciousness without being censored.

fluid   a continuous process.

mild transient   temporary interference, usually with abrupt onset. Specific symptoms depend on the cause.

nociceptor   a receptor preferentially sensitive to a noxious stimulus or to a stimulus that would become noxious if prolonged. Avoid use of terms like *pain receptor, pain pathway,* etc., because they reflect anachronistic concepts and can mislead. Pain is a complex perception that takes place only at higher levels of the central nervous system.

noxious stimulus   stimulus that is potentially or actually damaging to body tissue. In some instances there is no lasting tissue damage (e.g., muscle pain due to excessive exercise).

obsessions   irrational thoughts that frequently recur and cause great anxiety.

obsessive   a neurotic mental state of having an uncontrollable desire to dwell on an idea or an emotion.

pain threshold   the least experience of pain that a subject can recognize.

panic   acute anxiety, terror, or fright that is usually of sudden onset.

phobia   uncontrollable, irrational, and persistent fear of a specific object.

psychodynamics   the scientific study of mental action forces.

ritual   a routine that the individual feels is essential and should not fail to be carried out.

startle response   the uncontrollable startle reaction that follows any stimulus for which there is usually no adaptation, such as a sudden noise.

stimuli   any factor that increases functional activity.

stranger anxiety   an anxiety or fear caused by the presence of a strange person. Children develop this at about age 6–8 months.

suffering   a state of emotional distress associated with events that threaten the biological and/or psychosocial integrity of the individual. Suffering often accompanies severe pain, but can occur in its absence; hence pain and suffering are phenomenologically distinct.

survey   a comprehensive appraisal of an area of study.

$\mathcal{B}$IBLIOGRAPHY

AGBOLOSU, N. B., CUEVAS, L. E., MILLIGAN, P., BROADHEAD, R. L., BREWSTER, D., AND GRAHAM, S. M. Efficacy of tepid sponging versus paracetachol in reducing temperature in febrile children. *Annals of Tropical Pediatrics* 17:283–288, 1997.

AKSOYLAR, S., AKSIT, S., CAGLAYAN, S., YAPRAK, I., BAIKILER, R., AND CETIN, F. Evaluation of sponging and antipyretics medication to reduce body temperature in febrile children. *Acta Pediatrics* 39:215–217, 1997.

BAKER KLEIMAN, M. Feverish children, frightened parents. *Contemp Pediatr* 6(3):161, 1989.

BARLOW, D. H. *Anxiety and Its Disorders.* New York: Guilford, 1988.

BECK, A. T. *Cognitive Therapy and Emotional Disorders.* New York: New American Library, 1976.

BURGS, R. *Art of Fear Management.* Singapore: WPC, 1994.

CLUM, G. A., CLUM, G. A., AND SURLS, R. A meta-analysis of treatments for panic disorder. *Journal of Consulting and Clinical Psychology* 61: 317–326, 1993.

FRIEDMAN, A. D., AND BARTON, L. L. Efficacy of sponging versus acetaminophen for reduction of fever. *Pediatric Emergency Care* 6(1):6–7,
1990.

GARBER, S. H., GARBER, M. D., AND SPIZMAN, R. F. *Monsters under the
Bed and Other Childhood Fears: Helping Your Child Overcome
Anxieties, Fears, and Phobias.* New York: Villard Books, 1993.

GITTELMAN, R. Anxiety disorders in children. In Lester Grinspoon (ed.),
*Psychiatry Update. The American Psychiatric Association Annual
Review, Vol. III.* Washington, D.C.: American Psychiatric Press, 1984.

GRAZIANO, A. M., AND MOONEY, K. E. Night fears in children: Maintenance of improvement at two-and-a-half to three-year follow-up.
Journal of Counseling and Clinical Psychology 50:598–599, 1982.

HALL, J. *Confident Kids: Helping Your Child Cope with Fear.* Port
Melbourne: Lothain, 1993.

HANSEN, B. D., AND EVANS, M. L. Preparing a child for procedures.
Maternal Child Nursing 6(6):392–397, 1981.

HYSON, M. Lobster on the sidewalk: Understanding and helping with
fears. *Young Children* 34:54–60, 1979.

JERSILD, A. T., MARKEY, P. V., AND JERSILD, C. L. Children's fears, dreams,
wishes, daydreams, likes, dislikes, pleasant and unpleasant memories.
Child Development Monographs 12:1–172, 1991.

KING, N. J., OLLIER, K., LACUONE, R., SCHUSTER, S., BAYS, K., GULLONE, E.,
AND OLLENDICK, T. H. The fears of children and adolescents in
Australia: A cross-sectional study using the Revised-Fear Survey
Schedule for Children. *Journal of Child Psychology and Psychiatry* 30:
775–784, 1989.

LOPEZ, J., MCMILLIN, K., TOBIAS-MERRILL, E., AND CHOP, W. Managing
fever in infants and toddlers. *Post Med* 101(2):241, 1997.

LORIN, M. *The Febrile Child.* New York: John Wiley and Sons, 1982.

LORIN, M. When fever has no localizing signs. *Contemp Pediatr* 6(2):14,
1989.

MAURER, A. What children fear. *Journal of Genetic Psychology* 106:
265–277, 1971.

MCCARTHY, P. *The Evaluation and Treatment of Febrile Children.* Vol. 1.
Norwalk, CT: Appleton-Century-Crofts, 1985.

MCNALLY, R. J. *Panic Disorder: A Critical Analysis.* New York: Guilford,
1994.

MEAHTENIA, P. S. An experience with fear in the lives of children.
Childhood Education 48:75–79, 1971.

MIDDLETON, D. B. An approach to pediatric upper respiratory infections.
Am Fam Phys 44(5 suppl):33s, 1991.

MORRIS, R. J., AND KRATCHOWILL, T. R. *Treating Children's Fears and
Phobias: A Behavioral Approach.* New York: Pergamon Press, 1983.

NEINSTEIN, L. S. *Adolescent Health Care: A Practical Guide.* 3rd ed.
Baltimore: Williams and Wilkins, 1996.

NEWTON, D. A. Sinusitis in children and adolescents. *Primary Care* 23(4):
535, 1996.

NIZET, V., VINCI, R., AND LOVEJOY, F. Fever in children. *Pediatr Rev* 15(4):
127, 1994.

NORDON, C., GILLESPIE, W. J., AND NADE, S. *Infections in Bones and Joints.* Cambridge, MA: Blackwell Scientific, 1994.

OSKI, F., DE ANGELIS, C., FEIGN, R., AND WARSHAW, J. *Principles and Practice of Pediatrics.* 2nd ed. Philadelphia: Lippincott, 1990.

OTTO, M. W., AND POLLACK, M. H. Treatment strategies for panic disorder: A debate. *Harvard Review of Psychiatry* 2:166–170, 1994.

PARROTT, T. Cystitis and urethritis. *Pediatr Rev* 10(7):217, 1989.

POLLACK, M. W., AND SMALLER, J. W. The longitudinal course and outcome of panic disorder. *Psychiatric Clinics of North America* 18: 785–801, 1995.

POZNAMSKI, E. O. Children with excessive fears. *American Journal of Orthopsychiatry* 43(3):428–438, 1973.

ROBINSON, E. H., ROBINSON, S. L., AND WHETSELL-VELASCO, M. The study of children's fears. *Journal of Humanistic Education and Development* 27:84–95, 1988.

ROBINSON, E. H., ROTTER, J., VOGEL, K., AND FEY, M. S. *Helping Children Cope with Fear and Stress: An Activity Guide.* Nairobi: Association of International Schools in Africa, 1988.

SCHLECUPNER, C. J. Urinary tract infections: Separating the genders and the ages. *Post Med* 101(6):231, 1997.

SCHWARTZ, R. A practical approach to chronic otitis. *Patient Care* 21(12):91, 1987.

SMART, M. S., AND SMART, R. C. *Preschool Children—Development and Relationships.* New York: Macmillan Co., 1973.

STEELE, R., TANAKA, P., LARA, R., AND BASS, J. Evaluation of sponging and of oral antipyretic therapy to reduce fever. *Journal of Pediatrics* 2: 824–828, 1990.

STERN, R. Pathophysiologic basis for symptomatic treatment of fever. *Pediatrics* 59(1):92, 1977.

SURVEY SCHEDULE FOR CHILDREN. *Journal of Child Psychology and Psychiatry* 30:775–784, 1970.

THEODORSON, G. A., AND THEODORSON, A. G. (1970). *A Modern Dictionary of Sociology.* New York: Thomas Y. Crowell, 1970.

TRESELER, K. M. *Clinical Laboratory and Diagnostic Tests: Significance and Nursing Implications.* 3rd ed. Norwalk, CT: Appleton and Lange, 1995.

WALLACH, J. *Interpretation of Diagnostic Tests.* 6th ed. Boston: Little, Brown, 1996.

WILSON, D. Assessing and managing the febrile child. *Nurs Pract* 20(11):59, 1995.

WOLMAN, B. B. *Children's Fears.* New York: Grosset and Dunlap, 1979.

WOODS, E. R., et al. Bacteremia in an ambulatory setting. *Am J Dis Child* 144(5):1195, 1990.

ZASTOWNY, T., KIRSCHENBAUM, D., AND MENG, A. Coping skills training for children: Effects on distress before, during, and after hospitalization. *Health Psychology* 5:231–247, 1986.

*H*ELPFUL INTERNET SITES

PEDINFO: An Index of the Pediatric Internet at http://www.pedinfo. org   An excellent site that covers nearly all topics within this review. It has a wealth of information and is worth a visit. It is written for health care professionals but others could also use the information.

The Virtual Hospital at http//www.vh.org   A good place to start looking for information concerning pain and fever, as well as many other issues about caring for the pediatric patient. A good site for lay persons and health care professionals. The Virtual Hospital site is a product of the University of Iowa.

Virtual Naval Hospital Information for Providers at http://www.vnh. org/Providers.html   This site is part of the University of Iowa's health care site and is linked to a large set of databases that can be used by health care providers. The site covers a larger number of links to other sources on health care issues and problems. This is an excellent starting place to discover information on various common diseases and their treatments.

University of Iowa Family Practice Handbook at http://www.vh.org/ Providers/Providers.html   This is an excellent resource for the health care professional. This Family Practice Handbook is an on-line 20-chapter resource that would be used by a physician in family practice.

166

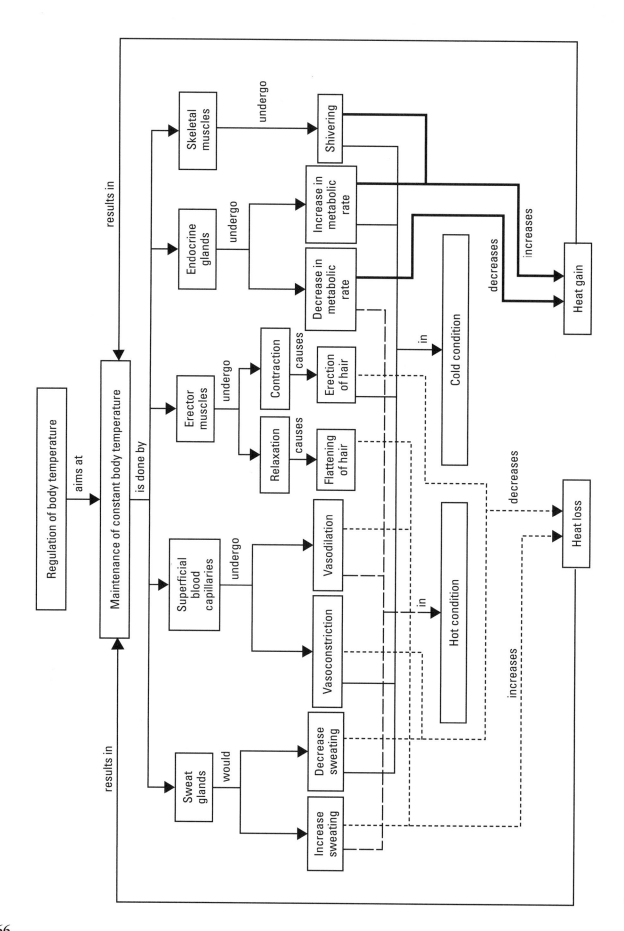

Concept Map 5-1

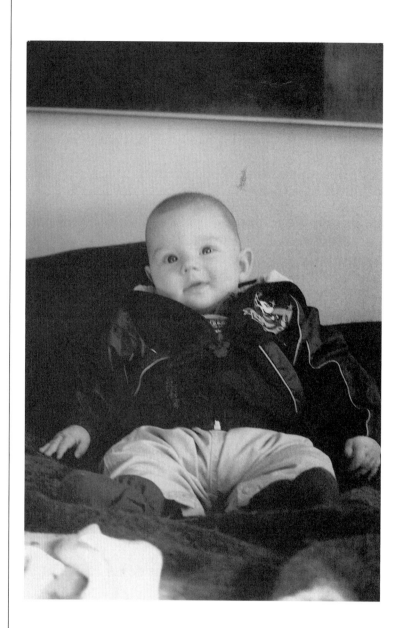

ℰYES, EARS, NOSE, THROAT, AND MOUTH

ℰYES

Human beings rely heavily on their sense of sight, but they don't see with their eyes. It is the brain that does the "seeing." The **eye** is just the sight information-gathering organ in the body; until it transmits the information to the brain via the optic nerve, one doesn't see anything. Light passes through the cornea, the pupil, and the lens, and falls on the light-sensitive surface of the retina. The images created by the light are reflected upside down on the retina. Several layers of cells make up the retina, and those closest to the back of the eye, called rods and cones, are the receptor cells that actually detect light. The other layers of the retina make sense out of what the rods and cones reflect, interpreting the information into a format that the brain can use. All the retina's cells feed into many optic nerves, which converge at the back of the eye to the point known as the optic disk, and then go on to the brain.

The eye is an outpocket of the brain, which has a rich supply of blood during fetal **development**. By the fourth week of fetal development, the optic vessel can be noted, and by the fifth week, the lens vesicle is formed.

The eyeball itself rests in an enclosed area in the skull, the eye socket, and is surrounded and protected by fat and bone. The accessory structures of the eye include the eyebrows, eyelids, conjunctiva, lacrimal apparatus, and intrinsic eye muscles.

The eyeball is a hollow sphere composed of three coats or tunics and an interior filled with fluids called humors. The lens is the focusing apparatus of the eye and is supported vertically. Lenses are biconvex, transparent,

Eye. The organ of sight. Parts of the eye include: eyeball or ball, conjunctiva, pupil, retina, iris, cornea, ciliary body, eye muscles, optic nerve, aqueous humor, fovea, sclera, vitreous body, choroid, white, lens, optic nerve.

Development. An increase in capability or function.

flexible vascular structures that can change shape to allow precise focusing of light onto the retina. With age the lens enlarges and becomes denser, more convex, and less elastic, which interferes with the ability to focus light properly.

The sclera forms the posterior portion and the bulk of the fibrous tunic (the white of the eye). Posteriorly, the sclera is secured by the optic nerve and is continuous with the dura matter of the brain. The anterior portion of the eye is modified to form the transparent cornea. The cornea should have perfect clarity, which is maintained by the excretion of sodium ions. The cornea has the ability to regenerate and repair itself. It may be transplanted from one person to another without fear of rejection, because it has no blood vessels and is beyond the reach of the immune system.

The vascular tunic or the middle coat of the eye is called the uvea. It is divided into the choroid, the ciliary, and the iris. The choroid is a vascular, deeply pigmented membrane that occupies the posterior part of the eyeball. The ciliary is a thickened ring of tissue that encircles the lens, which controls shaping. The iris is made up of circular and radial smooth muscle fibers, both sympathetic and parasympathetic, and acts as a reflectively activated diaphragm to vary pupil size. Pupil size is controlled by the sympathetic and parasympathetic fibers.

The internal chambers of the eyeball are called the anterior and posterior chambers. The posterior chamber is filled with vitreous humor, and the anterior chamber is filled with aqueous humor or clear fluid. Fluid balance inside the eyeball is maintained by constant production and drainage, through Schlemm's canal, of an aqueous solution supplying nutrients and oxygen to the lens and cornea and carrying away the metabolic wastes.

Visual Disturbances in Children

The etiology of impaired vision can be divided into two general categories: refractive or nonrefractive errors. Refractive errors in vision are those that can be alleviated with corrective lenses. Examples are myopia, hyperopia, anisometropia, and astigmatism. Nonrefractive errors in vision, on the other hand, are retinal abormalities, including glaucoma, cataracts, retinoblastoma, eye muscle imbalance, and systemic disease with ocular manifestations, which cannot be fixed with corrective lenses alone.

Refractive Errors in Children

In order to have clear vision, light must focus precisely on the retina. In *myopia,* or nearsightedness, light is focused in front of the retina. A child with myopia can see objects held close, usually has no problems with reading, but would have difficulty reading the chalkboard in a classroom. Myopia is the most common clinically significant refractive error seen in childhood.

In *hyperopia,* or farsightedness, light is focused behind the retina. The child's distance vision is very good, but he/she has difficulty seeing objects that are close. This condition is relatively rare in children and usually does not require corrective lenses unless it causes the child's eyes to cross, or results in reduced vision.

Astigmatism is a condition in which the curvature variations of the optical system result in unequal light refraction. It can begin in either childhood or adulthood, and can easily be corrected if it causes blurred vision or eye discomfort.

Anisometropia is a condition in which there is a difference in the refractive error of both eyes. Corrective lenses are indicated.

Refractive errors remain the most common cause of decreased visual acuity. Refractive errors requiring the use of corrective lenses exist in almost 20% of the pediatric population.

Nonrefractive Errors in Children

Children and adults with nonrefractive errors in vision have impaired acuity at both near and far distances.

Legal blindness, in the United States, is defined as requiring corrective lenses to 20/200 or less in both eyes, or visual fields less than 10 degrees centrally. The history you take from the child's caregiver should determine:

1. If vision is affected in one or both eyes, and if near and/or far vision is affected.
2. If associated symptoms have been noted, such as eye discomfort, increased tearing, cloudy vision, or flashing lights.
3. If the caregiver thinks the child's vision appears normal. The nurse should note the level of development of eye-hand coordination.
4. In school-age children, if the caregiver thinks school performance and reading ability are equal to others in the child's class.
5. If there are any past eye problems or treatments, and how the child reacted to them.
6. What, if any, family eye disease history exists.

The physical examination by the nurse should reveal any external swelling, ptosis, or discharge. Note the clarity of the cornea. Determine extraocular movement. Measure peripheral vision and perform a cover test along with a corneal light reflex test. The nurse should elicit a red reflex and perform a fundoscopic exam. Visual acuity should be determined.

If the history and the eye exam indicate a refractive error in the child's vision, the child should be referred to an optometrist or an ophthalmologist. If, however, nonrefractive error is diagnosed, the chance of the acute onset of visual impairment requires emergency care.

Blepharitis is a common inflammation that produces a red-rimmed appearance on the margin of the eyelids. It is frequently chronic and may affect both upper and lower eyelids. Clinical presentation includes itching and burning of the eyelids, or the sensation of a foreign body in the eye. The eyelids are sticky and encrusted upon waking. Blepharitis begins in childhood and continues throughout adulthood. Both types of blepharitis, seborrheic and ulcerative, can be caused by lice infestation.

Seborrheic blepharitis results from seborrhea of the scalp, eyebrows, and ears. Seborrheic blepharitis is often caused by an infection, most often *Staphylococcus aureus*. Cosmetics, smoke, and smog may aggravate the problem. Hypertrophy and desquamation of the epidermis near the margin of the eyelid result in scaling and erythema. The main complaint from the child or his/her caregiver will be redness of the eyelid margin and its accompanying burning and discomfort. There may also be flaky scales on the eyelashes or even loss of lashes.

In *ulcerative blepharitis*, there is a chronic inflammation of the follicles of the lashes and the associated glands of the eyes. The most likely causative pathogen is *S. aureus* or *S. epidermidis*. Ulcerative blepharitis begins with a purulent inflammation of the glands of the eyelid margin, resulting in the formation of small ulcers. As the condition progresses, lashes are lost and a distortion of the eyelid margin may develop (*ectropion*). Presentation may be with dilated blood vessels in the eyelid margin, loss of lashes, recurrent *chalazia*, and *hordeolums*, and may result in secondary *conjunctivitis* and *keratitis*.

The nurse's diagnosis will depend on the child's history and characteristic symptoms. The nurse should inquire about the child's chronic exposure to irritants such as smoke, cosmetics, and/or chemicals, and should take a culture of the eyelid to determine the presence of *S. aureus*. The physical examination should determine the child's visual acuity. The nurse should perform a complete eye examination, especially of the eyelid, **palpating** the eyelid margin for masses. The differential diagnosis could include chalazion, sty, conjunctivitis and keratitis, or sebaceous cell carcinoma.

The care plan should include early treatment, which is essential to prevent recurrence and complications. The treatment depends on the type of blepharitis, either seborrheic or ulcerative. Treatment for seborrheic blepharitis would be daily shampooing of the eyelashes and frequent shampooing of the scalp and eyebrows. Apply warm moist compresses 3 to 4 times a day and apply antibiotic ointment 3 to 4 times a day as follows: (1) sulfacetamide sodium ophthalmic ointment 10%, rubbed into the lid margin for 7 days; (2) Polymyxin B-Bacitracin ophthalmic ointment to the lid margin qid (4 times a day) for 7 days. Vibramycin 100 mg bid (2 times a day) for 6 weeks may be needed for deep-seated infections, tapering off according to the severity of the child's symptoms. Treatment of eyelashes infested with lice would include: (1) shampooing the scalp with Dwell, Nix, or Rid shampoo; (2) applying a thick layer of petrolatum to the eyelashes; (3) after 5 to 8 days, mechanically removing the nits and lice. Treatment must continue for several weeks until the child is completely free of the infection, to prevent recurrences. For mild cases no follow-up is needed; however, for severe cases, follow-up in 10 to 14 days is indicated.

A *cataract* is a decrease in the transparency of the crystalline lens to the point of disturbed vision. Cataracts commonly occur bilaterally with each eye progressing independently. Exceptions are traumatic cataracts, which

Palpation. The technique of touch to identify characteristics of the skin, internal organs, and masses. Characteristics include texture, moistness, tenderness, temperature, position, shape, consistency, and mobility of masses and organs.

are usually unilateral and congenital, and may remain stationary. Most cataracts occur as a natural part of the aging process; however, children are also affected. Causes of cataracts, other than the aging process, include metabolic, congenital, or drug-induced problems; ocular trauma; or ocular conditions such as chronic anterior *uveitis*. Risk factors for the development of cataracts include ultraviolet B radiation exposure, diabetes mellitus, drugs (certain major tranquilizers and diuretics), alcohol use, and low antioxidant vitamin intake.

The clinical presentation of cataracts includes:

1. Painless, gradual loss of vision.
2. Pupil becomes milky.
3. Complaints of blinding glare from headlights and poor reading vision.
4. Poor vision in bright sunlight.
5. Children may not verbalize their vision deficiency. Behavioral changes must be observed, such as not catching a ball, decreased ability to see the chalkboard in class, etc.

The medical history should include information regarding the onset of the decrease in vision and if it has occurred in one or both eyes. An ophthalmoscopy or slit lamp examination will confirm the diagnosis if it reveals a dark area in the normal homogeneous red reflex. It is important to include a list of medications being taken and report of any recent eye injury. The differential diagnosis could be macular degeneration or diabetic retinopathy.

The nurse's care plan should include referral to an ophthalmologist. Surgery would be indicated based on the severity of the child's functional impairment. Corrective lenses may have to be adjusted. Progression may be decreased by reducing risk factors such as exposure to sunlight or smoke, and increasing antioxidant vitamin ingestion.

The nurse should give instruction on postoperation plans and activities if surgery is performed, and there should be a follow-up visit on the day following surgery.

Chalazion is a chronic inflammation lipogranuloma of a meibomian gland. This is a common eye disorder characterized by localized swelling, which usually develops slowly over several weeks. This disorder is the result of an obstruction to the meibomian gland duct. A secondary infection of the surrounding tissues may also develop.

Chalazion clinically presents as a hard, nontender nodule away from the eyelid border. If it becomes infected, a painful swelling of the entire lid may develop. Some may resolve without treatment; however, large chalazia may decrease vision and cause pressure on the eyeball.

The history should note the onset and duration of the symptoms. **Pain** or tenderness should be noted. A complete eye examination is needed, as is a vision test to determine visual acuity. Determine if there have been any other such episodes. The differential diagnosis could include sebaceous cell carcinoma, or the chalazion may be associated with a hordeolum and blepharitis.

Pain. An unpleasant sensory and emotional experience associated with actual or potential tissue damage. Pain exists when the patient says it does.

Treatment for small, asymptomatic chronic chalazia is not required because they usually disappear spontaneously within a few months. However, large chalazia or a secondary infection would require treatment, including application of warm, moist compresses for 15 minutes several times throughout the day, and a prescription for sulfacetamide sodium ophthalmic ointment 10%, qid for 7 days. If they do not respond to the preceding treatment, excision should be performed and antibiotic ointment continued for 1 week. Small chalazia require no follow-up; large ones should be reevaluated in 2 to 4 weeks.

Congenital nasolacrimal duct obstruction is a defect of the lacrimal drainage system in which a lack of patency affects drainage function. An imperforate membrane at the distal end of the nasolacrimal duct is the usual cause of the obstruction. It is the most common abnormality of the infant's lacrimal apparatus. It presents within the first few weeks of life with persistent tearing, crusting of the lashes, and mucopurulent discharge. Tears spill over the lower eyelid in the involved eye. Material may be elicited by pressing over the nasolacrimal sac of the involved eye. Most obstructions clear spontaneously within 1 year.

The history should include when the symptoms first started and if it occurs in one or both eyes. The caregiver should provide information about the color and consistency of any discharge and also any visual abnormalities that have been observed. It is important to assess visual acuity. Do a complete examination of the eye. Palpate the tissue around the eye and inspect and palpate the lacrimal apparatus. Also, gently press over the nasolacrimal sac on the affected side to elicit material. The differential diagnosis could include conjunctivitis, blepharitis, and dacryocystitis.

A conservative treatment is recommended. Instruct parents to massage the lacrimal sac several times a day in an effort to rupture the membrane at the lower end of the duct. If there is evidence of secondary infection, a topical antibiotic is indicated: (1) apply sodium sulfacetamide, 1 to 2 drops, qid for 7 days; (2) apply erythromycin ointment, 0.05-cm strip in lower lid, qid for 7 days; and (3) instruct the parents that the antibiotic will reduce the infectious component of the discharge, but not cure the blockage. Controversy exists about when to surgically treat the condition.

Amblyopia is a marked decrease in visual acuity in one eye due to an interruption of normal visual development during a critical period in the first few years of life, usually before the age of 7. The exact mechanism for the development of this condition is not known, but there appears to be a microscopic defect in the retina-to-brain connection that results in the disuse of one eye. Three main causes for this condition appear to be physical occlusion, refractive errors, and *strabismus*.

Amblyopia affects about 5% of the population. Children with this problem test better with single letters than with rows of letters. The condition is reversible when identified before visual development is complete.

Ask caregivers about the child's visual history. For infants, ask if the child can fixate on and follow objects. Determine if the fine motor development is at appropriate level for the child's age. Inquire if the child has any abnormal face or head positioning postures. For older children, ask if development was achieved at an appropriate age. Finally, inquire about any other eye problems the child may have had and the treatments used.

The physical examination requires a test for visual acuity. Inspect eyelids, conjunctiva, cornea, and height and equality of the level of upper eyelids. Assess the pupils for shape, size, equality, and reaction to light. Assess extraocular movements using an appealing object, such as a teddy bear, for the child to follow. Perform the cover test and corneal light reflex test and assess for the presence of red reflex. The differential diagnosis could be optic nerve hypoplasia, abnormalities of the retina, cortical blindness, cataract, anisometropia (unequal refractive error between the eyes), or strabismus.

Recognition and treatment of underlying causes is the first step in treatment. The care plan should include referral to an ophthalmologist and treatment with an occlusive therapy by a specialist. The nurse should be certain the caregivers realize the importance of a follow-up visit with the ophthalmologist.

Conjunctivitis is an inflammation of the conjunctiva. Noninfectious conjunctivitis is the result of hypersensitivity to allergens. Eight types of conjunctivitis will be described here.

Bacterial conjunctivitis (Figure 6-1; Color Insert 1) is characterized by acute onset of mucopurulent discharge and the sensation of a foreign body in the eye. Eyelids are often edematous with matting of the eyelashes upon awakening. Typically, the infection begins in one eye and then becomes bilateral in 2 to 5 days. Usually the condition is self-limiting but it may become chronic with associated blepharitis and/or hordeolum. Corneal infiltration and ulceration may occur, particularly if the pathogen is *Neisseria gonorrhoeae*.

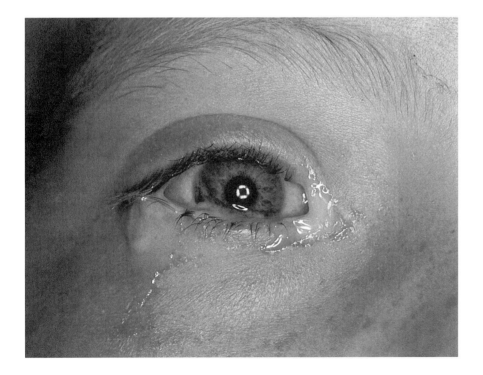

FIGURE 6-1

◈

Bacterial conjunctivitis. Mucopurulent discharge, conjunctival injection, and lid swelling, in a 10-year-old with *Haemophilus influenzae* conjunctivitis. (See also Color Insert 1.) (Courtesy of Frank Birinyi, MD.)

Chlamydial conjunctivitis is primarily transmitted through sexual contact with an infected person. It is typically an indolent infection that is characterized by a thin mucoid discharge. The child may have photophobia and enlarged, tender preauricular nodes. The infection may persist for 3 to 12 months.

Viral conjunctivitis is often accompanied by a systemic infection, characterized by marked conjunctival injection, large preauricular nodes, and a watery discharge. The course of the virus is self-limiting and usually resolves within 2 weeks after onset.

Viral conjunctivitis due to herpes simplex is often accompanied by a fever blister on the face or lips. Typically, it presents with vesicles on the skin of the eyelids and dendritic corneal herpes lesions. This condition may lead to permanent corneal ulceration, which can result in permanent visual loss from scarring.

Allergic conjunctivitis (Figure 6-2; Color Insert 2) is characterized by itchy, red eyes and rhinorrhea, which are often seasonal. Discharge is watery and bilateral, and eyelids may have a cobblestone appearance. Vernal catarrh is a serious form of allergic conjunctivitis, seen most often in children and adolescents. It could result in severe corneal ulceration and loss of vision.

Ophthalmia neonatorum from gonococcal infection (Figure 6-3, Color Insert 3) is the most dangerous and virulent cause of ophthalmia neonatorum. A decreased incidence of the condition has been seen since the instillation of nitrate into the eyes of the newborn has become a common procedure. Onset of a serosanguineous discharge is rapidly followed by a purulent exudate, which occurs 24 to 48 hours after birth. Corneal destruction and perforation are the major complications.

Ophthalmia neonatorum from chlamydial infection occurs 5 to 14 days after birth to infants born to mothers with chlamydial cervicitis. It begins

FIGURE 6-2 Allergic conjunctivitis. Conjunctival injection, chemosis, and a follicular response in the inferior palpebral conjunctiva in this patient with allergic conjunctivitis secondary to cat fur. (See also Color Insert 2.) (Courtesy of Timothy D. McGuirk, DO.)

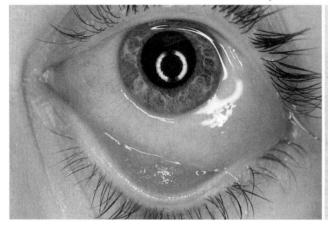 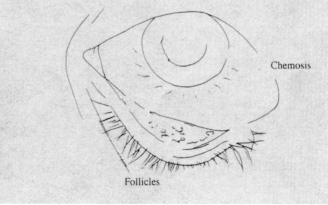

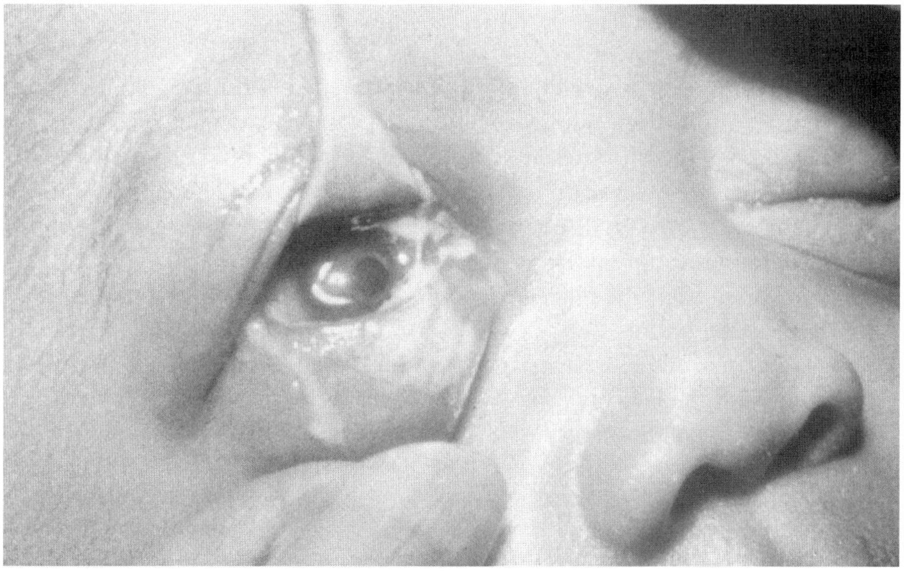

FIGURE 6-3

⌧

Ophthalmia neonatorum from gonococcal infection. Copious and purulent drainage in a newborn with neonatal gonococcal conjunctivitis. (See also Color Insert 3.) (Reprinted with permission of American Academy of Ophthalmology. *Eye Trauma and Emergencies: A Slide-Script Program.* San Francisco, 1985.)

with a watery discharge that later becomes purulent. The condition usually resolves spontaneously in 3 to 4 weeks without complications if left untreated. Complications include conjunctival scarring, formation of a pseudomembrane, and the development of amblyopia and strabismus from lid swelling and closure.

Ophthalmia neonatorum due to herpes simplex is seen more and more frequently because of the rising incidence of genital herpes infections. This condition can have local or disseminated infection. Complications include keratitis, cataracts, chorioretinitis, and optic neuritis.

Diagnosis Diagnosis requires a through history. Inquire regarding the onset and duration of the symptoms, whether there have been past episodes, and if so, what treatments were given, and if they were effective. Ask about the family history of allergies and eye infections. Determine if the child has been in contact with any person who had "pink eye." Ask the caregiver or the child to describe the discharge. Determine any changes in visual acuity, photophobia, and/or pain. With regard to pain, inquire about any associated pain, especially in the ear. Ask if there are any respiratory problems. Finally, if the client is an infant, ask the mother about any exposure to sexually transmitted disease during her pregnancy.

Physical Examination The physical examination should determine visual acuity, visual fields, pupillary function, and extraocular movement. Examine the eyelids for inflammation or tenderness. Evert the eyelid and examine it for foreign bodies. Examine sclera and conjunctiva for hyperemia and edema. Check the cornea for clarity. Determine the type of discharge present. In older children, instill topical anesthetic, stain the eye with fluorescent paper, and observe it under an ultraviolet lamp to rule out abrasion or herpes simplex. Palpate for preauricular adenopathy. Viral conjunctivitis often is accompanied by upper respiratory symptoms, so perform a complete examination of the ears, nose, throat, and lungs, too.

Differential Diagnoses

1. In conjunctivitis, redness of the conjunctiva is diffuse, pain is minimal, and vision, pupil size, and reactivity are normal.
2. Acute glaucoma presents with pain, considerably decreased vision, cloudy cornea, and sluggishly reacting pupils. There is moderate injection, usually bulbar, near the limbus.
3. Iritis presents with pain, moderate decreased vision, dull and swollen iris, and sluggish-reacting pupils. Injection is usually bulbar near the limbus.
4. Lacrimal duct obstruction produces pain, redness, and edema around the lacrimal sac. Pressure over the lacrimal duct will express purulent material from the upper and lower canaliculi.
5. Blepharitis may have a presentation similar to conjunctivitis with burning and itching of the conjunctiva, but with blepharitis there is inflammation of the lid margin.
6. Corneal abrasions often have a history of trauma with mild to moderate bulbar injection.

Diagnostic Testing Diagnostic testing could include a culture. The specimen should be collected prior to any instillation of medication. Most often, however, cultures and/or smears of the discharge are not recommended.

Management Management of the different types of conjunctivitis is as follows.

1. Bacterial conjunctivitis: Use warm compresses as well as a prescription for (1) sodium sulfacetamide ophthalmic ointment 10% 0.5 to 1.0 cm in the conjunctival sac bid for 7 to 14 days; (2) Bacitracin ointment 0.5 to 1.0 cm in the conjunctival sac bid for 7 to 14 days; (3) if accompanied by acute otitis media, treat with oral β-lactamase-resistant drugs Septra or amoxicillin. Topical antibiotics are not recommended. A poor clinical response after 48 to 72 hours indicates that the bacteria are resistant to the topical agent or that the conjunctivitis was not caused by a bacteria.
2. Chlamydial conjunctivitis: (1) Prescribe doxycycline 100 mg bid for 10 days; topical erythromycin ophthalmic ointment applied 1 or more times per day should be considered. (2) Any sexual partner should also be treated.
3. Viral infection, primarily due to adenovirus: This is usually self-limiting and may require only symptomatic treatment such as warm compresses. Typically, topical antibiotics are prescribed to prevent a secondary bacterial infection.
4. Viral infection due to herpes simplex: Refer the client to an ophthalmologist. Steroid medication should never be prescribed if there is a possibility of herpes simplex. Steroid preparations can enhance the proliferation of the virus and result in permanent eye damage.
5. Allergic conjunctivitis: Cool compresses may alleviate symptoms. Prescribe cromolyn ophthalmic solution 4% 1 to 2 drops 4 to 6 times a day for 4 days. Systemic antihistamines are also recommended.

6. Ophthalmia neonatorum: If caused by *N. gonorrhoeae*, treat with Rocephin 25 to 50 mg/kg intravenous or intramuscular in a single dose not to exceed 125 mg. For chlamydia infection, prescribe oral erythromycin 50 mg/kg day divided into 4 doses for 14 days. Treatment of the mother and her sexual partner is recommended: doxycycline 100 mg bid for 10 to 14 days. Consult the physician and usually refer the infant with herpes simplex infection to a pediatric ophthalmologist.

Follow-up The client should return to the clinic in 48 hours if no improvement is noted. No follow-up is necessary for mild cases. For severe cases, however, schedule a return visit in 10 to 14 days.

Other Eye Problems

Hordeolum is an acute inflammation of the follicle of an eyelash or the associated gland, a "sty." It is a localized purulent staphylococcal infection, which if left untreated can lead to cellulitis of the eyelid.

Age is not a factor, because a sty can occur in infants as well as adults, but it is more common in children and adolescents. Clients often present with a sudden onset of localized tenderness, redness, and swelling of the eyelid. The infection may occur in crops because the infecting pathogen may spread from one hair follicle to another.

The history should determine the onset and duration of the symptoms. Inquire about any pain or visual disturbances, and document any past episodes and previous treatments.

The physical examination should assess the client's visual acuity. Inspect the eyelids for inflammation, swelling, and drainage. Palpate the eyelids for induration and/or masses. Evert the eyelid and examine the inner surface for pointing. Examine sclera and conjunctiva for any abnormalities. Palpate for preauricular adenopathy.

No diagnostic tests are necessary. Treatment with warm moist compresses for 15 minutes throughout the day will make the client more comfortable. The eyelids should be cleansed daily with a neutral soap. Prescribe topical application of one of the following antibacterial ointments into the conjunctival sac:

1. Sulfacetamide sodium ophthalmic ointment, 10%, 0.5 to 1.0 cm qid for 7 days or 10% drops, 2 every 3 to 4 hours for 7 days.
2. Polymyxin B-Bacitracin ophthalmic ointment, 0.5 to 1.0 cm, qid for 7 days. If not responsive to therapy, consult an ophthalmologist for incision and drainage.
3. If crops of sties occur, diabetes mellitus must be ruled out. Advise the client to refrain from rubbing the eyes.

Teach the client and/or the caregiver that appropriate periorbital hygiene will prevent recurrence of sties. Advise clients to avoid using makeup and to discard any old cosmetics.

Usually, no follow-up visits are required.

Strabismus is defined as abnormal ocular alignment. Strabismus may be divided into two general types according to the underlying pathophysiology: nonparalytic strabismus, a condition caused by muscle weakness, focusing difficulties, unilateral refractive error, nonfusion, or anatomical differences in the eyes; and paralytic strabismus, a motor imbalance caused by paresis or paralysis of an extraocular muscle. Because visual axes are not parallel, the brain receives two images, thereby interfering with binocular vision. Familial tendencies toward strabismus have been well documented, but no clear-cut genetic mode of inheritance has been identified.

Whereas the eyes of the newborn infant are rarely aligned during the first few weeks of life, by the age of 3 months, normal oculomotor behavior is usually established, and an experienced examiner may be able to document the existence of abnormal alignment by that time. Strabismus involves a number of complex clinical entities and only the common patterns are listed here. This discussion is limited to nonparalytic strabismus. Convergent deviation is a crossing or turning in of the eyes and is designated by the prefix *eso-*. Divergent deviation is a turning outward of the eyes and is designated by the prefix *exo-*. Vertical deviations are designated by the prefixes *hyper-* (upward) and *hypo-* (downward).

Pseudostrabismus is one of the most common reasons for asking a pediatric ophthalmologist to evaluate the infant. A false appearance of strabismus when visual axes are in reality aligned accurately may occur because of the flat, broad nasal bridge, prominent epicanthal folds, or narrow interpupillary distance, so the observer may see less white sclera nasally than expected.

Esotropia or nonparalytic strabismus is the condition of inward or convergent deviation of the eyes. It is the most common ocular misalignment, representing more than half of all ocular deviations in the pediatric population. Infantile esotropia occurs in infancy; whether it is congenital or has onset soon after birth is undetermined. Accommodative esotropia occurs between 6 months and 7 years, with an average age being 2.5 years, and may be intermittent or constant.

Exotropia or nonparalytic strabismus is characterized by divergent misalignment of the eyes that may be intermittent or constant. Intermittent exotropia, the most common type of exotropic strabismus, is characterized by an outward drift of one eye, most often occurring when the child is fixating on a distant object. Deviation is more frequent with fatigue or illness. Photophobia in the exotropic eye is common. Visual acuity tends to be good in both eyes with normal binocular vision. The age of onset is usually between infancy and age 4. Constant exotropia may be congenital, but most often results from deterioration of intermittent exotropia, significant loss of vision in one eye (usually after age 5), and overcorrection following surgery for esotropia.

When eliciting the history, ask when the symptoms were first noticed and what, in particular, was observed. For infants, ask if the child can fix his/her sight on an object and follow it when the object is moved, and ask if the fine motor coordination is at an appropriate level for the child's age. Inquire whether the child has abnormal face or head position. For older children, ask if developmental tasks have been achieved at an appropriate age. Also, document any other eye problems and their treatments.

Test for visual acuity, testing both eyes separately (use the illiterate E test or the Allen picture cards for preschoolers and school-age children; use fixation and following testing for infants). Inspect the eyelids, conjunctiva, cornea, and height and equality of the level of the upper eyelids. Assess pupils for shape, size, equality, and reaction to light. Perform a corneal light reflex test. Assess extraocular movement using an interesting target, assess for the presence of red reflex, and perform the cover test.

All children in whom strabismus is suspected must be evaluated by a pediatric ophthalmologist to rule out pseudostrabismus. When poor fixation is present, the preferred eye must be patched to allow vision to develop in the other eye. The decision to perform eye muscle surgery is based on the degree and frequency of deviation. Follow-up should be done by the ophthalmologist.

$\mathcal{E}$ARS

We hear with the brain. The ear is a sensory organ that interprets sound waves for the brain and also maintains the body's equilibrium. Sound travels along the auditory canal until it contacts the tympanic membrane, or ear drum, which begins vibrating. The incus and stapes, attached to the malleus on the other side of the ear drum, vibrate also. Once the vibrations pass through the oval window of the inner ear they travel by way of the fluid of the cochlea to the round window, where they dissipate. The delicate hair cells of the organ of Corti are set in motion by those same vibrations. The hairs contact the membrane of the organ of Corti, which in turn sends impulses to the sensory endings of the auditory cranial nerve. These impulses are sent to the temporal lobe of the brain for interpretation as sound.

Hearing Disorders

Hearing disorders are classified as conductive, sensorineural, or mixed. Conductive hearing disorders result from blockages of the transmission of sound waves from the external auditory canal to the inner ear. In children conductive losses are caused by middle ear effusion (filling with fluid). The major cause of **conductive hearing losses** is otitis media and its sequelae.

The American Academy of Pediatrics recommends that children who have had recurring otitis media, which persists for more than 3 months, be evaluated for hearing and language development deficits. The age at which to screen affected children is between 18 and 24 months, because most children begin the use of expressive language during that period of development. Helping parents to understand that early detection of hearing deficits will mitigate the likelihood of communication disorders is of vital importance. The screening tools used for hearing deficits vary according to

Conductive hearing loss. Hearing loss caused by inadequate conduction of sound from the outer to the middle ear.

age. Taking a thorough history of the child since birth is paramount, because a family history of hearing loss could place the child at risk for these problems. The nurse needs to include any evidence of perinatal infections such as rubella, herpes simplex, toxoplasmosis, syphilis, birth weight less than 1500 g, hyperbilirubinemia, bacterial meningitis, asphyxia at birth, and/or Apgar scores of 0 to 3.

Another important developmental milestone to consider is the infant's response to loud noises at 0 to 4 months. Normal responses at 4 months of age are widening of the eyes, slight turning of the head, and looking toward where the sound is coming from. A deaf child does not blink in response to loud noises. From 2 to 4 years of age, problems are evident if the child does not respond to his/her name or to a loud voice calling him/her.

At 3 years of age, a child's hearing can be tested with earphones. If the child does not respond to the test, it should be repeated within 1 week. After the second test, if the child still does not respond, he/she should be referred for audiologic evaluation, and to an otolaryngologist for evaluation and further treatment.

Otitis media (Figure 6-4; Color Insert 4) refers to a spectrum of diseases in which fluid is present in the middle ear space. In *acute otitis media,* signs and symptoms of acute inflammation accompany middle ear effusion. The most frequent symptom is otalgia (pain in the ear); fever, irritability, nausea, vomiting, or diarrhea may also be present. The tympanic membrane may be bulging and full, red or opaque. In otitis media with effusion, there are no signs or symptoms of acute inflammation. Otitis media with effusion is often noted at well-child checkups or at follow-up examinations after an episode of acute otitis media.

The diagnosis of otitis media is based on the history and physical examination findings. The preferred technique of examining the ear is pneumatic otoscopy, which allows evaluation of both the appearance and mobility of the tympanic membrane, thereby providing a more accurate assessment of middle ear status than with the otoscope alone. Tympanometry, which allows a quantitative assessment of tympanic membrane mobility, may have a role in confirming the diagnosis. Although the role of audiometry in the

FIGURE 6-4

⊠

Otitis media. The middle ear is filled with purulent material behind an erythematous, bulging tympanic membrane. (See also Color Insert 4.) (Courtesy of Richard A. Chole, MD, PhD.)

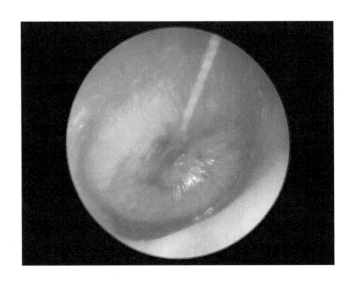

evaluation of otitis media in children should not be understated, it is useful mainly in determining the need for therapy rather than as a diagnostic tool.

Certain environmental and host factors predispose young children to acute otitis media. It is more common in male than in female children. Native American, Alaskan, and Canadian Eskimo children have a higher rate of acute otitis media than do Caucasian children. The age of the child at the first episode (before 4 months) is significantly and inversely associated with recurrent episodes. This relationship has been termed the "early and often" risk for otitis media. Children who have siblings and those in group day care with 7 or more children have a high incidence of otitis media, as do those who experience frequent upper respiratory infections. Infants and children who are exposed to tobacco smoke also have an increased risk of otitis media. Fall, winter, and spring are the peak seasons for acute otitis media. Breast-feeding offers a protective effect; studies indicate the incidence of otitis media in nursing infants is lower than in infants who are bottle-fed.

Infants Acute otitis media is common in children after the neonatal period, the first 28 days of life. Otitis media initially presents itself in a nonspecific manner in infants. The behaviors frequently noted are irritability, lethargy, decreased appetite or failure to thrive, mild respiratory symptoms, and a low-grade fever. Older infants may present with a history of tugging on one or both ears. Parents report crying increasing at night after the infant has been placed in the crib. This is due to the pain from increased pressure on the inner ear when the infant is placed in the supine position. Lack of sleep from the acute ear pain is a major problem for some infants and children with otitis media. These symptoms can be quite emotionally distressing to families and the afflicted infant.

Education is the foundation for adequate caretaking. Considering the large number of children affected by otitis media at some point in their life, it is important to educate all families during well-baby visits on risk factors and signs and symptoms of otitis media. The practitioner should encourage families to keep children in day care settings with a low turnover rate and which have fewer than 5 unrelated children. This precaution tends to decrease the organisms and infected children a child is exposed to, thus decreasing the risk of infection. The practitioner should also discourage smoking tobacco in the same household as the infant, which should decrease one of the risk factors for otitis media. There is some evidence that secondhand smoke not only increases the risk of otitis media, but increases the duration after onset of the condition. Mothers should be encouraged to breast-feed their infants during the first 6 months of life. If mothers choose to bottle-feed their infants, the parents should be taught to feed the baby in the upright position, and to keep the baby upright for 30 minutes after each feeding to prevent injection of milk and possible pathogens through an incompetent eustachian tube into the middle ear. During acute episodes of pain, parents can hold the infant upright to relieve some of the pressure on the middle ear. These techniques will help decrease the incidence of otitis media in infants and increase a parent's ability to meet the immediate needs of the infant.

Toddlers Children at this age with otitis media may verbalize ear pain, pull on the affected ear, or stick objects in the ear. The earache, which may be preceded by an upper respiratory infection at all ages, may present with a sudden onset of otalgia, fever, and hearing loss. The toddler may also present with disequilibrium manifested by falling, stumbling, or clumsiness. The major issue at this age is decreased hearing acuity from chronic otitis media, during the important developmental stage when language skills are being acquired. Developmental delays in receptive and expressive language are a complication of prolonged hearing loss resulting from otitis media with effusion. In reality, the child with otitis media with effusion is hearing through water, thus distorting and decreasing the sounds heard. This is a serious complication for the toddler who is just acquiring the skills to explore the environment both physically and verbally.

The toddler falls into the age category frequently affected by recurrent otitis media; thus it is important to educate family members on preventive techniques and presenting symptoms of otitis media. Family members should receive information on day care centers and smoking. Parents should be taught to wean the child from the pacifier by 10 months of age and wean the child from bottle-feeding as soon as possible. While still bottle-feeding, the child should be held in an upright position and should never be given a bottle while lying in bed. Eliminating bottle-feeding decreases the child's incidence of otitis media, and it also promotes independence with the new skills obtained drinking from a cup.

In order to prevent or decrease the problems of otitis media, it is important for the parent to be knowledgeable not only of the symptoms of otitis media, but of the importance of treatment and follow-up care to confirm resolution of the infection and effusion. Once an effusion has been identified, the practitioner is obligated to educate the family on the possible increase of conductive hearing loss because of otitis media. Material should be made available for the family to learn normal speech development stages for a toddler and clues for identifying any hearing deficits.

School-Age Children The school-age child will present with symptoms similar to those of infants and toddlers, but more specific. There is usually a history of upper respiratory infection for several days, sudden otalgia, fever, and hearing loss. The school-age child is usually able to localize the pain and verbalize which ear is involved.

Early hearing loss associated with otitis media is of great concern at this age because of language development. The parents should be aware of behaviors sometimes present with hearing loss, so that early intervention can be sought. Some of the behaviors that a parent may be taught to watch for are: the child responding only to people in his/her visual range; long delays in responding to verbal information; not responding to or localizing sounds; and social withdrawal. Parents should be made aware of potential complications of otitis media in order to improve compliance with follow-up. With early intervention during otitis media and consistent follow-up, the potential complications of otitis media can be prevented.

Foreign Body in the Ear Canal

Children tend to insert objects into their ear canals. A first attempt at removing the object from the ear canal should always be to straighten the ear canal by pulling on the pinna and gently shaking the child's head. If the object is a smooth bead, the removal could be done by using a cotton-tipped applicator with warm collodion. Coat the applicator with warm sticky solution and let it set. After a couple of minutes, when you touch the smooth surface of the bead with the treated applicator, the bead will stick to the applicator and can easily be pulled out of the ear canal. If, however, the object has an irregular surface, it should be removed at the doctor's office, where the nurses usually use irrigation or a suction machine. Caution is always important when removing foreign objects from the ear canal to prevent any risk of traumatizing the ear canal and causing edema. Edema would further embed the object into the ear canal, and it would then have to be removed surgically under anesthesia.

Impacted Cerumen

Impacted cerumen (ear wax) prevents visual access to the tympanic membrane. It can also cause itching, pain, and sometimes hearing loss. The most common cause of impacted cerumen is the use of cotton-tipped swabs by parents, who, in an effort to clean the ear canal, actually push the wax farther into the ear canal, eventually impacting it against the tympanic membrane. Parents should be instructed that wax in the ear protects the ear and any excess will come out by itself. The technique for removing impacted cerumen depends on the consistency of the ear wax and should be done by a nurse with the aid of an otoscope.

$\mathcal{N}$OSE

Rhinitis

The common cold is the most frequent infection in children and adults. The incidence of colds in early childhood is high, with an estimated 12 colds per year for children less than 5 years of age. Upper respiratory infections are caused by a variety of viruses and are more prevalent during the winter months.

Nose. The organ of smell. Syn.: nasal organ, nasal cavity, nares passages, nostrils, olfactory nerves.

The child with a cold usually has an onset of mucoid rhinorrhea and low-grade fever. The worst symptom is congestion in the **nose** and sinuses, which is sometimes accompanied by sore throat and cough. The major complication of rhinitis after 5 to 7 days is acute otitis media, which is always accompanied by fever. Other major complications can be sinusitis, conjunctivitis, or even pneumonia.

There is no cure for a cold, so the symptoms should be treated. Acetaminophen is helpful for the fever and pain and for sore throat and sore muscles. Parents sometimes worry about the number of colds that children come down with; however, parents should be assured that it is a normal part of childhood. Knowing how to treat mild upper respiratory infections can alleviate parents' concerns. A visit to the physician's office is often unnecessary. The prognosis is excellent, if no complications arise and the cold lasts for 4 days or less.

Two-thirds of all children will have recurrent rhinitis (inflammation of the mucosa), but only one-third of those will develop allergic rhinitis, which is defined as inflammation of the mucosa due to sensitivity of nasal mucosa to allergens. The difference between diagnosis and treatment of the common cold and allergic rhinitis is that the onset for a cold is usually after 6 months of age, and the bouts of rhinitis are always accompanied by low-grade fever, with cultures of the mucus negative for bacteria.

Allergic rhinitis usually has its onset after 2 years of age; there is no fever; and the attack includes frequent sneezing and profuse clear discharge. The nasal turbinate is swollen. A variety of oral decongestants and antihistamines are usually tried until the right one for the child is found. Avoidance of allergens such as tobacco, dust, and the hair and dander of cats and dogs should be encouraged. When symptoms persist, vasoconstrictor nose drops are prescribed. However, warn parents against using them for more than 7 days, which may result in chemical rhinitis, a rebound reaction, and secondary nasal congestion. Allergic rhinitis usually responds to antihistamines.

Another form of rhinitis is vasomotor rhinitis, in which children react to changes in the environmental temperature with congestions and rhinorrhea. The treatment for vasomotor rhinitis is the use of oral decongestants periodically as needed.

The most common clinical presentation in children with persistent nasal discharge or postnasal drip and daytime cough for longer than 7 to 10 days is acute sinusitis. It is the acute inflammation of the paranasal sinuses. The maxillary and ethmoidal sinuses are commonly involved with poor drainage related to anatomic features. When mucociliary clearance and drainage are further compromised by an upper respiratory infection, the risk of secondary bacterial infection increases.

Sinusitis is also seen during pollen season in children with allergic rhinitis. The bacteria usually found in sinusitis are *Streptococcus pneumoniae*, *Haemophilus influenzae*, *Moraxella catarrhal*, and *β-hemolytic streptococci*. The most common clinical presentation is the persistence of rhinitis, or postnasal drip, low-grade fever, bad breath, periorbital swelling, facial pain in percussion, and headache. Acute sinusitis is treated with oral antibiotics for 2 to 3 weeks. The usual antibiotic used is amoxicillin 15 mg/kg, 3 times a day. Also, topical decongestants and oral combinations are frequently used to promote drainage.

Epistaxis

Epistaxis, or nosebleeds, can be very alarming to parents, so it is important to teach parents that isolated nosebleeds are common during childhood, but recurrent episodes of more than once a day should be reported to the pediatrician. Nosebleeds in children occur for a variety of reasons. Among the most frequent causes are falls, fights, nose blowing, or nose picking. However, 5% of the nosebleeds are caused by bleeding disorders.

The majority of children have few nosebleeds. If there is a suspicion of a bleeding disorder in a child, a baseline hematocrit is indicated. Children from families with a history of bleeding disorders or a past medical history of bleeding should be screened. Children with allergic rhinitis are also prone to epistaxis because of inflamed mucosa and the itching and rubbing of their noses.

To treat a nosebleed, have the child sit down comfortably and lean forward so that he/she will not swallow the blood. Next, pinch the nose with pressure over the bleeding site for 10 minutes by the clock. Do this twice for a total of 20 minutes. If this treatment is not effective, the child should be taken to a health facility so he/she can be treated with 0.25% phenylephrine or 1:1000 epinephrine. Preventive treatment is the best approach to this problem. Parents should be instructed about the fragility of the nasal vessels and that nosebleeds can be decreased by the use of daily applications of petrolatum with a cotton applicator to the inside of the nostrils. The ointment should be applied for 5 days postnosebleed and then weekly for a month. Humidification in the child's room is also helpful.

THROAT AND MOUTH

Tonsillitis and Pharyngitis

More than 95% of the cases of sore throat and fever in children are viral in nature. Tonsillitis and pharyngitis (Figures 6-5; Color Insert 5 and 6-6; Color Insert 6) account for 10% of the infections in children with sore throat and fever. A **throat** culture should be obtained in order to confirm the diagnosis. The most common bacterial causes of pharyngitis and tonsillitis in children and adolescents are Group A beta-hemolytic streptococcal (GABHS), *N. gonorrhea,* and *Corynebacterium diphtheriae.* Children who have tonsillitis usually have an abrupt onset without nasal symptoms. They complain of malaise, fever, sore throat, nausea, abdominal pain, and headache. If untreated, the child could develop petechiae, beef-red uvula,

Throat. Syn.: neck, windpipe, larynx, trachea, esophagus, jugular region, gullet, gorge, jugulum.

red pharynx, exudate in the tonsils, or tender cervical lymph nodes. The goal of therapy is to prevent the development of rheumatic fever and glomerulonephritis. The management plan includes antimicrobial therapy. The medicine of choice is penicillin G, intramuscular, 600,000 units (if the child weighs more than 60 pounds, 1,200,000 units); or potassium penicillin V (oral), 125 mg 2 to 3 times a day for 10 days. If there is evidence of penicillin resistance or allergy, amoxicillin or dicloxacillin can be prescribed instead.

Along with antibiotic therapy, the child should be given supportive care with plenty of fluids and rest. The parents should be taught about the danger of noncompliance with the medicine. Continued failure to give the prescription for the entire prescribed time could result in the infection becoming resistant to the effects of the medication. In the case of a clinical relapse, a second round of antibiotics should be given. Parents also should be told that the child can go back to school 24 hours after he/she is afebrile.

Many parents ask about surgical removal of tonsils after tonsillitis. A tonsillectomy is usually unnecessary because there is the risk of postoperative bleeding and death. Contrary to what parents believe, big tonsils do not mean bad tonsils, and recurrent colds and sore throats will not disappear with a tonsillectomy. The indications for removal of tonsils are persistent oral obstruction, recurrent peritonsillar abscesses, recurrent pyogenic cervical adenitis, and suspected tonsillar tumor. Contraindications for a tonsillectomy are if the child has a short palate, bleeding disorder, and/or acute tonsillitis.

FIGURE 6-5

⊠

Pharyngitis. Exudative pharyngitis showing erythema and tonsillar exudate in patient with viral mononucleosis. (See also Color Insert 5.) Courtesy of George L. Murrell.)

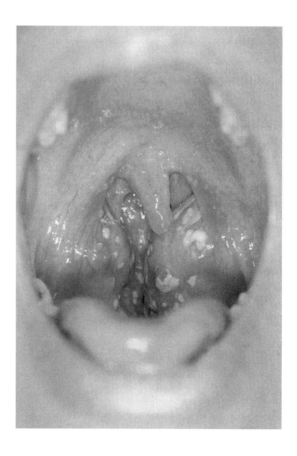

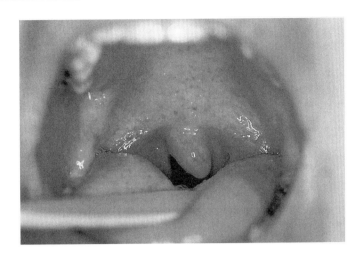

FIGURE 6-6

❖

Palatal petechiae. Palatal petechiae and erythema of the tonsillar pillars in a patient with streptococcal pharyngitis. (See also Color Insert 6.) (Courtesy of Kevin J. Knoop, MD., MS.)

Gingivitis

Gingivitis is the most prevalent lesion of the oral soft tissues in young children. It is estimated that 90% of young children have gingivitis at one time or another. Gingivitis results from poor hygiene or poor dexterity while brushing the teeth, causing plaque to accumulate in the soft tissues around the neck of the teeth, and thus causing inflammation of the gums. Usually children display red gums that bleed easily. The cure is good oral hygiene including the use of dental floss and visits to the dentist every 6 months. Parents/caregivers should help children with oral hygiene, especially if the child's dexterity is insufficient to thoroughly clean his/her own teeth. If not treated, gingivitis can cause loss of bone and teeth. Educate parents about dental diseases and their consequences. The best time to introduce parents to the importance of their child's dental hygiene is during the prenatal visits. The American Academy of Pediatrics recommends that the first visit to the dentist should be at 12 and 18 months of age.

Oral Candidiasis

Oral candidiasis or thrush (Figure 6-7; Color Insert 7) is caused by *Candida albicans*, a common inhabitant of the oral cavity. Candidiasis is sometimes mistaken for milk left in the oral cavity. *C. albicans* reproduces rapidly when the child has lowered resistance, and is seen in immunosuppressed children or after a child has had antibiotic therapy. In nurseries, especially neonatal nurseries, oral candidiasis or thrush is common. The tongue displays raised furry white patches, and the palate bleeds when it is scraped with a tongue blade. The condition is treated with nystatin, 1 cc, applied to the mouth after feedings.

FIGURE 6-7

🔯

Oral candidiasis or thrush. Whitish plaques are seen on the buccal mucosa. These plaques are easily removed with a tongue blade, differentiating them from lichen planus or leukoplakia. (See also Color Insert 7.) (Courtesy of James F. Steiner, DDS.)

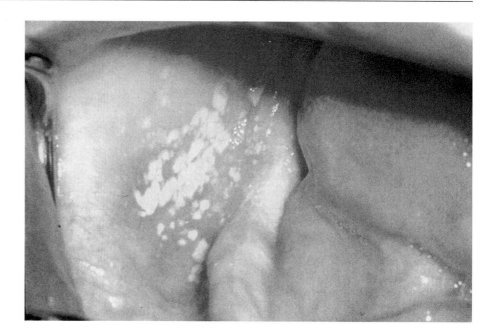

Acute Stomatitis

Acute stomatitis is the presence of single or multiple small ulcers on the inside of the lips, throat, and/or mouth. There is usually no association with fever. The ulcers are very painful and usually last 2 weeks. The cause may be *Candida* (Figure 6-8; Color Insert 8), viral, as in herpes simplex, or unknown, as in aphthous ulcers. Therapy is guided toward avoidance of foods or substances that may cause stomatitis. The treatment consists of the use of antacids or sucralfate as a mouthwash several times a day. Pain is treated symptomatically with 2% viscous lidocaine or protective dental paste (oral base). Diet should be bland since acid foods may cause irritation.

FIGURE 6-8

🔯

Candidiasis. The angles of the mouth are also places where intertriginous conditions favor the overgrowth of ubiquitous *Candida albicans*, streptococci, staphylococci, and other ordinarily saprophytic but facultatively pathogenic microorganisms. The condition produced at the angles of the mouth is called *perlèche* or *angular stomatitis*. From such a beginning or even without it, the lips themselves may become involved. (See also Color Insert 8.)

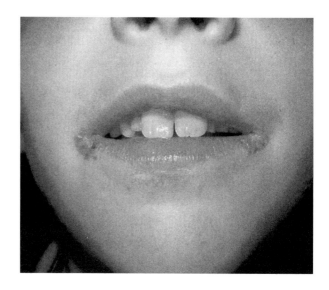

S UMMARY

This chapter encompasses a comprehensive view of problem prevention in relationship to growth and development. It stresses the early identification of problems rather than the treatment of illness. Special attention is given to the examination of subjective data and physical examination. The chapter presents a thorough overview of the diagnostic tests used throughout infancy, toddlerhood, school age, and adolescence. The nurse is encouraged to make a diagnosis based on objective data and observation of differential diagnoses. Special attention is given to the teaching and counseling of parents as it relates to prevention and management of the conditions. The chapter also addresses when the nurse needs to do follow-up of the patients and ask for consultations and referrals.

C RITICAL POINTS IN THE MANAGEMENT OF CONDITIONS OF THE EYES, EARS, NOSE, THROAT, AND MOUTH

The most important intervention in the treatment of conditions of the eyes, ears, nose, throat, and mouth is to help parents identify the risk factors over which they have control. Such factors include a well-balanced, healthy diet; control of environmental irritants such as tobacco smoke in the child's home; and, most important, close observation of the developmental milestones with regard to what is considered normal for the child's age.

Parents are the best source for observing the child's growth and development. The parents' observations are invaluable when the nurse is doing a health assessment. If the nurse suspects vision deficits, questions to parents about the child's responsiveness to visual stimulation can provide important clues for the diagnosis and care of the child. Such questions might include: When the parent smiles at the child, does the child respond? If the parent approaches the child in his/her crib, does the child turn to see who it is? Does the child readily reach or search for objects or special toys? Does the child appear overly clumsy? Each of these questions provides evidence toward a diagnosis for or against vision deficit. Also, these questions illustrate to the parents what types of behaviors to look for in their child. If the child is diagnosed with vision problems, it is the nurse's responsibility to apprise the parents of the cause of the condition and the appropriate care for the child. Most importantly, the nurse should empower the parents with the knowledge of how they can help the child to fully utilize his/her level of vision.

Observation is only one of the methods of information gathering that the parents possess that can aid in caring for their child. Ear infections, for instance, require that parents realize the importance of compliance with the directions for completion of antibiotic prescriptions and follow-up visits to the doctor's office. Prenatally, mothers should know that ear infections occur less frequently in breast-fed infants than in bottle-fed infants. If the mother chooses not to breast-feed the child, she should be instructed to keep the baby's head elevated when feeding with a bottle, so that milk cannot leak into the normally underdeveloped eustachian tube, thus preventing one of the causes of ear infections. Tobacco smoke in the house is another contributor to ear and upper respiratory infections, and the use of a pacifier after 8 months of age is discouraged. Knowledge about the prevention of ear infections should be taught to parents early in their child's development.

Special attention should be given to the birth order of the child and the age of the parents. Parenting is challenging at any age, but teenage parents are especially vulnerable because of their inexperience. In addition, many times teenage parents lack both social support and expert support systems in caring for a child. The nurse's goal should be to help the parents, no matter what their age, to develop parenting skills and coping levels that will best benefit the individual growing child and that will maximize the parent/child relationship.

A child with upper respiratory problems and difficulty breathing can cause parents to panic, no matter what age they are. Educating parents about the distinction between problems with respiration because of an infection and because of an anatomical problem will go a long way in preventing unnecessary visits to the doctor's office. The nurse should instruct the parents of children prone to respiratory infections to watch out for respiratory distress, dehydration, and, most important, what strategies the parents can utilize in the event of an emergency at home. The nurse should stress to the parents that the best intervention is to recognize the effect of stress on the respiratory system and the importance of environmental control in order to avoid illness in the child.

No child gets through childhood untouched by sore throat or pharyngitis. So it is important that all parents be taught about the risk factors that contribute to their child getting sick, such as exposure to others who have colds. By far, the most important lesson that a parent can learn is compliance with the instructions for taking antibiotics and repetition of throat cultures to rule out strep infections, which can lead to rheumatic fever and acute glomerulonephritis if left untreated.

The nurse needs to remember that empowering parents with essential knowlege about prevention and care is an ongoing process of evaluating the child and the child's environment. Families have a tremendous impact on the treatment of any condition or disease. The parents' knowledge and confidence in dealing with a sick child can be enhanced by the nurse who helps them understand through teaching.

$\mathcal{Q}$UESTIONS

Diagnosis: Strabismus

History: Baby Barbara was born with deviations in her eye alignment. After bringing her home, her parents became concerned about the condition of her eyes. The doctor told them that she was not concerned, and that the condition would be checked when they brought Barbara back for regular check-ups.

Plan: The child goes home with parents and the condition of the eye alignment will be checked during the regular visits. At this point, the doctor decided that the baby did not need referral to the ophthalmologist.

Nursing problems: Risk of amblyopia; repeated evaluations required; close monitoring needed during therapy; surgery may be needed if nonsurgical methods are ineffective.

Chief concerns of the nurse: For the baby, the chief concern is to achieve the best binocular vision. For the parents, the chief concern is to relieve them of anxiety due to possible impending surgery, and to reassure them that the prognosis is good if the infant is treated early.

1. Why is the treatment for strabismus delayed in the case of baby Barbara?

   A. All babies are born with strabismus.
   B. Her nervous system is still immature.
   C. Coordinated eye movements normally occur at 8 months of age.
   D. She should see an ophthalmologist during the first month of life.

2. In doing the history and physical examination of baby Barbara, the nurse must pay special attention to:

   A. Family history
   B. Mother's prenatal care
   C. Family's history of diabetes
   D. Barbara's eye movements

3. Barbara's mother tells the nurse she is worried that the reason that Barbara has developed strabismus is because of the prophylactic eye care that Barbara received in the nursery after she was born. The nurse explains to the mother that the classification of strabismus is complex, but that congenital strabismus is caused by:

   A. Birth trauma
   B. Intracranial tumor
   C. Presence of red reflex
   D. Absence of trigeminal nerve

4. Barbara's mother asks the nurse what tests are used in the office to evaluate strabismus. The nurse tells her that the tests are:

   A. Pinpoint and transillumination tests
   B. Corneal light reflex and cover tests
   C. Alternate cover and confrontation tests
   D. Amblyopia and field of vision tests

5. While doing the examination, the nurse thoroughly explains the ocular deviation to Barbara's parents. The reason she does this is because:

   A. The parents need to perform the light reflex test at home.
   B. It is a legal responsibility.
   C. It is the policy of the clinic.
   D. Parents are in the best position to observe misalignment.

Diagnosis: Otitis Media

History: Jorge, a 7-month-old baby boy, was seen in the emergency room with a fever of 101°F with signs of irritability. On physical examination, the nurse realized that the baby's right middle ear was inflamed and Jorge cried louder when that ear was examined. His mother was a 19-year-old college student who appeared scared and exhausted. The mother told the nurse that she and Jorge's father were college students, and that they were not married. On examination, the nurse also realized that the baby was underweight and slightly dehydrated. Further history revealed that the mother was bottle-feeding the infant and that in order to study while feeding him, she propped up the bottle. Although the mother was very concerned, on observation it was obvious that she had not bonded with Jorge, and that the baby lacked stranger anxiety.

Plan: Jorge was sent home with his mother, who was given instructions about follow-up visits and arrangements for parenting classes and emotional and financial help.

Nursing problems: Otitis media; bonding; emotional support for the mother; economic support; parenting skills classes.

Chief concern of the nurse: The immediate concern for the baby is to take care of the otitis media and to start the baby on a regular schedule of feeding and support. For the mother, the immediate concern is to relieve her of some stress, help her find economic support, and provide referrals for counseling and parenting skills classes.

1. The nurse makes the diagnosis of otitis media based on:
   A. Laboratory results
   B. Ear cultures
   C. Otoscopic findings
   D. Throat cultures

2. Older children may complain of pain in the ear, stuffy nose, and cough. Younger children demonstrate their symptoms by:
   A. Increased irritability and difficulty in feeding and sleeping
   B. Lethargy and presence of loose stools
   C. Crying and lethargy
   D. Lethargy and the presence of discharge from the affected ear

3. Jorge's mother tells the nurse that her neighbor told her the best medicine for otitis media is vasoconstrictor ear drops, because they are a decongestant. The best response is:
   A. Is your friend a nurse or a doctor?
   B. We used them years back, but we have better medications now.
   C. They are of no value, because it is impossible to instill them in the auditory tube.
   D. They are of no value in the treatment of otitis media.

4. In planning Jorge's treatment, the nurse knows that his treatment should consist of:
   A. Amoxicillin p.o. qid, visit to the office 48 hours later, and a follow-up visit in 3 weeks
   B. Amoxicillin p.o. qid, and a visit to the office 10 days later
   C. Amoxicillin p.o. tid, and a visit to the office 7 days later
   D. Amoxicillin p.o. for 7 days, and then a call to the office

5. Jorge's mother wants to know the essential symptoms for the diagnosis of an unresponsive otitis media. In addition to a lack of response to antibiotics, which other findings are present?
   A. Red or yellow immobile tympanic membrane
   B. Earache, irritability, and anorexia
   C. Loss of appetite, malaise, anorexia, and irritability
   D. Irritability, loss of appetite, and diarrhea

Diagnosis: Epistaxis

History: Douglas, a 3-year-old boy, is brought to the doctor's office with a nosebleed. Douglas's mother is concerned because the nosebleeds happen during the night and also because Doug has many colds with running nose and cough. She further states that she usually treats the nosebleeds and they stop, but this time, she just wanted to make certain that Douglas is okay. Upon examination, the nurse notices that Douglas exhibits a few scratches and bruises especially on his lower extremities. There is no history of blood diseases in the family, and otherwise Douglas is in good health.

Plan: Douglas is to go home with his mother. She will be taught the management of nosebleeds in children and will be able to seek help in dealing with her anxiety and fears.

Nursing problems: Parent education; child education.

Chief concern of the nurse: The nurse realizes that, at this time, the most important intervention is teaching and clarifying beliefs that the mother has. Nosebleeds are common in school-age children but very rare in teenagers. Most children with nosebleeds have a history of having them at home, but almost all are nonexistent at the time of the visit to the doctor's office. Nosebleeds are seen in the anterior or posterior part of children's noses. Anterior bleeding is more easy to control than posterior bleeding.

1. Douglas's mother wants to know the common causes of nosebleeds in children. Which of the following is most accurate?
   A. Trauma, rhinitis, colds, cold weather
   B. Medications, lack of vitamin K
   C. Heredity, lack of vitamin C
   D. Trauma and heredity

2. What is the most important question that the nurse must ask Douglas's mother while assessing Douglas?

   A. Does the child take Tylenol?
   B. What medications are given for Douglas's cold?
   C. What measures were used to stop the bleeding?
   D. Is there a family history of nosebleeds?

3. For how long should pressure be applied to the nose?

   A. 10 minutes
   B. 20 minutes
   C. 5 minutes
   D. 3 minutes

Diagnosis: Group A β-Hemolytic Streptococcus

History: Melissa, a 9-year-old girl, has had a sore throat and fever for 3 days. She has been complaining of sore throat, difficulty swallowing, and malaise. Melissa has no breathing difficulty or drooling, and otherwise appears to be in good health. A week ago she spent the weekend at her grandmother's home because her grandmother was sick with the flu. On examination, Melissa has a temperature of 101.6°F. She does not have adenopathy, but her tonsils are red and display exudate bilaterally.

Plan: Melissa is to go home with her parents. The management of her condition will be based on its etiology.

Nursing problems: Compliance with treatment; hydration; use of analgesics; prevention of rheumatic fever; prevention of acute glomerulonephritis.

Chief concern of the nurse: For the child, the chief concern is the resolution of the infection and return to normal health. For the family, the chief concern is compliance with medication and follow-up visits. Melissa displays tonsillar exudate, which is a sign of streptococcal infection. A throat culture was done immediately. If positive, she will be treated accordingly.

1. The nurse suspects that Melissa has group A β-hemolytic streptococcus. Which subjective data help the nurse arrive at this conclusion?

   A. Acute onset of sore throat, high fever, rash
   B. High fever, vomiting, malaise
   C. Rash, high fever, malaise
   D. Sore throat, vomiting, malaise

2. Melissa is diagnosed with group A β-hemolytic streptococcus infection. Which objective data support this diagnosis?

   A. Appears toxic, enlarged anterior cervical lymph nodes, Pastia sign
   B. High fever, stridor, malaise, nausea, vomiting
   C. Chronic cough, nausea, vomiting, anorexia
   D. Periorbital edema, tachypnea, diaphoresis, stridor

3. The nurse is concerned with treatment compliance once the child goes home. The best medication to give in this case is:
   A. Benzathine penicillin G, intramuscular
   B. Potassium penicillin B, intramuscular
   C. Erythromycin ethyl succinate
   D. Tetracycline, intramuscular

Answers

Strabismus

1. *B.* Children do not develop coordinated eye movement until about 3–5 months of age. Infants often exhibit temporary deviation of the eyes followed by subsequent realignment. Any child who has constant deviation of the eyes, particularly after 6 months of age, should be evaluated for strabismus.

2. *A.* Strabismus affects approximately 3% of the population, and the condition affects children less than 6 years of age. About 50% of the affected children have a positive family history.

3. *A.* Congenital strabismus may result from birth trauma, muscle anomalies, or congenital infections affecting the eyes, but has nothing to do with prophylactic eye care.

4. *B.* The two basic tests for strabismus are the corneal light reflex test and the cover test.

5. *D.* Parents see their children move often. They are in the best position to observe misalignment.

Otitis Media

1. *C.* The diagnosis of otitis media is based on otoscopic findings, which include the appearance of the tympanic membrane and the assessment of its mobility.

2. *A.* Irritability may be related to pain and hearing loss. Because of the fever, the child may have anorexia and sleeping difficulties.

3. *C.* The anatomy of the ear makes it impossible to deliver any drops to the entrance of the auditory tube.

4. *A.* At the initial visit the child is given amoxicillin 250 mg qid for at least 10 days. If symptoms persist after 48 hours, the child should be evaluated for meningitis versus an unresponsive meningitis.

5. *A.* Antibiotic therapy that results in a good clinical response usually is effective in 48 hours. The other symptoms may persist but they can be treated on an outpatient basis.

Epistaxis

1. *A.* Trauma from nose picking, inflammation of the nasal mucosa from dry cold weather, rhinitis, and allergies are the most common causes of nosebleeds.

2. *C.* Application of pressure to the nose for 10 minutes is the best treatment for nosebleeds. Parents are also instructed to apply petroleum with an applicator to the nose for a period of 1 week and to maintain humidity in the child's bedroom.

3. *A.* The child should sit up and lean forward so that he/she will not swallow the blood. The nose should be pinched, with pressure over the bleeding site for a period of 10 minutes.

Group A β-Hemolytic Streptococcus

1. *A.* The parent or the child will report to the nurse that he/she has a sore throat, high fever, rash, abdominal pain, and malaise.

2. *A.* On physical exam the nurse reports that the patient has an elevated temperature of 102°F, appears toxic, the tongue is white-furred, has red pharynx, and exhibits Pastia sign (Pastia sign is the presence of red lines of rash in flexor surfaces that do not blanch with pressure).

3. *A.* Benzathine penicillin G is given once. If the child weighs less than 60 lbs., 600,000 units are given; 61–90 lbs., 900,000 units; more than 90 lbs., 1.2 million units. The child should remain for a period of 30 minutes to 1 hour in the doctor's office for observation.

$\mathcal{G}$LOSSARY

conductive hearing loss   hearing loss caused by inadequate conduction of sound from the outer to the middle ear.

development   an increase in capability or function.

eye   the organ of sight. Parts of the eye include eyeball or ball, conjunctiva, pupil, retina, iris, cornea, ciliary body, eye muscles, optic nerve, aqueous humor, fovea, sclera, vitreous body, choroid, white, lens, optic nerve.

nose the organ of smell. Syn.: nasal organ, nasal cavity, nares passages, nostrils, olfactory nerves.

pain an unpleasant sensory and emotional experience associated with actual or potential tissue damage. Pain exists when the patient says it does.

palpation the technique of touch to identify characteristics of the skin, internal organs, and masses. Characteristics include texture, moistness, tenderness, temperature, position, shape, consistency, and mobility of masses and organs.

throat syn.: neck, windpipe, larynx, trachea, esophagus, jugular region, gullet, gorge, jugulum.

ℬIBLIOGRAPHY

ALHO, O., OJA, H., KOIVU, M., AND SORRI, M. Risk factors for chronic otitis media with effusion in infancy. *Archives of Otolaryngology Head Neck Surgery* 121: 839–843, 1995.

BATES, B. *A Guide to Physical Examination and History Taking.* Philadelphia, PA: Lippincott, 1995.

BEHRMAN, R. Disorders of the ear. In R. Kliegman, W. Nelson, and V. Vaughan, III (eds.), *Nelson Textbook of Pediatrics* (pp. 1608–1618). Philadelphia: W. B. Saunders, 1992.

BLUESTONE, C. *Current Concepts.* Kalamazoo, MI: Upjohn, 1993.

BURNS, C. E., BARBER, N., BRADY, M. A., AND DUNN, A. M. *Pediatric Primary Care: A Handbook for Nurse Practitioners.* Philadelphia: W. B. Saunders, 1996.

DUNCAN, B., ELY, J., HOLBERG, C., WRIGHT, A., MARTINEZ, F., AND TAUSSIG, L. Exclusive breast-feeding for at least 4 months protects against otitis media. *Pediatrics* 91: 867–872, 1993.

ETZEL, R., PATTISHALL, E., HALEY, N., FLETCHER, R., AND HENDERSON, F. Passive smoking and middle ear effusion among children in day-care. *Pediatrics* 90: 228–232, 1992.

FACIONE, N. Otitis media: An overview of acute and chronic disease. *Nurse Practitioner* 15: 11–35, 1990.

HARDY, A., AND FOWLER, M. Child care arrangements and repeated ear infections in young children. *American Journal of Public Health* 83: 1321–1325, 1993.

HAY, W. W. JR., GROOTHUIS, J. R., HAYWARD, A. R., AND LEVIN, M. J. *Current Pediatric Diagnosis and Treatment.* Norwalk, CT: Appleton and Lang, 1995.

HOLBERG, C., WRIGHT, A., MARTINEZ, F., MORGAN, W., TAUSSIG, L., AND GROUP HEALTH MEDICAL ASSOCIATES. Child day care, smoking caregivers, and lower respiratory tract illness in the first 3 years of life. *Pediatrics* 91: 885–892, 1993.

MALASANOS, L., BARKAUSKAS, V., AND STOLTENBERG-ALLEN, K. *Health Assessment.* Chicago: C. V. Mosby, 1990.

MARIEB, E. N. *Human Anatomy and Physiology*. Redwood City, CA: Benjamin/Cummings, 1989.

MCMAHON, E., NEAL, R., HODGSON, B., AND NORRIS, C. (ed). *Professional Guide to Diseases*. 5th ed. Springhouse, PA: Springhouse, 1995.

MERENSTEIN, G. B., KAPLAN, D. W., AND ROSENBERG, A. A. *Handbook of Pediatrics*. New York: Lange, 1991.

SIEDEL, H., BALL, J., DAINS, J. E., AND BENEDICT, G. W. *Mosby's Guide to Physical Examination*. St. Louis, MO: Mosby-Year Book, 1995.

UPHOLD, C. R., AND GRAHAM, M. V. *Clinical Guidelines in Family Practice*. 2nd ed. Gainesville, FL: Barmarrae, 1994.

WEITEN, W. *Psychology: Themes and Variations*. 3rd ed. Pacific Grove, CA: Brooks/Cole, 1995.

WONG, D. L., AND WHALEY, L. F. *Nursing Care of Infants and Children*. 5th ed. St. Louis, MO: C. V. Mosby, 1995.

$\mathscr{H}$ELPFUL INTERNET SITES

PEDINFO: An Index of the Pediatric Internet at http://www.pedinfo. org   An excellent site that covers nearly all topics within this review. It has a wealth of information and is worth a visit. It is written for health care professionals but others could also use the information.

Virtual Naval Hospital Information for Providers at http://www.vnh. org/Providers.html   This site is part of the University of Iowa's health care site and is linked to a large set of databases that can be used by health care providers. The site covers a larger number of links to other sources on health care issues and problems. This is an excellent starting place to discover information on various common diseases and their treatments.

FACE NOSE ORAL CAVITY ASSESSMENT

includes the → **MOUTH ORAL CAVITY**

requires

- Inspect lips for color, symmetry, moisture, swelling, sores, and fissures.
- Inspect buccal margins, gingivae, tongue, and palpate for moisture, color, intactness, and bleeding.
- Visualize any abnormalities.
- Observe for odor or halitosis.
- Inspect tongue for movement and size.
- Observe movement of tongue in infants and younger children.
- Inspect teeth for number, type, condition, and occlusion.
- Inspect tonsils in older children.
- Observe movement of uvula during examination of tonsils.
- Observe quality of voice.

includes the → **FACE AND NOSE**

requires

- Observe the spacing and size of facial features.
- Observe facial expression, especially eyes and mouth.
- Observe symmetry of nasolabial folds as child cries and smiles.
- Observe size and shape of the nose.
- Observe external nares for flaring, discharge, excoriation, and odor.
- Test patency of nares.
- Inspect and visualize internal nasal cavity.
- Assess sense of smell in older child.
- Palpate eyebrows.

includes understanding → **ANATOMY AND PHYSIOLOGY**

change over time and with development

- The infant's face is clearly different from the adult's.
- The nose warms, filters, and moistens air as it enters the respiratory tract.
- Sense of taste is immature at birth but develops and becomes acute by 2 to 3 months.
- Full sense of taste is not fully developed until 2 years of age.
- Dentition begins at approximately 6 months of age.
- Tonsils are found in the pharyngeal cavity and are part of the lymphatic system.
- Tonsils begin to shrink at approximately 7 years of age.

support for is found in → **RATIONALE FOR ASSESSMENT**

support by the fact that

- Emotional status and clues to neurologic, congenital, and allergic conditions can be assessed through an inspection, palpation, and ascultation of the face, nose, and oral cavity.
- Examination of the nose, mouth, and sinuses provides information as to the functioning of the respiratory and digestive tracts.
- Common disorders and occurrences of tonsilitis provide a primary reason for including the face, nose, and oral cavity in assessment.

Concept Map 6-1

201

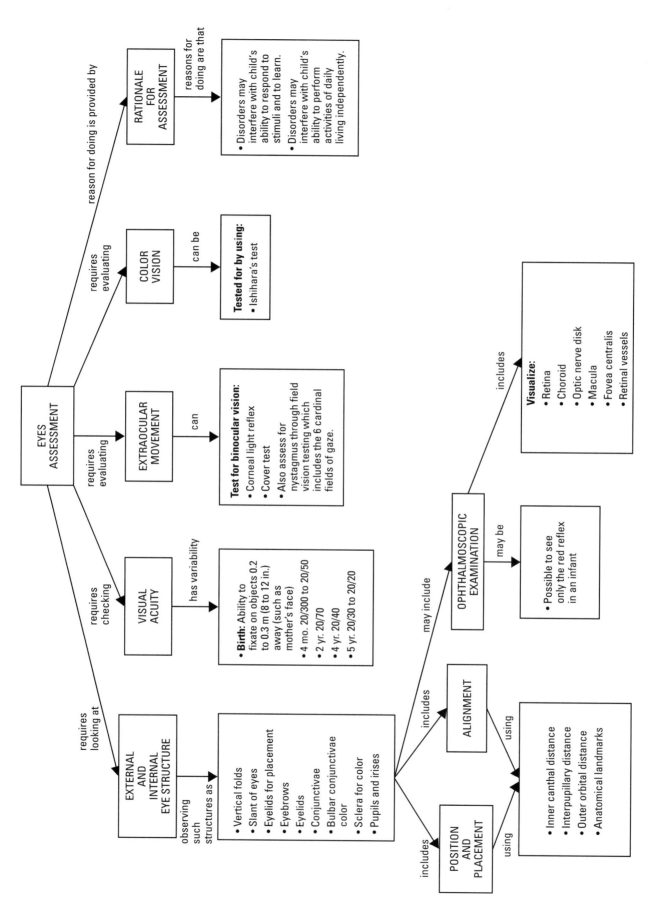

EYES ASSESSMENT

reason for doing is provided by → **RATIONALE FOR ASSESSMENT** → *reasons for doing are that*
- Disorders may interfere with child's ability to respond to stimuli and to learn.
- Disorders may interfere with child's ability to perform activities of daily living independently.

requires evaluating → **COLOR VISION** → *can be*
Tested for by using:
- Ishihara's test

requires evaluating → **EXTRAOCULAR MOVEMENT** → *can*
Test for binocular vision:
- Corneal light reflex
- Cover test
- Also assess for nystagmus through field vision testing which includes the 6 cardinal fields of gaze.

requires checking → **VISUAL ACUITY** → *has variability*
- **Birth:** Ability to fixate on objects 0.2 to 0.3 m (8 to 12 in.) away (such as mother's face)
- 4 mo. 20/300 to 20/50
- 2 yr. 20/70
- 4 yr. 20/40
- 5 yr. 20/30 to 20/20

requires looking at → **EXTERNAL AND INTERNAL EYE STRUCTURE** → *observing such structures as*
- Vertical folds
- Slant of eyes
- Eyelids for placement
- Eyebrows
- Eyelids
- Conjunctivae
- Bulbar conjunctivae color
- Sclera for color
- Pupils and irises

includes → **ALIGNMENT** → *using*
- Inner canthal distance
- Interpupillary distance
- Outer orbital distance
- Anatomical landmarks

includes → **POSITION AND PLACEMENT** → *using*
- Inner canthal distance
- Interpupillary distance
- Outer orbital distance
- Anatomical landmarks

may include → **OPHTHALMOSCOPIC EXAMINATION** → *may be*
- Possible to see only the red reflex in an infant

includes →
Visualize:
- Retina
- Choroid
- Optic nerve disk
- Macula
- Fovea centralis
- Retinal vessels

Concept Map 6-2

202

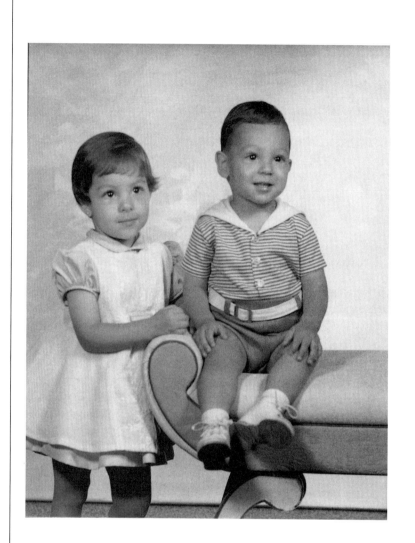

NEUROLOGIC DISORDERS

INTRODUCTION

The neurologic system is the central processing unit of the body, which integrates, receives, and responds to stimuli from the internal network of organs and subsystems and/or the environment. It consists of three major parts that are intimately connected for normal functioning: (1) the central nervous system (CNS)—the brainstem, cerebellum, and spinal cord; (2) the peripheral nervous system; and (3) the autonomic nervous system.

Neurons develop between 15, 20, and 30 weeks of gestation. Head circumference, which is measured in children up to 3 years of age, averages 33 to 35 cm (13 to 14 inches) and should be 2 to 3 cm larger than chest circumference at birth. Brain growth is 50% achieved in the first year of life, 75% by age 3, and 90% by age 6. It comprises 12% of body weight at birth, doubles in weight the first year, and is tripled by age 5 or 6. In embryo, the brain and the spinal cord are the first to be recognized, and are the last to finish developing after birth.

The mastery of gross and fine motor skills is related to the myelination of the nervous system and follows the law of cephalocaudal-proximodistal development. Infants are guided primarily by primitive reflexes, but with myelination and development, a growing child progressively performs complex tasks requiring coordinated movements.

The brain is protected by the skull, and at birth, the anterior and posterior fontanels are separated for brain expansion. The posterior fontanel closes at 8 weeks and the anterior fontanel closes at 18 months. By 12 years, the sutures are inseparable by **intracranial pressure**. Within the skull

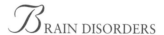

intracranial pressure. Pressure in the intracranial cavity.

are 3 more protective membranes, or meninges: the dura mater, arachnoidea mater, and pia mater. The brain is further protected by the blood-brain barrier, an anatomic-physiologic feature that separates blood from the brain parenchyma. Eighty percent of the cranium is filled by the brain; 10% is cerebrospinal fluid; and another 10% is blood—all of which must maintain constant levels, guided by the Monro-Kellie hypothesis, which states that a change in volume in one of the brain's components must be followed by a change in another.

The brain depends on oxygen-rich blood to function efficiently and works on the principle of autoregulation. The blood supply is carried by the internal carotid arteries, which branch out to supply all the other brain segments. A disturbance in the structure or function of any part of the nervous system results in impairment of its integrative and regulatory mechanisms.

$\mathcal{B}$RAIN DISORDERS

Seizure Disorders

Seizure is a sudden episode of involuntary motor activity, sensory overload, or autonomic changes that may occur alone or in any combination, often accompanied by an altered level of consciousness, or loss of consciousness, caused by temporary changes in metabolic or autonomic functioning, anoxia, trauma, or infectious disturbances in the brain. Epilepsy or seizure disorder is characterized by repeated seizures and the cause may be strongly identified. Idiopathic or genetic epilepsy usually appears between ages 4 and 16. The onset of seizure varies. Between 3 and 8 months, infantile spasms usually occur. Between 4 and 11 years of age, typical petit mal absence seizures occur, and complex partial seizures usually occur before age 15. Seizures are classified as partial, simple partial, and complex partial, absence, generalized tonic-clonic, or hysterical.

A complete history and a thorough assessment is the key to diagnosing and treating seizure disorders. Status epilepticus is a seizure lasting at least 30 minutes without complete recovery and is a medical emergency. This is commonly caused by noncompliance with seizure medications.

Electroencephalogram. Useful tool to provide specific answers to neurologic disorders.

Diagnostic evaluation of seizures includes complete cell blood count (CBC), electrolytes, glucose, calcium, magnesium, urine, and blood toxicology. A lumbar puncture is warranted for central nervous system infection or inflammation, or if a child presents with fever. An **electroencephalogram** (EEG) is also helpful in determining the type of seizure. Skull films, computerized axial tomography (CAT) scan of the brain, positron emission tomography (PET), and magnetic resonance imaging (MRI) are also helpful in diagnosing seizure disorders.

Pharmacological management of seizure disorder depends on the patient's specific seizure type and cause. It is administered and titrated depending on response and drug blood levels and works to decrease the level of neuronal excitability below the threshold of seizures. The most common drugs used are carbamazepine (Tegretol), 10 to 25 mg/kg/day p.o.; clonazepam (Clono-pin), 0.1 to 0.35 mg/kg/day p.o.; ethosuximide (Zarontin), 20 to 50 mg/kg/day p.o., phenobarbital (Luminal), 3 to 5 mg/kg/day p.o.; phenytoin (Dilantin), 3 to 8 mg/kg/day p.o.; primidone (Mysoline), 5 to 20 mg/kg/day p.o.; and valproic acid (Depakene), 15 to 60 mg/kg/day p.o.

The treatment for seizures is generally based on the cause. Protection from self-injury and from aspiration of vomitus is of primary concern. With young epileptics, however, nurses should educate the parents and the child about the disease and encourage compliance. Normal living is within reasonable bounds; precautions should be taken with daily activities. Adolescents should avoid alcohol because it may trigger a seizure. Driving restrictions vary depending on the state, but the law usually allows epilep-tic teenagers to drive if they have been seizure-free for 2 years and treat-ment does not interfere with driving abilities. Pregnant teenagers are also at risk for having a child with birth defects because of the teratogenic effects of anticonvulsant therapy. As soon as a pregnancy is confirmed, the physician should be notified.

Compliance is one of the major problems with the use of anticonvul-sant medications. Parent education should include the effects of anticon-vulsant therapy. Anticonvulsants will not produce permanent damage and are given to prevent seizure activities. Since dosage requirements are titrated according to needs, parents should be encouraged to have peri-odic reevaluations. Blood levels are often drawn and anticonvulsants are titrated based on the results. Therapy is gradually tapered off, not with-drawn abruptly.

Febrile Seizures

Febrile seizures usually occur in 2 to 3% of children between the ages of 6 months and 3 years, manifested by temperatures of 38.8° C or higher. Febrile seizures are diagnosed only when nervous system infection has been ruled out. The fever is usually caused by an accompanying infection—otitis media, adenitis, or pharyngitis. Ninety percent of febrile seizures are gener-alized and last less than 5 minutes. Only 2 to 4% lead to epilepsy, which is frequently outgrown. Recurrent episodes of febrile seizures are usually associated with a positive family history. Initial treatments are aimed at controlling the fever with acetaminophen 10 to 15 mg/kg every 4 hours p.o. or p.r. and stopping the ongoing seizure. Electrolytes, glucose, calcium, magnesium, skull x-rays, or CAT scan can also help if the focus of infection is unidentified. However, a white blood count (WBC) greater than 20,000 with an extreme shift to the left warrants ruling out of meningitis.

Children with epilepsy may have seizures in the absence of fever. Febrile seizures are benign when the child is neurologically normal, fever is pres-ent, and central nervous system infection is ruled out. The benign seizure activity should occur only once in a 24-hour period, last less than 15 min-utes, and be generalized with no residual postictal focal neurologic deficits observed, and the EEG should be normal.

A febrile seizure that lasts more than 20 minutes and/or occurs more than once within 24 hours is considered an "atypical" seizure. Therapy is prescribed on a long-term basis and the usual drug of choice is phenobarbital.

Prevention of recurrent febrile seizures includes educating the parents on fever prevention tasks, i.e., tepid water sponging, antipyretics, compliance with prescribed antibiotics, and/or anticonvulsant therapy. Tepid water sponging—applying cool compresses to the child's skin or tepid baths in the bathtub for 20 to 30 minutes with warm, gradually cooled water—can lower the core temperature if the temperature is above 38.5°C (101.4°F). Chilling should be avoided because it can make the child shiver, hence increasing heat production and increasing the core temperature. Acetaminophen is the antipyretic drug of choice; aspirin should be discouraged because of its possible association with Reye's syndrome. Ibuprofen is also used for children older than 6 months and is sometimes alternated with acetaminophen. Caution parents about medication frequency and dosages and to avoid overdosing their children with fever medications.

Intracranial Infections

Infections are caused by bacteria, viruses, or other microorganisms. The causative agent may affect the meninges (meningitis), brain (encephalitis), or spinal cord (myelitis). Infections usually manifest with generalized malaise, fever, and impaired heart, lung, liver, or kidney function. With CNS infections, headaches, stiff neck, hypothermia, altered mental status, seizures, and motor and focal sensory deficits are usually present alone or in any combination.

Carefully evaluate patients with a change in level of consciousness, including hyperirritability with a progression to lethargy and coma. Positive Brudzinski and Kernig signs also manifest meningeal irritation. The port of entry of the microorganism should be sought in the initial assessment. Sinuses, the ears or other structures in the head, face, and neck region, open head injuries, postneurosurgical procedures, presence of shunts and immunodeficiencies, Reye's syndrome, and animal bites, all must be carefully considered. A CBC, cultures, and cerebrospinal fluid (CSF) should be obtained. Lumbar puncture must be performed to obtain the CSF and should be examined for white and red blood cells, glucose, protein, bacteria, and other microorganisms, and should be cultured. High protein and low glucose usually suggest bacterial infection as well as fungi mycobacteria and some viruses like herpes simplex, mumps, choriomeningitis virus, or arboviruses. **Computed tomography** (CT) scans, MRIs, and EEGs are effective in ruling out the presence of meningeal inflammation, brain abscesses, infarction, hemorrhages, and subdural effusions.

The most common type of CNS infection is meningitis. Bacterial meningitis is usually caused by pus-forming bacteria, especially meningococcus, influenza bacillus, and pneumococcus, and is a fatal disease if left untreated. Ninety percent of cases occurs in infants from 1 month to 5 years old, and infants from 6 to 12 months old are at greatest risk.

Computed tomography. Commonly used noninvasive imaging procedure, which provides useful information about acquired and congenital lesions.

Bacterial meningitis is commonly caused by *Haemophilus influenzae,* *Streptococcus pneumoniae,* and *Neisseria meningitidis.* These organisms are usually seen in 95% of children age 2 months and older. The most predominant organism seen in children age 3 months to 3 years, however, is *H. influenzae.*

Pharmacological treatment depends on the causative organism. Children younger than 3 months are initially treated with cefotaxime and ampicillin. Ceftriaxone, cefotaxime, or ampicillin plus chloramphenicol for 7 to 10 days are the antibiotics of choice for children older than 3 months in whom *H. influenzae* is identified as the causative microorganism. For other infections it usually takes 14 to 21 days. The treatment of viral infections is usually limited to supportive and symptomatic measures. But if the causative agent is herpes simplex virus, the choice of treatment is acyclovir.

Encephalitis occurs with the postinfectious involvement of the CNS after a viral disease, i.e., HIV and herpes simplex, or direct invasion of the CNS by a virus. Viral encephalitis may also involve arthropod vectors and those associated with hemorrhagic fevers. Mosquitoes are one of the most common vector carriers. Rabies is also an acute infection and is transmitted via wild animals like skunks, raccoons, bats, foxes, or even dogs. If rabies is suspected, immunization with human rabies immune globulin (HRIG) is given, followed by human diploid cell rabies vaccine (HDCV) intramuscularly at 3, 7, 14, and 28 days after the first dose.

With Reye's syndrome, cerebral edema is present, but there is no direct association with the microorganism or inflammation; instead, it is accompanied by the fatty infiltration of the liver and liver dysfunction. Since Reye's involves the inflammatory process in all intracranial structures, careful monitoring of cerebral pressure, hydration, and water and electrolyte balance and prevention of seizures should be initiated.

$\mathcal{S}$PINA BIFIDA

Spina bifida is caused by the developmental defect of the neural tube, which fails to close at the end of the fourth week of gestation. Spina bifida is the most common developmental defect of the CNS and most commonly occurs in the lumbar or lumbosacral region. There are 3 types: (1) spina bifida occulta—when the posterior vertebral arches fail to fuse, and no herniation of the spinal cord or meninges is noted; (2) meningocele—a form of spina bifida that consists of a saclike cyst of meninges filled with spinal fluid; and (3) myelomeningocele—a hernial protrusion of a saclike cyst containing spinal fluid, meninges, and a portion of the spinal cord with its nerves.

The degree of neurologic dysfunction can be determined by the anatomic level of the defect and the nerves involved. Neurogenic bladder and bowel, urinary retention, rectal or vaginal prolapse, foot deformities, flexion contractures, dislocated hips, or total flaccid paralysis may occur.

Assessment is usually with inspection. Malformation can manifest by a dimple on the back. Motor and sensory disturbances in the lower extremities include deformity or weakness of a foot or bladder and bowel sphincter control disturbances. Signs and symptoms may be invisible and may become more pronounced during the adolescent growth years. A radiograph is also used for diagnosis. No treatment is needed, unless the spinal cord is involved, in which case surgery is needed.

In meningocele the sac is seen protruding over the vertebrae, and if transilluminated, light easily passes through. Head circumference is frequently measured to determine the development of hydrocephalus. After birth, the sac is usually closed surgically within the first 24 hours. Prognosis is good if hydrocephalus is not evident.

In meningomyelocele, hydrocephalus may occur in neonates. Physical manifestations may be seen when a neonate is born with talipes valgus or varus deformities or hip dislocations. In adolescence, scoliosis or kyphosis may develop. When transilluminated, light cannot pass through. Flaccid paralysis of the legs with sensory loss, functional bowel and bladder impairment, and development of hydrocephalus may occur, depending on the level of damage. Assessment also includes a radiography of the skull, hips, chest, and spine. The presence of infection can be obtained from urine cultures and a CAT scan can be done to confirm hydrocephalus.

Pregnant women can be screened routinely via amniocentesis or ultrasound studies, because 90% of neural tube defects can be detected. Research and studies have also shown that daily doses of folic acid (0.4 mg) can help lower the incidence of neural tube defects.

CEREBRAL PALSY

Cerebral palsy (CP) is the lack of voluntary muscle strength or control in which posture and movement are impaired at birth or in early infancy. Causes, prognosis, and manifestations vary widely. Ischemia, hypoxia, hemorrhage, trauma, congenital malformation, intrauterine bleeding, infections, toxins, and obstetric complications are some of the causes, but asphyxia is the most important causative factor in full-term neonates. CP is nonprogressive and nonhereditary.

CP is classified by the predominant motor deficit. Spastic forms account for 75% of the cases. Quadriplegia involves the four extremities; diplegia, the legs more than the arms. Hemiplegia refers to one-sided involvement; paraplegia, only the legs are involved; monoplegia, one extremity is involved; and triplegia, three extremities involved. Ataxia is the other form, which involves about 15% of cases. It can also occur in combination with other forms. Dyskinesia, which accounts for 5% of the cases, often occurs with spastic quadriplegia or diplegia. Hypotonic forms occur in less than 1% of cases.

Associated deficits include seizures; mental retardation, which ranges from mild to moderate depending on the severity of CP; and speech and sensory deficits. Varying degrees and combinations of speech, hearing, vision, and perceptual function impairment are also seen.

CP is assessed on history and physical examination. The infant usually appears floppy and tendon reflexes may appear abnormally increased. The primary complaint is usually the delayed acquisition of gross motor milestones. Toe walking, shuffling gait, obligatory fisting in infants older than 3 months, excessive extension or trunk, hips, and legs with fine voluntary motor movements usually decreased, and an overflow of associated movements are seen. A child may also lie with legs crossed or scissored and elbows flexed and fists clenched, but this is seen in extreme cases. Rigidity is associated with cerebral palsy.

Treatment of CP should be to help achieve and maximize the child's potential rather than focusing on making the child "normal." It also requires a multidisciplinary approach involving the parents, physical therapist, occupational therapist, neurologist, and orthopedist. Diazepam is usually used in treating seizures, which are dealt with the same way as in other children. Death due to recurrent infection is seen in patients with severe CP. Average- and below-average-intelligence children with CP usually lead a fairly normal life.

Hydrocephalus

Hydrocephalus is an increase in CSF volume because of an interference in its absorption or circulation, and progressive ventricular dilatation. It is classified as communicating or noncommunicating. In communicating hydrocephalus, communication between the ventricles and subarachnoid space is normal. There is no obstruction. Noncommunicating hydrocephalus involves an obstruction in the flow between the ventricular and subarachnoid systems. Hemorrhage, infection, tumors, and congenital malformations, i.e., spina bifida, play major etiologic roles in the development of hydrocephalus

Children with hydrocephalus usually have large heads. An increase in head growth is measured by the occipital frontal circumference and is used as a diagnostic gauge. Irritability, hypertonia, loss of appetite, vomiting, hyperflexia, and impaired extraocular movements are also some of its clinical features. CT scan, MRI, and radionuclide scans are used to diagnose hydrocephalus. The goal of treatment is to establish a balance between the resorption and production of CSF and to provide an alternative outlet for the CSF. In providing this alternative route ventriculoperitoneal shunt, ventriculoatrial shunt, and ventriculopleural shunt are performed surgically. Acetazolamide (Diamox) is sometimes used to reduce the production of CSF.

Survival rate is 85 to 90%, but IQ levels in one-third of these children are 75 or below.

$\mathcal{H}$EAD INJURY

One of the most common causes of emergency department visits is closed head injury. Most deaths are caused by head injury following multiple trauma, as seen in child abuse, accidents, and shaken-baby syndrome. In children this may be classified as mild, moderate, or severe.

In assessing a child with head injury, a thorough health history should include the mechanism of injury: how, where, when, how high was the fall, on what surface? Was the child awake after the fall or were there any changes in the level of consciousness, or loss of consciousness? What does the child remember about the incident and after? Was there any vomiting, headaches, blurred vision, gait problems, lethargy, and discharge from the ears or nose? Neurologic assessment should be detailed with the mechanism of injury always in mind. The vital signs and level of consciousness by Glasgow coma scale (GCS) in children older than 3 years are some of the neurologic tools used to assess the severity of the injury. The child's behavior should be noted. Irritability, speech, pupillary equality size and reaction, reflexes, body posture, and bruises should all be observed and should be consistent with the complaint and history.

If a child is presented awake, alert, oriented, with no loss of consciousness or amnesia, asymptomatic, with dizziness and slight headache, then he/she probably suffered from mild head injury. Moderate head injury presents with a history of loss of consciousness. The child may not remember the incident. Vomiting more than once, restlessness, headache, or lethargy may be present. A concussion is an example, but in this injury, there is no anatomic damage and the child returns to his/her normal state. A skull x-ray is often ordered to diagnose the extent of the injury. The child is sent home and parents are instructed to observe the child closely at home every 3 to 4 hours for the next 24 to 36 hours. Any changes or concerns warrant mandatory return to a hospital. A contusion, on the other hand, is a bruise and may manifest with local hemorrhage. There is alteration in the level of consciousness with focal findings related to the area of the brain that has been injured. A CT scan is usually done and the child is admitted for observation and neurologic consults. Severe head injury is classified when a child is disoriented and the level of consciousness is deteriorating, or unconscious with a depressed skull fracture or penetrating skull injury. With this injury there is usually an increase in intracranial pressure (ICP). It should be treated immediately and aggressively. This is where pediatric advance life support comes into play. Focus will be on the ABCs (airways, breathing, circulation): rapid-sequence intubation with the use of sedatives and muscle relaxants, hyperventilation, and avoidance of hypoxemia, to acutely lower the ICP. Peripheral perfusion should also be maintained with fluid infusions. Mannitol (0.5 g/kg intravenous) and Lasix (1 to 2 mg/kg intravenous) will aid in reducing the water in the brain. Giving pain and fever medications, raising the bed 30°, and keeping head midline will also aid in the therapy for increased ICP. Remember, bradycardia, hypertension, and irregular respirations, otherwise known as Cushing's triad, and papilledema are late signs. With severe head injury and increased ICP, the focus is on preventing precipitating herniation; otherwise, death occurs.

Teaching the child to wear protective gear like a helmet in potentially hazardous sports or hobbies, and to wear a seatbelt, also aids in preventing head injuries.

HEADACHES

Headache is one of the most frequent complaints and symptoms in neurologic disorders. A careful history with the child's age, sex, past medical history, chronic illness, current medications, and treatment should be noted. Duration, severity, presence of fever, history of trauma, other general symptoms, or CNS symptoms with symptom patterns should also be considered. In very young children, headache is not usually a psychosomatic symptom, as it may be in adolescents and older children.

In adolescents, tension headache is the most frequently seen. It varies in location—frontal or occipital—and occurs alone as a symptom. Neurologic and physical examination is normal, and headache is usually treated with minor analgesics and avoiding stress precipitants. Despite the head pain, adolescents usually function.

Chronic progressive headache in children, with worsening severity and frequency, and morning headache with vomiting but without nausea indicate brain tumor requiring neurologic evaluation. Headache with deteriorating school grades and athletic coordination, or important positive neurologic examination, are warning signs and need further evaluation. An MRI is usually done for tumor visualization. If tumor is not suspected, a CT scan can be performed instead, less expensively.

MIGRAINES

Migraine attacks are described as pounding, pulsating, and throbbing with pain being described as frontal, bilateral, or unilateral. The severity varies. Migraines occur twice as much in girls as in boys after age 10. School stresses, motion sickness, positive family history, and food are some factors that precipitate the onset, but migraine attack is brief. Sleep, acetaminophen, ibuprofen, and a quiet, darkened room often result in comfort. If the migraine is severe and a child is more than 12 years old, Fioricet or Midrin, 2 capsules every 4 hours, is used. If this pharmacologic treatment is ineffective and migraine becomes severe, frequent, and disabling, prophylaxis is recommended: propanolol, 10 to 40 mg tid; cyproheptadine, 2 to 4 mg every 8 to 12 hours; or calcium channel blockers. Imipramine, an antidepressant, 25 to 50 mg at bedtime, is also found to be useful, but is not recommended in children.

ℬRAIN TUMORS

Brain tumors account for 1500 to 2000 new malignancies—25 to 30% of all childhood cancers—and are the most common solid tumor of childhood cancers in the United States. The cause remains unknown. Because of their rarity, they are often misdiagnosed or diagnosed late. In childhood tumors range from low-grade localized lesions to high-grade tumors with neuraxis dissemination and are histologically and biologically heterogenous. In young children with high-grade tumors, high-dose systemic chemotherapy is used to delay or avoid cranial irradiation.

Clinical manifestation is age specific and depends on the location of the tumor. Children less than 2 years old commonly have infratentorial tumors. They usually present with lethargy, irritability, vomiting, unsteadiness, ataxia hyperreflexia, and cranial nerve palsies. With tumors located in the hypothalamic region, extreme weight loss and emaciation with paradoxical alertness are usually seen. Optic glioma is usually associated with neurofibromatosis in children, and symptoms are usually related to defects in the eye. With this tumor, difficulty tracking and visual disturbances occur. In older children, supratentorial tumors are more prevalent. Children usually present with visual symptoms, headaches, seizures, and neurologic deficits. Infratentorial tumors are usually noted with symptoms of progressively worsening headache, vomiting, double vision, unsteady gait, and papilledema. Tumors in the brainstem manifest with extraocular and facial palsies, hemiparesis, and ataxia. In approximately 25% of these patients, hydrocephalus is present.

The most common pediatric brain tumors are located above the tectorium and in the posterior fossa. They are classified by the cell of origin into glial tumors (astrocytomas and ependymomas) or nonglial tumors like medulloblastoma and neuroectodermal tumors. Astrocytomas are low-grade tumors found in the posterior fossa. This is the most common brain tumor in childhood; medulloblastomas and related primitive neuroectodermal tumors are the most common high-grade tumors. Third in frequency are the brainstem tumors, which are frequently high grade.

Treatment of childhood brain tumors requires a multidisciplinary team approach including neurosurgery, neuro-oncology, endocrinology, neurology, neuropsychology, radiation therapy, rehabilitation medicine, specialized nurses, social workers, physical therapy, and occupational therapy.

If cerebral edema is present dexamethasone (0.5 to 1 mg/kg initially, then 0.25 to 0.5 mg/kg/day qid) is started. Phenytoin, 4 to 8 mg/kg/day, is also given if the child has had seizures. The goal of treatment is to eradicate the tumor. If surgical removal is too risky, open or stereotactic biopsy, radiation therapy, or chemotherapy can be used.

Despite surgical technology and radiation therapy techniques, however, the prognosis for a normal life-style is poor for children with high-grade brain tumors.

Summary

In this chapter, common congenital abnormalities involving the central nervous system were discussed. Congenital neurologic defects are described according to the anatomic abnormality that is present. The associated changes that result from those structural abnormalities, including the differences in normal versus abnormal growth and development, and the resulting pathophysiology of motor dysfunction and cerebrovascular diseases, were also discussed.

Critical Points in the Care of Neurologic Conditions

The most important nursing interventions in the evaluation of the child with neurologic symptoms are the history and physical evaluation. The purpose of the history is to obtain information that enables a tentative diagnosis to be made. Information obtained from the history should allow the time of illness to be assessed and the findings to be interpreted. Based on these findings the nurse determines if the disease process is acute or chronic, and whether the onset was abrupt or insidious. The formal neurologic examination is used to confirm the information obtained by observation. The nurse needs to be aware of all the laboratory tests frequently used in the evaluation of these children in order to educate the parents and recognize differences that may make great differences in the children's care.

Many conditions can cause acute brain dysfunction in children, which can result in progressive alterations of consciousness. Many of these conditions can be corrected quickly if a timely diagnosis is done. The nurse needs to be keenly aware that associated abnormalities with developmental delays may mean retardation. The treatment of these conditions needs to be handled by an interdisciplinary team; often it is the nurse who coordinates the efforts of the team. The nurse also needs to emphasize the support and education of the parents. It is vital not to take away all their hope, and also to help them arrive at a realistic expectation about the condition of their child. Children with neurologic conditions present a very complicated picture. It is essential that the nurse help to optimize their growth and development and at the same time support the child and the family.

QUESTIONS

Diagnosis: Febrile Seizures

History: Jason is an 18-month-old who was brought to the emergency department via rescue. According to rescue, his mother called because the child started shaking, but when rescue got there, Jason was already crying and no seizure activity was observed. According to his mother, this is the first time it happened. Jason was well all day, but felt a little warm after lunch. The seizures lasted for approximately 3 minutes and involved the whole extremities. The eyes rolled back and some drooling was observed. His mother also reported that Jason has a history of ear infection, which was diagnosed 3 months ago, in which he finished the 10-day course of amoxicillin. Jason is presently awake and alert, crying and clinging to his mother. Jason weighs 13 kg. He is diagnosed with febrile seizures and left otitis media.

1. Upon assessment, the vital signs are as follows: temperature 40°C rectally, respirations 26, pulse 100, blood pressure 90/60. The nurse should:
   A. Administer a tepid sponge bath.
   B. Administer Dilantin.
   C. Do an Accu-Chek.
   D. Hydrate the child.

2. Which of the following questions is not relevant in obtaining a thorough history in Jason's case?
   A. What did he eat this morning for breakfast?
   B. Does seizure or epilepsy run in the family?
   C. Did Jason hit his head anywhere?
   D. Did the mother give any fever medications today?

3. The doctor starts ordering lab tests. Which test would the nurse question?
   A. CBC, BCP 7, blood culture
   B. Calcium and magnesium
   C. Urinalysis and urine culture
   D. Stool culture

Diagnosis: Seizure Disorder

History: Jason is diagnosed with febrile seizures. The doctor ordered Rocephin, 700 mg intramuscular, which was given. He is to go home on antibiotics and fever prevention measures are emphasized to his mother. Three days later, Jason comes back to the emergency room and presents with a seizure that lasted longer than 5 minutes. Vital signs show an elevation of temperature (39°C). Jason is postictal, but comes around and starts recognizing people. According to his mother, he has been taking his medicines religiously. The last dose of antibiotics was given after lunch, and the fever subsided yesterday.

Plan: Admit Jason for observation and further evaluation; find the cause of seizures; pharmacologic treatment.

Nursing problems: Compliance with medication, refills, visits, lab values; teaching parents about disease process and progress; teaching emergency treatment for seizures.

1. What is most likely to happen to Jason?

    A. Nothing; he likely will be sent home again.
    B. He will be admitted to the hospital for further neurological workup.
    C. Jason will continue having seizures because Dilantin wasn't administered.
    D. He will be intubated, paralyzed, and sedated and will be in the PICU.

2. When Jason starts seizing at home his parents should:

    A. Allow the seizure without interference.
    B. Restrain the child or use force.
    C. Put a tongue depressor in the child's mouth.
    D. Place Jason on his back.

Diagnosis: Bacterial Meningitis

History: Anderson is a 3-week-old first child, born via normal vaginal delivery with no complications. He was brought to the clinic with complaints of fever, irritability, and vomiting. Upon assessment, rectal temperature was 101°F.

Plan: Child is to go to the emergency room for diagnostic evaluation, blood work, CSF analysis, and CT scan, with possible admission for intravenous antibiotics.

Nursing problems: Explanations of diagnostic evaluations, disease, and causes; fear and anxiety of parents, for first-born baby; use of antibiotic prophylaxis.

1. A lumbar puncture is done. The CSF result(s) that would suggest bacterial meningitis is/are:

    A. High protein, low glucose
    B. High glucose, low protein
    C. Clear CSF
    D. No red blood cells seen

2. Initial treatment of suspected bacterial meningitis include(s):

    A. Vancomycin
    B. Cefotaxime and ampicillin
    C. Acyclovir
    D. Vancomycin and amphotericin

3. The most common organism in bacterial meningitis is:

A. *N. meningitidis*
B. *H. influenzae*
C. *S. pneumoniae*
D. Herpes simplex

Diagnosis: Head Trauma

History: Sam, a 10-year-old girl, was riding her bike without a helmet, when a car hit her. She was thrown to the sidewalk. She sustained severe head injury and was airlifted to the nearest hospital. She is now unconscious and intubated, with ICP, in the PICU. In observing Sam's condition, the nurse considers the significance of Cushing's triad.

1. Which of the following is in the triad?

A. Bradycardia, hypertension, and irregular respirations
B. Hypotension, tachycardia, increase in ICP
C. Hypertension, tachycardia, decrease in ICP
D. Bradycardia, increase in ICP, hypotension

2. In acutely managing and helping decrease the ICP, the nurse should:

A. Put the bed at reverse Trendelenburg and increase fluids.
B. Raise the head 30°C, keep head midline, administer Mannitol as ordered.
C. Keep the bed flat, head to the side, and administer Lasix as ordered.
D. Maintain head of bed at 15 degrees with the head turned to the side.

3. All of the following are appropriate for checking the neurologic status except:

A. Glasgow coma scale
B. AVPU
C. Pupillary reaction
D. Snellen chart

Diagnosis: Seizures

1. Sam suddenly develops seizures. What do seizures indicate?

A. Sam is getting better and will soon regain consciousness.
B. There is a continuing increase in ICP.
C. Sam has bacterial meningitis.
D. There is a sudden drop in ICP.

Diagnosis: Headaches

History: Joshua is a 15-year-old A− student, who suddenly develops headaches increasing in frequency and duration. His mother has noticed that he has been staying home more often in bed and refuses to go out with his friends.

1. The most frequent type of headache in adolescents is:
   A. Migraine
   B. Tension headache
   C. Psychosomatic headache
   D. Psychological headache

2. Joshua should be taken to the doctor because:
   A. His complaints should be further evaluated.
   B. He might fail school and not go to college.
   C. He may be depressed and a psychologist is needed.
   D. He may be on drugs.

3. Which of the following is the most frequent symptom of brain tumor?
   A. Headache relieved by Tylenol or ibuprofen.
   B. Headache with reading.
   C. Morning headache increasing in frequency and duration with vomiting.
   D. Vomiting.

Diagnosis: Hydrocephalus

1. Susan is born with hydrocephalus. The most objective assessment is based on:
   A. Birth weight
   B. Chest circumference
   C. Head circumference
   D. Length

2. Hydrocephalus may be communicating or noncommunicating: Which of the following is present in communicating hydrocephalus?
   A. There is no obstruction between the ventricles and subarachnoid space.
   B. There is obstruction between the ventricles and subarachnoid space.
   C. There is communication between the ventricles and dura mater.
   D. CSF is leaked to the abdomen.

Diagnosis: Cerebral Palsy

History: Carlos is a 5-year-old who has cerebral palsy from a near drowning episode.

1. Cerebral palsy is:
   A. A musculoskeletal disorder that can be cured.
   B. Nonhereditary and nonprogressive.
   C. The same as muscular dystrophy.
   D. The same as Parkinson's disease.

2. The most probable cause of Carlos's cerebral palsy is:
   A. Child abuse
   B. Hypoglycemia
   C. Abruptio placentae
   D. Hypoxia from the near drowning episode

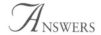

$\mathcal{A}$NSWERS

Febrile Seizures

1. *A.* A tepid sponge bath and antipyretics would help reduce the fever that is causing the seizures.

2. *B.* All the other questions are relevant in neurologic examinations, and letter *D* would also aid if fever intervention was initiated. It would also assist in determining the prior frequency of antipyretic administration.

3. *D.* All of the other tests are necessary to find the focus of infection.

Seizure Disorder

1. *B.* Jason could have "atypical" seizures and should be further evaluated by a neurologist.

2. *A.* Seizures should be observed and should be allowed without interference.

Bacterial Meningitis

1. *A.* C and D are normal findings; B is indicative of viral meningitis.

2 *B.* Cefotaxime and amoxicillin are the drugs of choice for bacterial meningitis.

3. *B. H. influenzae* is the most common, although *A* and *C* could also be the causative microorganisms. *D* is viral.

Head Trauma

1. *A.* Cushing's triad is bradycardia, hypertension, and irregular respirations.

2. *B.* All these interventions may help in reducing ICP.

3. *D.* The Snellen chart is used for visual acuity. All the other tests are neurologic tests.

Seizures

1. *B.* The brain isn't decompressing. The seizure indicates a continuing increase in ICP.

Headaches

1. *B.* Tension headaches are the most frequent type of headache in adolescents.

2. *A.* Further evaluation may be needed because he may have a neurologic disorder.

3. *C.* Morning headaches and vomiting indicate increase in ICP, tumor, or abscess.

Hydrocephalus

1. *C.* Hydrocephalus is manifested by a large head and head circumference is the objective measurement.

2. *A.* Communicating hydrocephalus has no obstruction between the ventricles and subarachnoid space.

Cerebral Palsy

1. *B.* Cerebral palsy is nonhereditary and nonprogressive.

2. *D.* The cause is hypoxia from the lack of oxygen from his near drowning episode. *A* and *C* may also be considered as causes for cerebral palsy, but the situation was already given.

Glossary

computed tomography commonly used noninvasive imaging procedure, which provides useful information about acquired and congenital lesions.

electroencephalogram useful tool to provide specific answers to neurologic disorders.

intracranial pressure pressure in the intracranial cavity.

Bibliography

ALTSCHULER, S. M., AND LUDWIG, S. *Pediatrics at a Glance*. Philadelphia: Appleton and Lange, 1997.

BETZ, C. L., et al. *Family-Centered Nursing Care of Children*. 2nd ed. Philadelphia: Saunders, 1994.

BOYTON, R. W., et al. *Manual of Ambulatory Pediatrics*. 3rd ed. Hagerstown, MD: Lippincott, 1994.

BURNS, E. C., et al. *Pediatric Primary Care*. Philadelphia: W. B. Saunders, 1996.

EISENBAUER, L. A., AND MURPHY, M. A. *Pharmacotherapeutics and Advanced Nursing Practice*. New York: McGraw-Hill, 1998.

FITZPATRICK, T. B., et al. *Color Atlas and Synopsis of Clinical Dermatology*. 3rd ed. New York: McGraw-Hill, 1997.

FOX, J. A. *Primary Health Care of Children*. St. Louis: Mosby, 1997.

GRODZIN, C. J., et al. *Diagnostic Strategies for Internal Medicine*. St. Louis: Mosby-Year Book, 1995.

HARRISON, T. R., et al. *Principles of Internal Medicine*. 14th ed. New York: McGraw-Hill, 1998.

HAY, W. W., et al. *Current Pediatric Diagnosis and Treatment*. Stamford, CT: Appleton and Lange, 1997.

JACKSON, P. L., AND VESSEY, J. A. *Primary Care of the Child with a Chronic Condition*. 2nd ed. St. Louis: Mosby, 1996.

KHER, K. K., AND MAKKER, S. P. *Clinical Pediatric Nephrology*. New York: McGraw-Hill, 1992.

KNOOP, K. J., et al. *Atlas of Emergency Medicine*. New York: McGraw-Hill, 1997.

LAGERQUIST, S. L. *Critical Thinking Exercises*. Boston: Little, Brown, 1996.

LORIN, M. I. *Review of Pediatrics*. Stamford, CT: Appleton and Lange, 1993.

OSKI, F. A., et al. *Principles and Practices of Pediatrics*. Hagerstown, MD: Lippincott, 1994.

PANSKY, B. *Review of Gross Anatomy*. 6th ed. New York: McGraw-Hill, 1996.

PIZZUTILLO, P. D. *Pediatric Orthopaedics in Primary Practice*. New York: McGraw-Hill, 1997.

WEINBERG, S., et al. *Color Atlas of Pediatric Dermatology*. 3rd ed. New York: McGraw-Hill, 1997.

WHALEY, L. F., AND WONG, D. L. *Nursing Care of Infants and Children.* 5th ed. St. Louis: Mosby, 1994.

*H*ELPFUL INTERNET SITES

PEDINFO: An Index of the Pediatric Internet at http://www.pedinfo. org   This is an excellent site that covers nearly all topics within this review. It has a wealth of information and is worth a visit. It is written for health care professionals but others could also use the information.

Pediatric Neurological Disorder at hyperlink http://ucneurology. uchicago.edu/Neurological_Disorders/Pediatric_Neuro_Disorders/ pediatric_neuro_disorders.html   This is a University of Chicago site geared to health care professionals. It has excellent information as well as links to similar sites.

NINDS Guide to Health Information about Neurological Disorders at hyperlink http://www.ninds.nih.gov   National Institute of Neurological Disorders and Stroke site that has a large amount of information about neurology disorders in general and specifically about stroke, epilepsy, and Parkinson's disease.

Neurological Disorders in Children at hyperlink http://www. wehealnewyork.org/inn/index.html   This is the index for a Web site developed by the Institute for Neurology and Neurosurgery, Beth Israel Medical Center, North Division, New York City. This site is an informational service for families of children with neurologic and neurosurgical illnesses.

Muscular Dystrophy Association at hyperlink http://www.mdausa. org   The Muscular Dystrophy Association Web site.

Muscular Dystrophy Association at hyperlink http://www.med.unc.edu   Alternate Muscular Dystrophy Association Web site.

National Clearinghouse for Alcohol and Drug Information at hyperlink http://www.health.org   This site is a clearinghouse and a wealth of information on drugs and alcohol, including associated neurologic disorders.

National Multiple Sclerosis Society at hyperlink http://www.nmss. org   National Multiple Sclerosis Society's Web site.

National Neurofibromatosis Foundation at hyperlink http://www. nf.org   National Neurofibromatosis Foundation's Web site.

Capitol Clinical Research Center at hyperlink http://www.centerwatch.com/pro218.htm   This site is dedicated to neurologic clinical trials and other research projects that deal with CNS disorders.

Lamm Institute for Child Neurology and Developmental Medicine at http://www.lich.org/lamm/lamm.html   Lamm Institute for Child Neurology and Developmental Medicine (Long Island, NY), specializing in the diagnosis and management of children with neurologic deficits and related problems of learning.

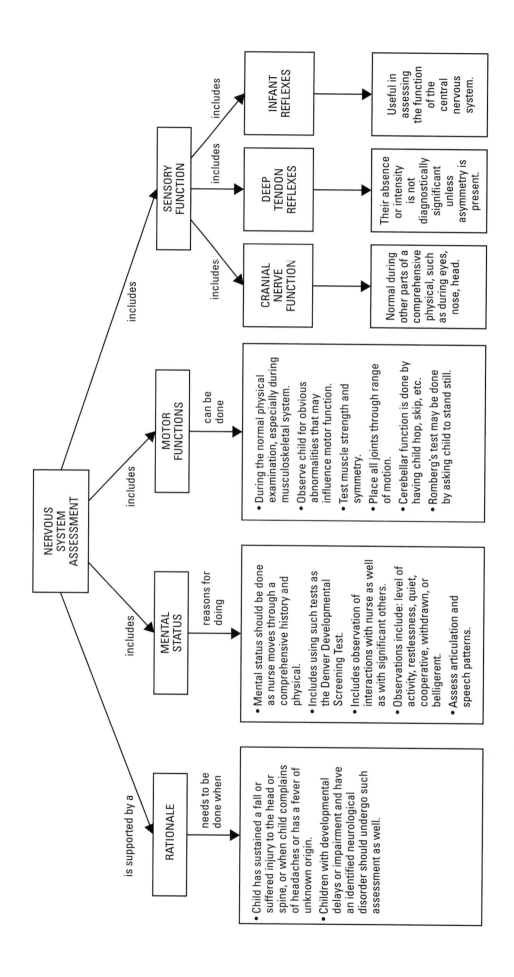

224

Concept Map 7-1

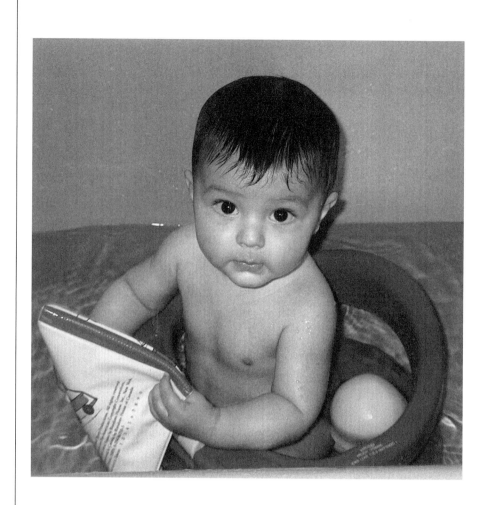

CARDIOVASCULAR DISORDERS

INTRODUCTION

Cardiovascular disorders in children are commonly caused by congenital abnormalities. These abnormalities result in hemodynamic changes in circulation, which eventually affect not only the heart and blood vessels but other organs as well. The cardiovascular diseases common to children will be presented in this chapter. More common congenital abnormalities and acquired conditions that involve the cardiovascular system will be discussed. To understand the physiologic changes related to circulation at birth, fetal circulation (that which occurs while the fetus is in utero) will be discussed first.

Fetal Circulation

Various readjustments to the in utero circulatory pattern occur shortly after birth (Figure 8-1). In utero, the lungs of the fetus do not function as they do after birth; i.e., they are not involved in ventilation (obtaining oxygen from ambient air). Oxygenation of the fetus depends on placental circulation. The circulation of the fetus follows this route: Blood from the inferior vena cava returns to the right atrium straight through the left atrium, through an opening between the right and left atria, the foramen ovale. The oxygenated blood received by the left atrium circulates to the left ventricle, where it is pumped mainly to the vessels of the head and forelimbs. Blood from the superior vena cava, which is mainly deoxygenated, returns to the

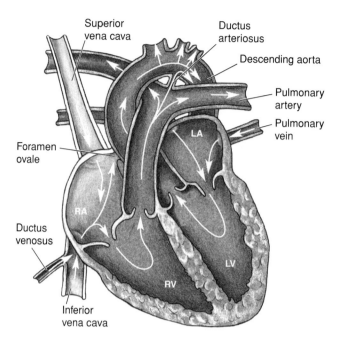

FIGURE 8-1

⬛

Prenatal circulation is different from postnatal circulation because of the structure of the fetal heart. During fetal life the lungs are nonfunctional and the liver is partially functional; therefore less blood supply is needed.

right ventricle through the right atrium, then to the pulmonary artery, and eventually to the aorta via the ductus arteriosus. Only 12% of fetal blood circulates through the lungs. Deoxygenated blood from the aorta circulates to the umbilical arteries, where it is eventually oxygenated.

Circulatory Transitions After Birth

In utero, only 45% of the blood circulates through the heart. The rest is circulated to the placenta. The liver of the fetus is only partially functional; the lungs are not functional. At birth, circulation shifts in the following manner: Once placental circulation no longer exists (when the cord is clamped and cut), systemic vascular resistance increases. These changes in resistance can be likened to crawling through a wide hole (placental circulation) to a little hole (newborn circulation; Figure 8-2). The left heart now has to pump harder against the resistance of the newborn's circulatory vessels. The lungs, which were nonfunctional in utero, now expand and therefore decrease the pulmonary resistance to flow. After birth, the right atrium and the left ventricle have lesser resistance to blood flow because of the resolution of pul-

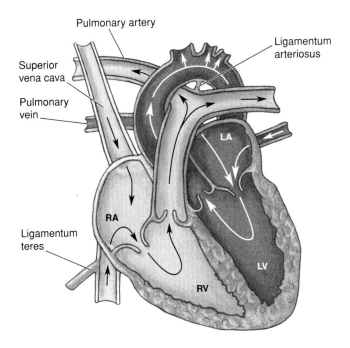

FIGURE 8-2

◙

In postnatal circulation, the circulation through the heart allows for oxygenation of venous blood by the lungs and delivers the saturated blood to the systemic circulation.

monary vasoconstriction and because of lung expansion. These shifts create a higher left atrial pressure and a lower right atrial pressure.

Closure of the Foramen Ovale

Because of the higher left atrial pressure and the lesser right atrial pressure, the valve of the foramen ovale (located on the left atrial side) is pushed shut. This mechanism eventually closes the foramen ovale permanently in two-thirds of all persons (Guyton, 1996).

Closure of the Ductus Arteriosus

It is believed that closure of the ductus arteriosus occurs because of the higher percentage of oxygen passing through the aorta after birth (Figure 8-3). During fetal life, blood passing through the ductus contains approximately 15 to 20 mm Hg of oxygen, compared to 100% saturation of oxygen after birth. This closure is almost complete at the end of the eighth day, eventually becoming a fibrous tissue in 4 months.

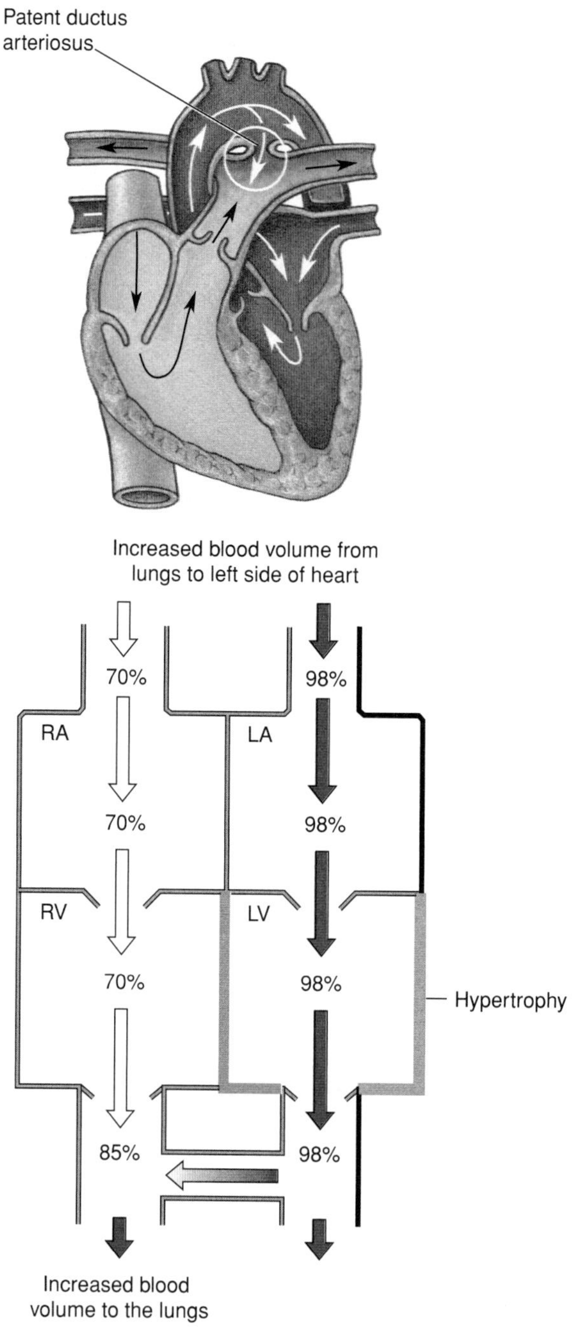

FIGURE 8-3 Patent ductus arteriosus is a function of the fetal ductus arteriosus, closing within the first weeks of life.

CONGENITAL HEART DEFECTS

There are many factors associated with the development of congenital heart defects. They include genetic and environmental factors such as maternal infections during pregnancy, maternal use of drugs, and complications associated with pregnancy and the birthing process (Table 8-1). Congenital heart defects may be described according to the anatomical abnormality that is present, the resulting changes in hemodynamics (flow of blood), or the resulting tissue oxygenation state.

Anatomical abnormalities may include nonclosure of the foramen ovale or the ductus arteriosus, communication between the ventricles resulting from a defect, or misplacement of the great vessels.

◙

TABLE 8-1

ENVIRONMENTAL FACTORS AND
ASSOCIATED CONGENITAL HEART DEFECTS

Cause	Type of Congenital Heart Defect
Infection:	
Intrauterine	PDA, pulmonary stenosis, coarctation of aorta
Systemic viral	PDA, pulmonary stenosis, coarctation of aorta
Rubella	PDA, pulmonary stenosis, coarctation of aorta
Coxsackie B	Endocardial fibroelastosis
Radiation	Specific cardiovascular effect not known
Metabolic disorders:	
Diabetes	VSD, cardiomegaly, transposition of great vessels
Phenylketonuria	Coarctation of aorta, PDA
Hypercalcemia	Supravalvular aortic stenosis, pulmonary stenosis, aortic hyperplasia
Drugs:	
Thalidomide	No specific lesion
Dextroamphetamine	One reported case of transposition
Alcohol	Tetralogy of Fallot, ASD, VSD
Peripheral conditions:	
Increased maternal age	VSD, tetralogy of Fallot (relationship unclear)
Antenatal bleeding	Various defects (relationship unclear)
Prematurity	PDA, VSD
High altitude	PDA, ASD (increased incidence)

PDA, patent ductus arteriosus; VSD, ventricular septal defect; ASD, atrial septal defect.
Source: Huether and McCance, 1996.

Hemodynamic abnormalities occur because of the changes in the circulatory patterns after birth. If structural defects are present, hemodynamic abnormalities are also likely to exist. These abnormalities include those conditions that alter blood flow to the pulmonary circulation.

Tissue oxygenation may also be compromised after birth as a result of congenital heart abnormalities. This is one reason why congenital heart defects may be classified as acyanotic (without cyanosis) or cyanotic. It must be noted, however, that children with acyanotic heart defects may exhibit cyanosis as one of the clinical signs.

OBSTRUCTIVE HEART DEFECTS

Coarctation of the Aorta

Coarctation of the aorta is a narrowing of the lumen of the aorta (Figure 8-4). It can occur in any part of the aorta and may be classified based on its location in relation to the ductus arteriosus. Any narrowing of the aorta causes higher pressures above the site and lower pressures below it (Table 8-2).

Medical Management The patient with coarctation of the aorta may undergo surgery to enlarge the narrowed lumen of the aorta, or to surgically resect the coarctation with eventual end-to-end anastomosis.

FIGURE 8-4

◙

Coarctation of the aorta consists of a flap of tissue that protrudes from the tunica media of the aortic wall. Postductal coarctation occurs after the insertion of the closed ductus arteriosus into the aortic arch. Preductal coarctation occurs before insertion of the patent ductus arteriosus.

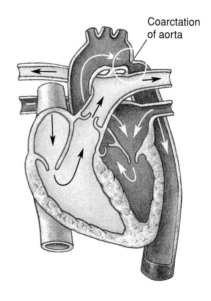

Coarctation of aorta

◙

TABLE 8-2

MANIFESTATIONS OF COARCTATION OF THE AORTA

Sign/Symptom	Hemodynamic Event
CHF	Occurs as a result of left ventricular failure. Blood pressure in the aorta is greater than in the pulmonary artery, causing blood to shunt from the aorta through the ductus and into the pulmonary circulation.
Upper extremity hypertension	Increased pressure in areas proximal to the coarctation.
Weak lower extremity pulses	Decreased pressure in areas distal to the coarctation.
Leg cramps with exercise	Tissue anoxia from decreased blood flow.

CHF, congestive heart failure.
Source: From McCance and Huether, 1998.

Aortic Stenosis

Aortic stenosis is a narrowing of the aortic valve or the aortic outflow tract (Figure 8-5). Normally, the aortic valve has three cusps, but in aortic stenosis there may only be two. This defect is more common in boys than in girls and accounts for 5% of congenital heart defects.

The physiologic changes that occur resulting from the obstruction of flow through the aorta include left ventricular hypertrophy and increased left atrial pressure. The ventricular hypertrophy occurs as a result of the

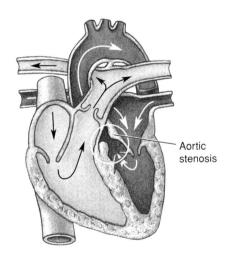

Aortic stenosis

FIGURE 8-5

◙

Aortic stenosis, narrowing of the aortic wall, causes resistance to blood flow in the left ventricle, decreases cardiac output, and causes left ventricular hypertrophy and pulmonary vascular congestion.

increased workload of the left ventricle against the obstruction. Increased left atrial pressure results from the backward pressure that occurs in the left ventricle. These dynamics predispose the child to congestive heart failure (CHF), mitral regurgitation, and in some cases infarction of the myocardium.

The clinical manifestations of aortic stenosis are similar to those found in coarctation of the aorta. In addition, chest pain, poor feeding, and dizziness may occur.

Pulmonic Stenosis

Pulmonic stenosis is a narrowing of the pulmonary outflow tract (Figure 8-6). Because of the narrowing, the right ventricle may hypertrophy and eventually also cause the right atrium to hypertrophy. If the right atrial pressure persists and exceeds left atrial pressure, shunting through the foramen ovale may occur.

In some instances, there may be no blood circulating to the lungs. This condition is known as pulmonary atresia.

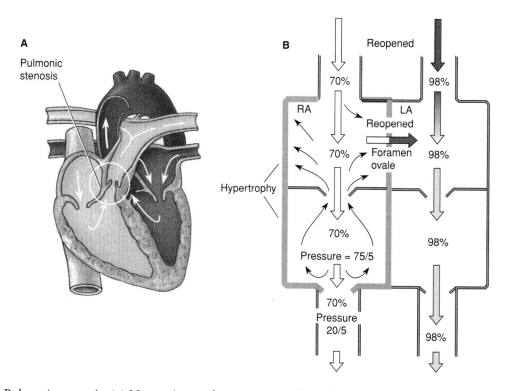

FIGURE 8-6 Pulmonic stenosis. (a) Narrowing at the entrance to the pulmonary artery causes resistance to blood flow, which results in right ventricular hypertrophy and decreased pulmonary blood flow. (b) Left-to-right shunt is caused by backup of ventricular afterload into the right atrium, which reopens the foramen ovale. Venous blood flows from the right atrium, causing left-to-right shunt. Percentages indicate level of O_2 saturation.

The signs of pulmonary stenosis include the presence of a **murmur** and an enlarged cardiac silhouette by x-ray. The child will be cyanotic and may progress to exhibiting the symptoms of left ventricular failure. Intervention includes surgical valvotomy or balloon angioplasty.

Murmur. Abnormal sounds that are heard during the cardiac cycle.

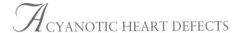

$\mathcal{A}$CYANOTIC HEART DEFECTS

Atrial Septal Defect

This cardiac abnormality, also known as ASD, is characterized by an abnormal opening between the right and left atria, which allows communication and shunting of blood (Figure 8-7). Since the pressure of the left heart is generally greater, a left-to-right shunt (see discussion on shunting) usually occurs.

Children with this cardiac abnormality may not have symptoms. Its diagnosis may be accidentally precipitated by auscultation of a murmur during routine physical examination.

Ventricular Septal Defect

Ventricular septal defect, also known as VSD, is a condition wherein there is a communication between the right and left ventricular compartments (Figure 8-8). VSD accounts for 25 to 33% of all congenital heart defects in children and thus is the most common abnormality.

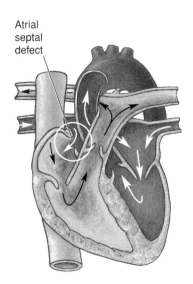

Atrial
septal
defect

FIGURE 8-7

◙

Atrial septal defect (ASD) is an abnormal opening between the atria, which causes blood from the left atrium to flow into the right atrium.

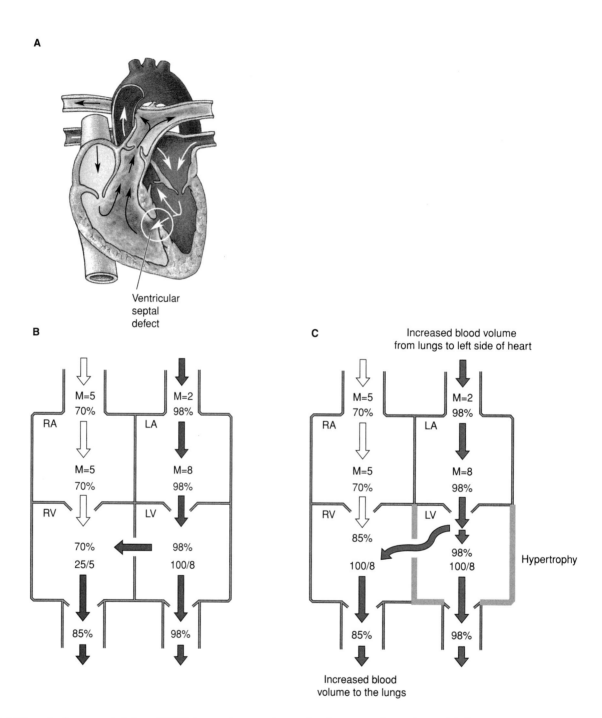

FIGURE 8-8 Ventricular septal defect (VSD) is an abnormal opening between the right and left ventricles. (a) VSD with left-to-right shunt. (b) Hemodynamics of a small VSD with left-to-right shunt. (c) Hemodynamics of a large VSD with left-to-right shunt. Percentages indicate levels of O_2 saturation.

The degree of shunting toward the pulmonary circulation depends on the size of the ventricular defect. Small VSDs have little effect on pulmonary circulation, whereas large VSDs eventually cause left-to-right shunting through the VSD and therefore increase pulmonary circulation through the pulmonary artery. If left untreated, the pulmonary vasculature becomes impaired, eventually leading to an increase in pulmonary resistance. When pulmonary hypertension occurs, the shunt reverses to a right-to-left shunt, a phenomenon called Eisenmenger syndrome. In this condition, venous mixing with arterial blood occurs, and cyanosis develops. Other symptoms associated with VSDs depend on the size of the defect. Large VSDs usually cause pulmonary hypertension, congestive heart failure, poor weight gain, dyspnea, and tachypnea. A physical finding in VSD is a systolic murmur and thrill at the left lower sternal border. This may radiate to the neck.

Electrocardiogram (ECG) examination may assist in evaluating the extent of the shunting that is present. Large VSDs may reveal enlargement of the right ventricle, the left atrium, and the left ventricle. Radiologic examination may also show cardiomegaly and signs of pulmonary hypertension. Echocardiography assists in evaluating the dimensions of the chambers of the heart and shunting patterns.

Some VSDs close spontaneously. Surgical intervention is usually performed during the first year of life on those exhibiting pulmonary hypertension and congestive heart failure.

Electrocardiogram. A noninvasive procedure used to obtain the graphic tracing of the electrical activity of the heart from different locations and in different planes.

Patent Ductus Arteriosus

In this condition, also called PDA, the ductus arteriosus remains patent after birth (Figure 8-9). As will be recalled, the ductus arteriosus is a duct that allows shunting of blood from the pulmonary artery to the aorta (see

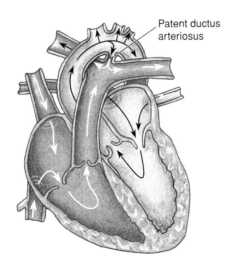

Patent ductus arteriosus

FIGURE 8-9

◙

Patent ductus arteriosus (PDA). Congenital failure of the fetal ductus arteriosus to close within the first weeks of life.

discussion on fetal circulation) during fetal life. Failure of this opening to close allows the greater pressures of the left side of the heart to shunt blood back into the pulmonary circulation. The ductus arteriosus functionally closes 10 to 15 hours after birth. The greater pressures of the aorta after birth allow shunting of blood to the pulmonary arteries. Because of this increase in pulmonary circulation, there will also be a corresponding increase in the workload of the left atrium. In addition, if pulmonary resistance continues to increase, the workload of the right ventricle is affected.

Exposure of the pulmonary vasculature to the higher pressures of the left atrium eventually will cause obstructive pulmonary disease. Because the shunting of blood is generally from an oxygenated source, the resulting manifestation in the child will not include cyanosis (Table 8-3).

Shunting When there is an abnormality in cardiac structure, blood is rerouted through a different pattern (shunt). Shunting may occur from left to right (as seen in patent ductus arteriosus), or right to left (as seen in tetralogy of Fallot). The direction of the shunt depends on which cardiac structure exerts the greatest pressure. The right-to-left shunt causes venous blood to enter the arterial system, thus causing cyanosis. Cyanosis is

🕉

TABLE 8-3

NONOBSTRUCTIVE LESIONS: PATENT DUCTUS ARTERIOSUS

Common congenital defect caused by persistent fetal circulation. When pulmonary circulation is established and systemic vascular resistance increases at birth, pressures in aorta become greater than in pulmonary arteries. Blood is then shunted from aorta to pulmonary arteries, increasing circulation to pulmonary system.

Clinical manifestations: Dyspnea; tachypnea; full, bounding pulses; poor development. Infant is at risk for frequent respiratory infections and subacute endocarditis. When a large PDS exists, congestive heart failure, intercostal retractions, hepatomegaly, and growth failure are also seen. A continuous systolic murmur is auscultated, and a thrill may be palpated in pulmonic area.

Diagnostic tests: When murmur is detected, diagnosis is confirmed by chest x-ray study, ECG, and echocardiogram. Chest x-ray film and ECG show left ventricular hypertrophy, PDA can be visualized, and left-to-right shunt can be measured on echocardiogram.

Medical management: Surgical ligation of PDA is the treatment of choice. Intravenous indomethacin often stimulates closure of the ductus arteriosus in premature infants. Transcatheter closure by obstructive device is sometimes attempted in children older than 18 months.

Prognosis: If PDA is not treated, child's life is shortened because pulmonary hypertension and vascular obstructive disease develop.

PDA, patent ductus arteriosus; ECG, electrocardiogram.

caused by an excessive concentration of deoxygenated **hemoglobin** in the capillaries and appears through the thin skin of the newborn. Cyanosis appears whenever the arterial blood contains more than 5 grams of deoxygenated hemoglobin (Guyton, 1996).

Left-to-Right Shunt The pattern of blood flow in this form of shunting is from the higher pressures of the left side of the heart to the right side. Blood from the left side, which is oxygenated, now shunts through an abnormal opening into the lesser resistance of the right side. The result is a decrease in the amount of blood ejected to the systemic circulation through the aorta. In this form of shunting, life is sustained by compensatory mechanisms to increase cardiac output. However, these mechanisms eventually impair the heart, causing it to fail.

Right-to-Left Shunt In this pattern of shunting, there is mixing of venous blood with the contents of the arterial side of the heart, thus causing cyanosis. The mechanics of how this occurs will be discussed in the section on tetralogy of Fallot.

Physical Findings and Treatment Physical findings in PDA usually include a widened pulse pressure, a continuous machinery-type murmur in the middle-to-left sternal border, and a thrill in the pulmonic area. As a consequence of the increase in pulmonary pressures, the child may exhibit dyspnea, tachypnea, congestive heart failure, poor weight gain, hepatomegaly, and frequent respiratory infections.

EKG examination may reveal chamber enlargement. In addition, radiologic examination may reveal increased pulmonary vascular markings. An **echocardiogram** may confirm the presence of a left-to-right shunt and reveal the PDA.

Indomethacin, a prostaglandin inhibitor, is usually administered to premature infants to stimulate closure of the duct. Surgical ligation of the PDA is usually recommended by age 2 to prevent further pulmonary hypertension and to decrease the risk of developing subacute bacterial endocarditis. The approaches to surgical correction of the PDA include transcatheter, transthoracic, and video-assisted thoracoscopic surgeries. In the transthoracic approach, cardiopulmonary bypass is not necessary because the lesion is extracardiac.

Atrioventricular Canal Defect

Also known as endocardial cushion defect, atrioventricular canal defect (AVC) accounts for 5% of cardiac abnormalities (Figure 8-10). This abnormality is frequently associated with Down syndrome. In AVC defect, the endocardial cushions fail to grow during fetal life, resulting in abnormalities in the septa, the structure that separates the atria and ventricles. Since the endocardial cushion is where the tricuspid and mitral valves grow, abnormalities in the formation of the atrioventricular valves will

Hemoglobin. Index used for diagnosis of anemia or polycythemia; can also reflect degree of desaturation and cyanosis.

Echocardiogram. A noninvasive procedure that reflects sound waves to identify intracardiac structures and their motion.

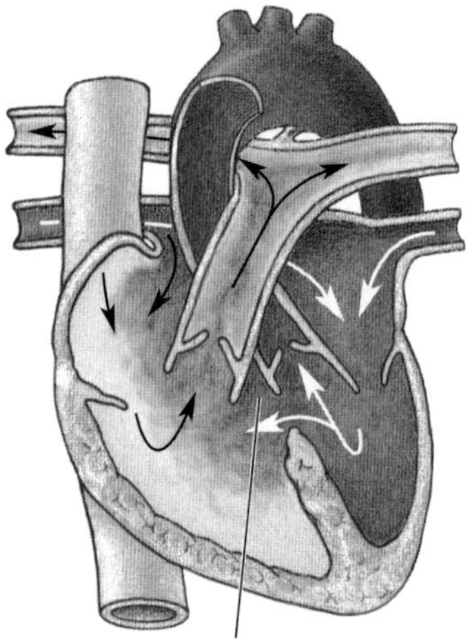

FIGURE 8-10

▣

Atrioventricular canal defect (AVC) is incomplete fusion of endocardial cushions during fetal life. It is the most common cardiac defect in children with Down syndrome.

Atrioventricular
canal defect

also be present. Three types of AVC defects may be seen: complex AVC, partial AVC, or transitional AVC.

Complex AVC defects involve a VSD, an ASD, and clefts in the tricuspid and mitral valves. Partial AVC defects consist of an ASD and a cleft in the anterior leaflet of the mitral valve. Transitional AVC defects involve abnormalities of the mitral and tricuspid valves, which result from partial closure of the endocardial cushions.

Hemodynamic changes associated with this defect depend largely on the type of structural abnormality present. It may mimic the changes seen in ASD or VSD and may result in enlargements of all cardiac chambers. In addition to the shunting that occurs as a result of unfused portions of the atrial and ventricular septa, the abnormalities of the valve structures also allow for regurgitation of blood to the atria.

Findings on physical examination are similar to those found in patients with ventricular septal defects. The regurgitation of blood to the atria may also cause a systolic murmur, which may be heard best at the apex. This murmur may also radiate to the back. Poor growth patterns, CHF, and frequent respiratory infections may also be present.

EKG findings include conduction and axis abnormalities, and ventricular hypertrophies. X-ray findings may include cardiomegaly, changes in the pulmonary vasculature, and a prominent pulmonary artery. Echocardiography reveals the hemodynamic defects, including the size of the chambers. Cardiac catheterization may be done to confirm the location of the defects.

Surgical correction to close the septal defects and to repair valvular defects is usually performed before the age of 1 to prevent pulmonary complications.

Cyanotic cardiac anomalies

Tetralogy of Fallot

The word *tetralogy* suggests that there are four defects present in this congenital condition. The four defects are right ventricular hypertrophy, pulmonary stenosis, usually a large ventricular septal defect (VSD), and overriding of the aorta. The embryonic error that causes these defects is not exactly known. It is a common abnormality, which occurs in 10% of all congenital cardiac defects.

Tetralogy of Fallot (Figure 8-11) does not have one definite pattern and direction of shunting. Although tetralogy of Fallot commonly causes a right-to-left shunt, other hemodynamic factors may produce little or no shunting, or the shunting may be from left to right. When there is no shunting, cyanosis is absent, and these infants are referred to as "pink tets." The major factor that influences the direction of shunting depends on the difference of systemic and pulmonary resistance to flow. In addition, the size of the VSD also influences the direction of shunting. Hypoxemia is usually present because of the mixing of unoxygenated and oxygenated blood leaving the aorta. The body compensates for the low oxygen levels by increasing the production of red blood cells (erythropoiesis). This leads to polycythemia. If cyanosis is chronic, clubbing of the fingers and toes may also be noted on physical examination. There will also be feeding difficulties, poor growth rate, failure to thrive, activity intolerance, and hypoxic spells. "Tet spells" are usually precipitated by crying or exertion. They usually result in dyspnea and cyanosis. These spells usually result from an increase in the shunting of blood from right to left. Older children with these spells usually assume a squatting position, which is a compensatory mechanism to relieve the symptoms. This compensatory mechanism delays venous return to the right heart (similar to applying a tourniquet to the extremities) and increases systemic resistance (or the pressure exerted by aortic flow to the general circulation). The hemodynamic changes that occur with squatting reverse the shunt to a left-to-right shunt.

Other signs of tetralogy of Fallot include a pulmonic systolic ejection murmur, which may radiate to the suprasternal notch. In addition, a ventricular heave may be palpable if right ventricular hypertrophy is present. Metabolic acidosis occurs from the hypoxemia.

Tricuspid Atresia

In this congenital anomaly, the opening between the right atrium and right ventricle is not patent or the tricuspid valve is absent (Figure 8-12). Because there is no opening between the right atrium and the right ventricle, blood from the right atrium circulates through an atrial septal defect to the left atrium, causing it to mix with oxygenated blood.

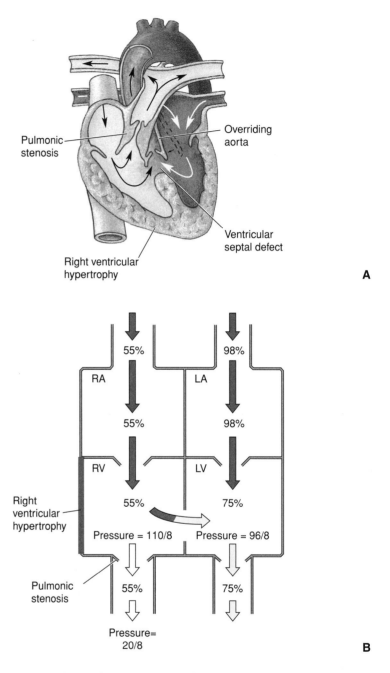

FIGURE 8-11 (a) Tetralogy of Fallot includes four defects: (1) ventricular septal defect, (2) pulmonary stenosis, (3) overriding aorta, (4) right ventricular hypertrophy. (b) Hemodynamics of tetralogy of Fallot with right-to-left shunt. Percentages indicate O_2 saturation levels.

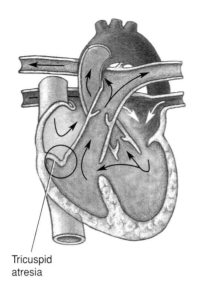

Tricuspid
atresia

FIGURE 8-12

◼

Tricuspid atresia is failure of
the tricuspid valve to develop,
resulting in no communication
between the atrium and the
right ventricle.

𝓜IXED CARDIAC ANOMALIES

Transposition of the Great Vessels

The transposition refers to the pulmonary artery being the outflow tract of
the left ventricle, and the aorta becoming the outflow tract of the right
ventricle (Figure 8-13). In this circulatory pattern, blood from the left ventricle repeatedly circulates into the pulmonary circulation. Therefore, oxygenated blood does not reach the systemic circulation. This lack of
oxygenation is incompatible with life. However, oxygen may be delivered
to the systemic circulation in the presence of any cardiac defect that allows
a communication between two circuits, allowing oxygenated blood to mix
with what is delivered to the general circulation. The presence of a PDA,
ASD, or VSD may allow for such mixing of oxygenated and unoxygenated
blood, which may permit extrauterine survival.

Total Anomalous Pulmonary Venous Return

In this anomaly, the pulmonary veins abnormally connect and empty into
the right atrium (Figure 8-14). The anomaly may also be caused by systemic
veins, which drain into the right atrium. This is an extremely rare condition.

A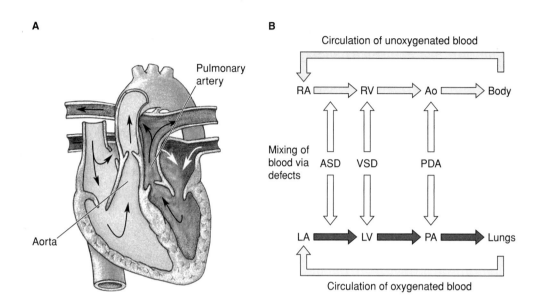

Pulmonary
artery

Aorta

B

Circulation of unoxygenated blood

RA → RV → Ao → Body

Mixing of
blood via   ASD   VSD   PDA
defects

LA → LV → PA → Lungs

Circulation of oxygenated blood

FIGURE 8-13 In transposition of the great vessels, the pulmonary artery leaves the left ventricle, the aorta exits from the right ventricle, with no communication between the systemic and pulmonary circulation.

FIGURE 8-14

◙

Hemodynamics of total anomalous pulmonary venous connections, or failure of the pulmonary veins to join the left atrium; conversely, the pulmonary veins are abnormally connected to the systemic venous circuit via the right atrium.

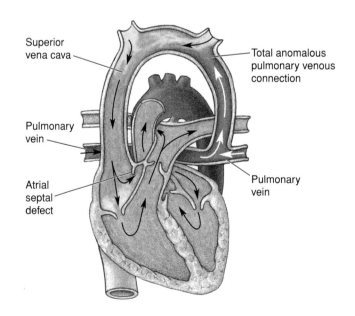

Superior
vena cava

Pulmonary
vein

Atrial
septal
defect

Total anomalous
pulmonary venous
connection

Pulmonary
vein

Truncus Arteriosus

This defect, caused by an embryonic error in which the truncus arteriosus fails to divide, creates a single vessel for the emptying of the right and left ventricles (Figure 8-15). The pulmonary artery and the aorta are therefore one vessel, which provides an outlet for both pulmonary and systemic circulation. Oxygenated and unoxygenated blood are mixed. This defect is usually associated with a VSD.

Hypoplastic Left Heart Syndrome

In hypoplastic left heart syndrome, also called HLHS, the left ventricle, the aorta, and the aortic arch are abnormally underdeveloped (Figure 8-16). This is accompanied by mitral and aortic atresia or stenosis. Survival from this anomaly depends on the presence of a PDA. Blood in the left atrium circulates through the right atrium through an atrial-septal communication and mixes with desaturated blood, then passes through the right ventricle and pulmonary artery to the ductus and finally the descending aorta.

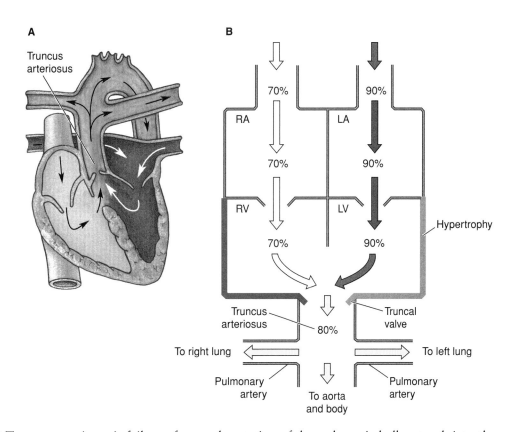

FIGURE 8-15 (a) Truncus arteriosus is failure of normal septation of the embryonic bulbar trunk into the pulmonary artery and aorta. The interventricular septum fails to close at the top. (b) Hemodynamics and alterations in the truncus arteriosus. Percentages indicate O_2 saturation levels.

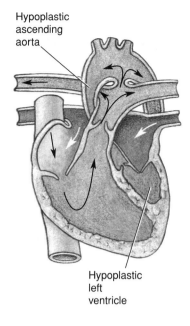

FIGURE 8-16

⬙

Hypoplastic left heart syndrome (HLHS). Underdevelopment of the left side of the heart, resulting in hypoplastic left ventricle and aortic atresia.

Hypoplastic ascending aorta

Hypoplastic left ventricle

$\mathcal{N}$URSING MANAGEMENT OF THE CHILD WITH CONGENITAL HEART DISEASE

The diagnosis of a congenital cardiac abnormality may be made from signs of hypoxia at birth or from the presence of physical signs such as murmurs that have no normal physiologic basis. Echocardiography, electrocardiography, and chest x-ray assist in identifying accompanying structural and hemodynamic changes associated with the abnormality. In addition, **cardiac catheterization** may be necessary to definitively identify the structural anomalies that are present.

The goals of nursing care for a child that has uncorrected cardiac abnormality may center on promoting cardiac output, diminishing respiratory distress, maintaining fluid balance, and promoting growth and development.

Cardiac catheterization.
Invasive procedure that provides information regarding oxygen saturation and pressure in the cardiac chambers, cardiac output, and function.

Cardiac Catheterization

If cardiac catheterization is indicated, the nurse must plan nursing care to assist the child and his/her family in minimizing complications that may arise from the procedure. This includes explaining the purposes of cardiac catheterization: to obtain information about the extent of structural cardiac and vessel abnormalities and the oxygenation levels in various cardiac structures, to assess electrophysiological patterns, and to identify hemodynamic pressures in the heart and great vessels. The procedure may include administration of heparin (to prevent thrombotic events), and the injection of a contrast medium to visualize cardiac structures. The cardiac catheter is usually threaded to the heart through the left femoral artery and/or vein. Local anesthesia is usually used to decrease pain associated with the catheter insertion.

Preparations for cardiac catheterization usually include obtaining the appropriate consent, adhering to institutional procedures for surgical preoperative preparation, putting the child on NPO status, and inserting an intravenous line. Because a dye may be used if angiography is included in the procedure, an accurate history including allergies must be obtained. Assessment of the peripheral pulses prior to the procedure is important because it offers a baseline for comparison after the procedure. Mark the peripheral pulses with a felt-tipped pen to make them more visible. Include the parents in these preparations. The child should be adequately prepared by utilizing developmentally and age-appropriate approaches.

Post–Cardiac Catheterization Care

After the procedure, the child's vital signs must be monitored. The vital signs and blood pressure are usually checked every 15 minutes for the first hour and at scheduled intervals thereafter (check each institutional or cardiologist's policy). Extremity checks, insertion-site checks for bleeding and hematoma formation, and level of consciousness must also be assessed at the same frequency as the vital signs. Because heparin or antithrombotic drugs are utilized prior to, during, or after the procedure, observe for signs of bleeding at the insertion site. Measures to prevent bleeding include maintaining the pressure dressing, applying a sandbag over the insertion site, and minimizing movement of the extremity to prevent disruption of hemostasis.

Other complications after the procedure include vascular occlusion resulting from thrombus formation or swelling. Monitor the quality of the pulse distal to the insertion site. Diminished or absent pulses, coldness and pallor of the distal surface, and diminished capillary refill may signal impaired or blocked arterial circulation. Report these findings immediately to the physician should they occur. Bleeding from the insertion site should be monitored. The pressure dressing is usually removed 24 hours after the procedure. Replace this dressing with a dry 2 × 2 dressing.

Other complications that need to be observed include untoward reactions to the dye, cardiac arrhythmias, cerebrovascular obstructive events, pulmonary emboli, hypotension, and infection. Since this procedure may be done on an outpatient basis, the parents should be taught the potential complications discussed previously and how to monitor the child's temperature (to watch for a fever of 101.3°F or higher), to observe for drainage or discharge at the insertion site, and to report these findings to their physician.

*A*CQUIRED DISORDERS OF THE CARDIOVASCULAR SYSTEM

Acquired disorders of the cardiovascular system in children include congestive heart failure, primary hypertension, rheumatic heart disease, and Kawasaki disease. These conditions are disorders that occur after birth and may result from congenital heart defects or other environmental factors.

Congestive Heart Failure

Congestive heart failure (Table 8-4) is a condition wherein the heart is unable to function effectively as a pump, resulting in its inability to meet the metabolic demands of the body. Since the function of the heart is to

◙

TABLE 8-4
CONGENITAL HEART DEFECTS CAUSING CONGESTIVE HEART FAILURE

Age	Congenital Heart Defect
Time of birth	Hypoplastic left heart syndrome
	Volume overload caused by tricuspid regurgitation
	Arterial venous fistula
Birth to 1 week	Hypoplastic left heart syndrome
	Aortic atresia
	Transposition of the great vessels
	Coarctation of the aorta
	TAPVC with obstruction
	PDA in premature infants
First 4 weeks	Coarctation of the aorta
	TAPVC
	Large left-to-right shunt caused by VSD, PDA in premature infants
	Tricuspid atresia
	All previously mentioned defects
4–6 weeks	Transposition of the great vessels
	Large left-to-right shunt caused by endocardial cushion defect
6 weeks to 6 months	VSD
6 months	Endocardial fibroelastosis
	Persistent truncus arteriosus with large left-to-right shunt

TAPVC, total anomalous pulmonary venous connection; PDA, patent ductus arteriosus; VSD, ventricular septal defect.
Source: McCance and Huether, 1998.

provide a mechanism for distribution of oxygen and nutrients to all parts of the body, its failure will have consequences in all major organs and systems. The most common cause of congestive heart failure in children is congenital cardiac abnormalities.

Congestive heart failure may be classified according to which side of the heart has "failed" (right versus left heart failure), by overall manifestations (backward failure versus forward failure), or by pathophysiology (systolic versus diastolic dysfunction).

Pathophysiology Shunting of blood resulting from cardiac anomalies results in inefficiency of the heart as a pump. The diminished cardiac output stimulates the release of compensatory mechanisms such as catecholamines. This results in increased heart rate and force of contraction. Like any other compensatory mechanisms, they eventually fail. With diminished cardiac output and subsequent decrease in renal flow, the renin-angiotensin mechanism is activated. This also results in the activation of aldosterone, which facilitates the reabsorption of sodium. Increased serum sodium in turn increases blood volume, which increases even more the workload of the already failing heart.

Clinical Manifestations The manifestations of congestive heart failure in the child include dyspnea, difficulty in feeding, failure to thrive, edema, and tachycardia. Dyspnea occurs primarily with activity such as feeding. Because of this difficulty, it might take a long time for the infant to complete feeding. This leads to a severe lack of nutritional balance. Respiratory findings such as tachypnea, cough, orthopnea, chest retractions, wheezing, rales, and rhonchi may all be caused by pulmonary interstitial accumulation of fluid resulting from left ventricular failure. Peripheral edema results from backward pressure and may even cause hepatomegaly, a condition wherein the liver becomes engorged. This may be evident on physical examination. Periorbital edema (edema around the eyes) may also be noted. Because of fluid retention, the child may demonstrate an increase in weight and head circumference. Tachycardia results as a compensatory effort to maintain the metabolic demands of the body.

Nursing Management Careful assessment of the physical signs of congestive heart failure will lead to early diagnosis and treatment. Observe the developmental pattern of the infant. Delays in growth may be attributable to poor feeding patterns due to congestive heart failure. Respiratory difficulty, especially with activity such as feeding, may be a classic sign. The respiratory rate may be increased to over 40 breaths per minute and may be accompanied by nasal flaring, cyanosis, wheezing, coughing, grunting, and rales on auscultation. Irritability may be present. Hepatomegaly and periorbital edema may also be evident. Weight gain and ascites may be a sign of fluid accumulation. In children, jugular neck vein distention may be present. However, this finding may not be visible in neonates because of their short necks.

Chest x-ray examination may reveal enlargement of the heart and the presence of increased pulmonary vascularity. An EKG may also help to determine the extent of cardiac enlargement.

The goal of treatment for children with congestive heart failure is to restore to some degree the heart's efficiency as a pump. This includes measures to improve cardiac output, improve tissue oxygenation, decrease venous return of blood to the right ventricle, and diminish cardiac demands for oxygen. In addition, the nurse implements actions to assist in breathing as well as to promote physical growth by ensuring proper nutrition.

The administration of digitalis in CHF is to increase the force of cardiac contraction and improve cardiac output. This therapeutic regimen is aimed at improving the forward flow of blood and therefore meeting the body's metabolic demands. Diuretics may also be administered to decrease the amount of fluid circulating through the heart. Decreasing the amount of volume circulating gives the heart an opportunity to pump more efficiently. Oxygen may also be administered to the child in congestive heart failure to ensure that tissues receive adequate amounts of oxygen. Feeding through a nasogastric tube may be necessary to maintain the child's nutritional status. High-calorie, low-sodium supplements may be prescribed to meet the child's caloric needs.

Positioning in a semi-upright position (such as in an infant seat), or held upright with the knees bent to decrease venous return assists in easing the breathing patterns of the child. Frequent, short feedings need to be included in the nursing care plan. The use of a soft nipple for infants who are bottle-fed may also reduce the energy required to suck. Also, plan to space nursing interventions so that the child has frequent rest periods, which helps to minimize cardiac demand for oxygen.

Careful monitoring of the effects of therapy (digitalis, diuretics, oxygen, and nutritional support) is an essential nursing measure. Daily weights and accurate intake and output should be measured to determine the effectiveness of therapeutic interventions. Weights should be taken at the same time each day. Weigh diapers to ensure an accurate output recording.

The use of diuretics may decrease serum potassium and therefore laboratory monitoring should be necessary. Digitalis can have toxic effects, so careful monitoring of serum digoxin levels is needed.

Parental support is essential in the management of infants and children with congestive heart failure. Allow parents the opportunity to verbalize their concerns. Listen to the parents' questions about the child's condition. Teach parents about the disease. Assist them in understanding the therapeutic regimen and coach them in the proper administration of medications, particularly the accurate measurement of diuretics and digoxin elixir. Instruct them on the monitoring of the patient's pulse prior to administration of digoxin (see guidelines for administering digoxin at home in Table 8-5). Instructions should also include monitoring of digitalis toxicity and hypokalemia. Digitalis toxicity may be difficult for parents to identify, particularly because the classic signs found in adults may not be manifested in the same manner in children. Typically, feeding difficulties may be associated with digitalis toxicity. Discuss with the parents the signs of congestive heart failure and instruct them to contact their medical provider immediately if these symptoms are noted.

◪

TABLE 8-5

GUIDELINES FOR ADMINISTERING DIGOXIN AT HOME

Give digoxin at regular intervals, usually every 12 hours, such as 8 AM and 8 PM.

Plan the times so that the drug is given 1 hour before or 2 hours after feedings.

Use a calendar to mark off each dose that is given or post a reminder, such as a sign on the refrigerator.

Have the prescription refilled before the medication is completely used.

Administer the drug carefully by slowly directing it on the side and back of the mouth.

Do not mix it with other foods or fluids, since refusal to consume these results in inaccurate intake of the drug.

If the child has teeth, give water after administering the drug; whenever possible, brush the teeth to prevent tooth decay from the sweetened liquid.

If a dose is missed and more than 4 hours has elapsed, withhold the dose and give the next dose at the regular time; if less than 4 hours has elapsed, give the missed dose.

Do not give a second dose if the child vomits.

Notify the practitioner if more than two consecutive doses have been missed.

Do not increase or double the dose for missed doses.

Notify the practitioner immediately if the child becomes ill.

Keep digoxin in a safe place, preferably a locked cabinet.

In case of accidental overdose of digoxin, call the nearest poison control center immediately.

Source: Oski, 1994

Primary Hypertension

The American Academy of Pediatrics identifies hypertension in children (Table 8-6) as an average systolic or diastolic blood pressure of 95 mm Hg or above in three consecutive readings. The pathophysiologic mechanisms of hypertension in children are not clear. However, risk factors such as obesity, hyperlipidemia, hypercholesterolemia, and smoking may influence the development of hypertension. Other risk factors are still under scrutiny, especially to determine if risk factors found in adults may also be true in children. It is recommended that children age 3 through adolescence should have their blood pressure checked at least once a year, especially those who have a strong familial history of the disease.

TABLE 8-6

CLASSIFICATION OF HYPERTENSION IN THE YOUNG BY AGE GROUP

Age Group	High Normal (90–94th Percentile) mm Hg	Significant Hypertension (95–99th Percentile) mm Hg	Severe Hypertension (>99th Percentile) mm Hg
Newborns (SBP)			
7 d	—	96–105	≥ 106
8–30 d	—	104–109	≥ 110
Infants (≤ 2 y)			
SBP	104–111	112–117	≥118
DBP	70–73	74–81	≥ 82
Children (3–5 y)			
SBP	108–115	116–123	≥124
DBP	70–75	76–83	≥84
Children (6–9 y)			
SBP	114–121	122–129	≥130
DBP	74–77	78–85	≥86
Children (10–12 y)			
SBP	122–125	126–133	≥134
DBP	78–81	82–89	≥90
Children (13–15 y)			
SBP	130–135	136–143	≥144
DBP	80–85	86–91	≥ 92
Adolescents (16–18 y)			
SBP	136–141	142–149	≥150
DBP	84–91	92–97	≥ 98

SBP, systolic blood pressure; DBP, diastolic blood pressure.
Source: Joint National Committee on Detection, Evaluation and Treatment of High Blood Pressure, 1993.

Kawasaki Disease

A mucocutaneous lymph node syndrome known as Kawasaki disease, although seen mainly in Japan, is the most common cause of acquired heart disease in children in the United States today. Its incidence in males is slightly higher than in females. Kawasaki disease also occurs in other ethnic groups and throughout the world. Kawasaki disease is characterized by systemic vasculitis and may present itself as a febrile illness. The diagnostic criteria for Kawasaki disease are given in Table 8-7.

During the acute phase of the illness, the nursing intervention should include monitoring for cardiovascular complications. These complications include pericarditis, myocarditis, and arteritis. Myocardial infarction may also occur, resulting from coronary artery aneurysms. Since fever is a characteristic of this disease during the acute phase, febrile seizures may occur. Medical treatment usually includes administration of antiplatelet agents (high doses of aspirin) and immune globulin.

⌖

TABLE 8-7

CRITERIA FOR DIAGNOSIS OF KAWASAKI DISEASE

---

1. Fever lasting ≥5 d
2. Bilateral conjunctivitis
3. Changes of lips and oral cavity
   a. Dry, red, fissured lips
   b. Strawberry tongue
   c. Diffuse erythema of mucous membranes
4. Changes of peripheral extremities
   a. Erythema of palms and soles
   b. Indurative edema of hands and feet
   c. Membranous desquamation from fingertips
5. Polymorphous rash (primarily on trunk)
6. Acute nonpurulent swelling of cervical lymph node to >1.5 cm in diameter

---

Source: Joint National Committee on Detection, Evaluation, and Treatment of High Blood Pressure, 1993.

SUMMARY

In this chapter, common congenital abnormalities involving cardiac structures were discussed. Congenital heart defects may be described according to the anatomical abnormality that is present or based on the resulting hemodynamic changes associated with those structural abnormalities. Understanding the structural and physiologic changes associated with these abnormalities, including the differences in cyanotic and acyanotic conditions, assists the nurse in identifying the appropriate nursing and medical interventions.

CRITICAL POINTS IN THE MANAGEMENT OF CARDIOVASCULAR DISORDERS

The most important intervention in the treatment of cardiovascular disorders is first to help parents acquire a basic understanding of their child's defect or condition, in order to recognize complications and relieve their anxiety. The child will probably have ongoing care from the health team, so it is essential that the family learn new coping strategies. The care of these children usually involves years of treatment, so the nurse must emphasize the normal aspects of the child's growth and development, as well as the limitations that these conditions present. Families should be encouraged to seek help from support groups that will provide additional information. Families also are faced with the reality that they have to make life-style changes regarding nutrition, exercise, and stress management. Medication management should be taught in detail, and often it is necessary to repeat these instructions more than once. Parents also need to be taught cardiopulmonary resuscitation (CPR). This is a process to which parents may not respond well, not because they do not want to learn, but because of its implications. If permitted by the parents, the nurse ought to make a community family referral. This helps families to assess their functioning and helps with health promotion.

Cardiovascular disorders always require specialized laboratory testing; therefore, it is very important for the nurse to have a thorough knowledge of all the tests and laboratory results. Families with children with heart problems often have a history of cardiac problems. The nurse must assess the anxiety that this causes parents. Issues of guilt or blame can destroy homes and relationships. The care of these children is multifaceted and multidisciplinary. If there is a critical phrase, it is that the medical team is dealing not with one broken heart, but with many broken hearts, and all of them need repair at the same time.

$\mathcal{Q}$UESTIONS

Diagnosis: Congenital Heart Defect

History: Baby Thomas was born 3 hours ago. The pediatrician noted that based on physical observations, the child likely has a congenital heart defect.

Plan: To stabilize Thomas hemodynamically and let him go home with his parents. The management of this condition is based on its seriousness.

Nursing problems: Crisis intervention for the parents. Medical management of medication to promote closure. Close assessment of the child to detect any critical changes. Reassurance and support of the parents.

Chief concerns of the nurse: To support the infant physiologically prior to, during, and after treatment. To reassure the parents and allow them to verbalize their fears and concerns. To promote bonding of parents and child.

1. The valve of the foramen ovale is pushed shut shortly after birth by which physiologic mechanism?
   A. The release of prostaglandins directly constricts the opening.
   B. Higher pressures in the left atrium after birth cause the valve to shut.
   C. Blood from the left ventricle regurgitates into the left atrium causing it to shut.
   D. Increased oxygen content of blood after birth allows adhesions to form over the ovale.

2. A newborn is diagnosed as having patent ductus arteriosus. Which physiologic event will most likely occur?
    A. A left-to-right shunt, which will cause mixing of arterial and venous blood.
    B. A right-to-left shunt, which will cause cyanosis.
    C. Pulmonary circulation will be bypassed.
    D. No significant shunting will occur.

3. A child is diagnosed with coarctation of the aorta. Which of the following signs or symptoms indicate shunting of blood from the aorta through the ductus and into the pulmonary circulation?
    A. Leg cramps with exercise
    B. Weak lower extremity pulses
    C. Upper extremity hypertension
    D. Congestive heart failure

4. An ECG was ordered for an infant diagnosed with ventricular septal defect. Which of the nurse's explanations to the mother is the most accurate?
    A. The ECG will identify the presence of arrhythmias.
    B. The ECG will assist in evaluating the extent of the shunting that is present.
    C. An ECG assists in evaluating the dimensions of the cardiac chambers.
    D. An ECG is most helpful in identifying the presence of congestive heart failure.

5. Tetralogy of Fallot is a combination of which four cardiac defects?
    A. Right ventricular hypertrophy, pulmonary stenosis, atrial septal defect, and overriding of the aorta
    B. Right ventricular hypertrophy, patent ductus arteriosus, transposition of the great vessels, and ventricular septal defect
    C. Right ventricular hypertrophy, pulmonary stenosis, ventricular septal defect, and overriding of the aorta
    D. Left ventricular hypertrophy, atrial septal defect, ventricular septal defect, aortic stenosis, and pulmonary stenosis

6. A child with tetralogy of Fallot squats to relieve a "tet spell." This compensatory mechanism relieves the symptoms by:
    A. Delaying venous return to the heart.
    B. Increasing venous return to the heart.
    C. Increasing the production of red blood cells.
    D. Allowing maximal chest expansion and oxygenation.

7. A child with congestive heart failure may have nutritional deficiencies associated with the condition. An appropriate intervention to include in the nursing care plan is to:
    A. Increase the daily oral intake of liquids.
    B. Position the infant flat to increase nutritional absorption.
    C. Encourage frequent and short feedings.
    D. Discourage breast-feeding.

8. Which physiologic response would be expected in a child with transposition of the great vessels?

    A. Decreased red blood cell count

    B. Clubbing of the fingers

    C. Petechiae

    D. Hyperkalemia

9. An 8-year-old child is scheduled for surgical correction of coarctation of the aorta. Which of the following assessment findings related to blood pressure would the nurse expect?

    A. A higher blood pressure in the upper extremity than in the lower extremity.

    B. No difference in readings between upper and lower extremities.

    C. A lower systolic pressure in the upper extremities.

    D. No audible blood pressure is audible in any extremity.

10. Ravella is diagnosed with congestive heart failure. She receives Lanoxin. Which of these findings indicates an early sign of digitalis toxicity?

    A. Sunken eyeballs

    B. Refusal to eat

    C. Loose stools

    D. Depressed respirations

$\mathcal{A}$NSWERS

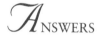

1. *B.* Shortly after birth, the right atrium and the left ventricle have lower resistance to blood flow because of the resolution of pulmonary vasoconstriction and because of lung expansion. Because of the higher left atrial pressure, the valve of the foramen ovale is pushed shut.

2. *A.* Shunting occurs from left to right due to the higher pressures of the left side of the heart. The shunting of blood from the left side, which is oxygenated, to the lesser resistance of the right side causes a decrease in the amount of blood ejected to the systemic circulation through the aorta. Because the shunting of blood is generally from an oxygenated source, the resulting manifestation in the child will not include cyanosis.

3. *D.* Since the blood pressure is greater in the aorta than in the pulmonary artery, the shunting of blood into the pulmonary circulation causes congestion in the lungs, which manifests itself in the classic signs of congestive heart failure resulting from left ventricular failure.

4. *B.* The ECG reveals manifestations of the cardiac structures that are enlarged and thus assists in identifying the degree of shunting that is present. Although ECGs also reveal the presence of arrhythmias, the primary reason for this procedure is to determine shunting patterns. To evaluate the dimensions of the chambers of the heart, echocardiography is more useful.

5. *C.* The word *tetralogy* suggests four defects, which include right ventricular hypertrophy, pulmonary stenosis, usually a large ventricular septal defect (VSD), and overriding of the aorta.

6. *A.* "Tet spells" usually result in dyspnea and cyanosis. Squatting delays venous return to the right heart and increases systemic resistance. These hemodynamic changes reverse the shunt to a left-to-right shunt.

7. *C.* Dyspnea occurs primarily with activities such as feeding, which causes feedings to be completed in a longer period of time. Short and frequent feedings decrease the cardiac demand for oxygen necessary for feeding. The child with congestive heart failure must be positioned semi-upright to decrease venous return and assist in breathing.

8. *B.* In this condition, there is chronic hypoxia due to cyanotic conditions. Chronic hypoxia causes the distal phalanges of the fingers to become rounded and bulbous, making the nail plate more convex. The proximal nail fold increases to 180° or more (clubbing).

9. *A.* A narrowing of the aorta causes higher pressure above the site and lower pressure below it.

10. *B.* Digitalis toxicity in children is manifested by feeding problems associated with nausea, which the child cannot verbalize.

$\mathcal{B}$IBLIOGRAPHY

BALL, J., AND BINDLER, R. *Pediatric Nursing: Caring for Children.* Norwalk, CT: Appleton & Lange, 1995.

GUYTON, A. C., AND HALL, J. E. *Medical Physiology.* 9th ed. St. Louis: Mosby, 1996.

HUETHER, S., AND MCCANCE, K. *Pathophysiology: The Biologic Basis for Disease in Adults and Children.* St. Louis: Mosby, 1996.

JACKSON, P. L. Digoxin therapy at home: Keeping the child safe. *American Journal of Maternal Child Nursing* 4(2):105–109, 1979.

Joint National Committee on Detection, Evaluation, and Treatment of High Blood Pressure (JNC V). *Archives of Internal Medicine* 153: 154–183, 1993.

MCCANCE, K. L., AND HUTHER, S. E. *Pathophysiology: The Biologic Basis for Disease in Adults and Children.* St. Louis: Mosby, 1990.

OSKI, F. *Principles and Practice of Pediatrics.* Philadelphia: Lippincott, 1994.

Task Force on Blood Pressure Control in Children. Report on the second task force of blood pressure control in children—1987. *Pediatrics* 79: 1–25, 1987.

WHALEY, L., AND WONG, D. *Nursing Care of Infants and Children.* St. Louis: Mosby, 1991.

*G*LOSSARY

cardiac catheterization   invasive procedure that provides information regarding oxygen saturation and pressure in the cardiac chambers, cardiac output, and function.

echocardiogram   a noninvasive procedure that reflects sound waves to identify intracardiac structures and their motion.

electrocardiogram   a noninvasive procedure used to obtain the graphic tracing of the electrical activity of the heart from different locations and in different planes.

hemoglobin   index used for diagnosis of anemia or polycythemia; can also reflect degree of desaturation and cyanosis.

murmur   abnormal sounds that are heard during the cardiac cycle.

*H*ELPFUL INTERNET SITES

PEDINFO: An Index of the Pediatric Internet at http://www. pedinfo.org   This is an excellent site that covers nearly all topics within this review. It has a wealth of information and is worth a visit. It is written for health care professionals but others could also use the information.

University of Michigan Congenital Heart Center at hyperlink http:// www.umchc.pdc.med.umich.edu/prof/bio_bove.html   This is a Web site for professionals as well as parents.

Galaxy at http://galaxy.einet.net/galaxy/Medicine/Health-Occupations/ Medicine/Medical-Specialties/Internal-Medicine/Cardiology.html This is a commercial site that has multiple links to a vast collection of information, including cardiovascular disorders.

Pediatric Cardiology Almanac at http://www.neosoft.com/~rlpierce/ pc.htm   This site has multimedia educational resources, a selection on pediatric ECG interpretation, and many other useful resources. It is geared more toward cardiologists than laypersons, but is a good resource for pediatric nurses as well.

Web Links of Interest to Pediatric Cardiology at http://www.bcm. tmc.edu/pedi/cardio/other-medical-links.html   This site has numerous links to pediatric cardiology sites as well as other general sites of interest to health care professionals.

Congenital Heart Defect Electrocardiograms at http://www.kumc.edu/ instruction/medicine/pedcard/cardiology/pedelectrocardiograms.html An excellent site for those who need electrocardiograms. It shows various heart defects in pediatric patients.

Pediatric Cardiology and Critical Care at http://www.kumc.edu/instruction/medicine/pedcard/cardiology/cardiology.html Teaching Resources for Health Sciences Faculty and Students Web site, maintained by the University of Kansas Medical Center. The site is aimed at faculty and medical students but is also an excellent resource for nurses.

CARDIOVASCULAR SYSTEM ASSESSMENT

includes the

VASCULAR SYSTEM

palpate the

Peripheral arteries for equality, rhythm, and pulse rate.
- Radial pulse
- Femoral pulse
- Popliteal pulse
- Dorsalis pedis pulse

includes the

HEART

includes

PALPATION:
- Anterior chest for apical pulse

includes

PERCUSSION:
- Used to estimate heart size by outlining cardiac borders.

includes

AUSCULATION:
- S_1 to S_2
- Additional sounds of S_3 to S_4

Assessing:
- Rate
- Rhythm

includes

INSPECTION:
- Observe child's body posture.
- Observe child for cyanosis, mottling, and edema.
- Observe for respiratory difficulty (grunting, costal retractions, flaring of nares, adventitious sound) and hacking cough.
- Inspect nailbeds for clubbing, lengthening, or widening.
- Examine anterior chest from an angle. Observe for symmetry of chest movement, visible pulsations, and diffuse lifts or heaves.

Concept Map 8-1

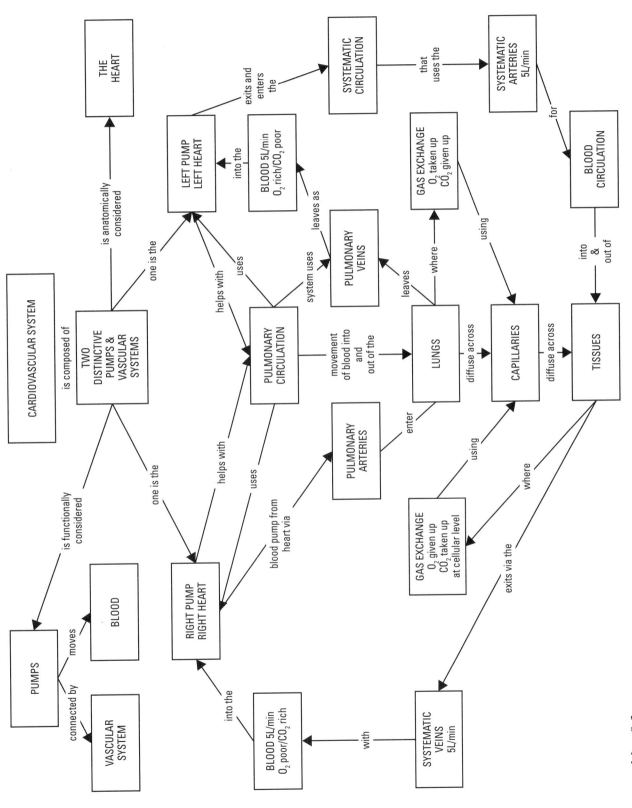

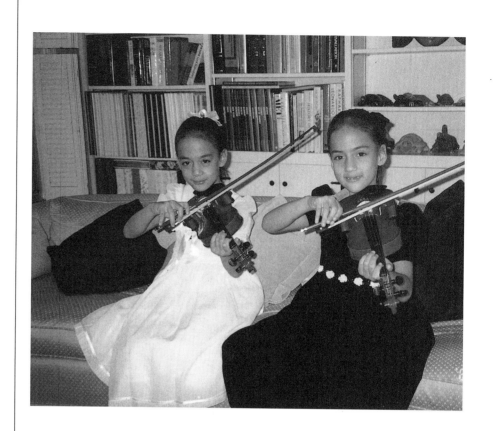

RESPIRATORY DISORDERS

INTRODUCTION

Respiratory disorders are the most common health problem in children. Most upper airway infections are caused by viruses and may be acute or chronic. The etiology and clinical manifestations of the respiratory disorders are influenced by the age of the child, the size of the anatomical structures of the respiratory system, the underlying pathophysiology, the part of the respiratory tract that is affected (upper or lower tract), and the seasons.

A respiratory assessment is basic to the care of the child with respiratory disorder. First, a complete health history is taken, followed by a physical examination. The rate, depth, and ease of respiration are assessed and documented; lung sounds are auscultated; and the child's skin color is noted.

RESPIRATORY ASSESSMENT

Observe the rate, depth, ease, and rhythm of respirations:

Rate—tachypnea (increased rate), bradypnea (slowed rate), or normal for child's age.
Depth—hypopnea (shallow respirations) indicates exchange of small volumes of air; hyperpnea (deep respirations) indicates exchange of large volumes of air; or normal for child's size and age.

Ease—dyspnea (shortness of breath or difficulty breathing) or effort-free breathing.

Rhythm—variation in depth and rate of respirations.

Other findings may include:

Adventitious breath sounds—wheezing, crackles, or rhonchi may indicate airway obstruction or bronchial obstruction.

Absent or diminished breath sounds—may indicate atelectasis (alveolar collapse) or bronchial obstruction.

Cyanosis—blue-colored tinge to skin, mucous membranes, and nail beds may indicate hypoxia (oxygen deficit).

Circumoral cyanosis—bluish ring around the mouth may indicate respiratory failure.

Retractions—inspiratory or "sinking in" of the soft tissues of the thorax may indicate respiratory difficulty.

Cough—may be dry or moist, nonproductive or productive; note frequency and character.

Sputum—note amount, color, viscosity, and odor; green- or yellow-tinged sputum signals infection.

Chest pain—pain on inspiration may indicate cardiac or pulmonary disease; some children experience referred abdominal pain.

Nasal flaring—may indicate respiratory distress.

Grunting—sounds during expiration which may indicate respiratory distress.

Restlessness—may indicate hypoxia and impending respiratory failure.

NASOPHARYNGITIS (COMMON COLD)

The common cold is the most frequent respiratory infection of childhood. Colds are usually caused by any one of a number of viruses. The principal viruses are respiratory syncytial virus (RSV), adenovirus, or rhinovirus. Symptoms of nasopharyngitis tend to be more severe in infants and children, and young children are more prone to develop complications than adults. The young infant is as susceptible as the older child, but is not as frequently exposed.

Clinical Manifestations

Young infants are usually afebrile. Infants older than 3 months develop fever in the course of infection, often as high as 104°F (40°C). The infant sneezes and is restless. Congested nasal passages interfere with feeding, increasing irritability. Infants may have accompanying vomiting and diarrhea caused by mucus entering the gastrointestinal tract. The older child may be febrile and may have severe pharyngitis (red, inflamed throat), sometimes a cough, nasal secretions, anorexia, and headache.

Diagnosis

Nasopharyngitis is diagnosed by the history and presenting clinical manifestations. The condition may precede many childhood contagious diseases and needs to be evaluated carefully. Common colds should be differentiated from allergic rhinitis.

Therapeutic Management

The child with uncomplicated nasopharyngitis does not require hospitalization. Antibiotic therapy and antihistamines are usually ineffective. Increased oral fluids, adequate nutrition, rest, normal saline nose drops, nasal suction with a bulb syringe for infants, and a humidified environment are usually all that is necessary. Antipyretics are administered for fever. Decongestants, to decrease swelling of the nasal passages, may be ordered for children older than 6 months. If symptoms persist for longer than 7 days, the child needs to be medically reevaluated to rule out complications such as otitis media or sinusitis.

$\mathcal{B}$RONCHIOLITIS

Bronchiolitis is an acute respiratory viral infection mainly affecting the bronchioles. It occurs with greatest frequency during the first 6 months of life and is rarely seen after the age of 2 years. Respiratory syncytial virus (RSV) is the causative agent in more than half of all cases of bronchiolitis. The virus is predominant in the late fall and winter months and is easily spread by droplet and hand-to-nose transmission.

Pathophysiology

The mucosa of the bronchi and bronchioles become swollen and inflamed. Thick respiratory secretions accumulate, plugging the bronchiolar lumen. The narrowing of the small airways compromises expiration, trapping air in the alveoli. The infant can breathe air in, but has difficulty expelling it. This trapped air causes lung hyperinflation and may lead to atelectasis. Inadequate gas exchange results in **hypoxemia** and **hypercapnia**.

Hypoxemia. Abnormally decreased arterial blood oxygen in the blood.

Hypercapnia. Greater than normal amounts of carbon dioxide in the blood.

Diagnosis

Diagnosis of bronchiolitis is made on the clinical findings, the age of the child, and the season. Bronchiolitis begins with symptoms of a mild upper respiratory infection accompanied by clear nasal secretions, sneezing, cough, poor appetite, and possibly a low-grade fever. Infants who are still bottle- or breast-fed are unable to suck because of increased respiratory effort. As these mild symptoms worsen, the child develops increasing respiratory distress with **tachypnea**, shallow respirations, wheezing, **retractions**, dyspnea, and a productive, congested cough. **Apnea** (cessation of breathing for longer than 20 seconds) may be a serious manifestation in very young infants.

Therapeutic Management

Most children with bronchiolitis can be treated at home. The infant with serious respiratory symptoms is usually hospitalized. Medical treatment involves giving oxygen if necessary, high humidity, fluids, and rest. Monitoring of oxygenation is done by pulse oximetry. Administration of oxygen is by tent, mask, or nasal cannula to keep oxygen saturation above 95%. Chest physiotherapy (CPT), which includes percussion, vibration, and postural drainage, helps to clear the lungs of excess mucus. The child receives intravenous (IV) fluids to maintain hydration and thin secretions. Bronchodilators and corticosteroids may be ordered. Antibiotics are not prescribed because the causative organism is usually viral.

Ribavirin (Virazole), an antiviral drug that speeds recovery, may be used to treat certain infants with RSV. It is administered as an inhalant by hood, mask, or tent. Ribavirin is prescribed cautiously because it may be a health hazard to health care personnel and pregnant women and is expensive. The American Academy of Pediatrics states the use of ribavirin is limited to those infants with known cardiac disease, chronic lung disease, premature infants, or with conditions of immunosuppression.

Nursing Management

Nursing care of the infant or child with bronchiolitis focuses on preventing the spread of infection, promoting gas exchange and effective airway clearance, maintaining hydration, and easing the work of breathing.

Respiratory droplets can transmit RSV for up to 9 days, so the infant is placed in a respiratory isolation room or with other RSV-infected children. Careful handwashing is important. Wearing gowns while holding or feeding the infant may help decrease transmission.

To promote airway clearance and effective gas exchange, the infant is repositioned every 2 hours. Chest physiotherapy is performed as ordered.

Tachypnea. An abnormally rapid rate of respirations.

Retractions. A visible drawing in of the skin of the neck and chest, which occurs on inhalation in children and young infants.

Apnea. Cessation of respiration lasting longer than 20 seconds.

PNEUMONIA

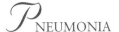

Pneumonia is an inflammation of the lung parenchyma. It occurs throughout childhood, but more frequently in infancy and early childhood.

Etiology

The cause of pneumonia is often a viral or bacterial agent (Table 9-1). Causative agents vary with the child's age and sometimes the season.

Pathophysiology and Classification

In all types of pneumonia the lungs, including the smallest alveoli, become inflamed, and exudate accumulates within the alveoli. Pneumonia is classified as follows:

Lobar pneumonia—all or part of a lung lobe is involved. If both lungs are affected the condition is known as bilateral or double pneumonia.

Lobular pneumonia or bronchopneumonia—starts in the bronchi, which become clogged with exudate to form consolidated patches of infection in nearby lobes.

Interstitial pneumonia—inflammation of the alveolar walls with diffuse bronchiolitis and peribronchiolar and interlobular tissues.

⊠

TABLE 9-1

ETIOLOGY OF PNEUMONIA

Type	Agent	Age of Child	Season
Bacterial	*Staphylococcus pneumoniae* group A	Infants from birth to 3 months	Any season
	Streptococcus		
	Klebsiella pneumoniae		
	Escherichia coli		
	Chlamydia		
	Haemophilus influenzae	Children ages 3 months to 5 years	Any season
	Streptococcus pneumoniae		
Viral	Respiratory syncytial virus	Children ages 2 months to 5 years	Winter and spring
	Parainfluenza virus	Children ages 4–6 years	Fall and winter
Mycoplasma	*Mycoplasma pneumoniae*	Children ages 5–12 years	Fall and winter

Clinical Manifestations and Therapeutic Management

Viral Pneumonia Viral pneumonia occurs more frequently than bacterial pneumonia. Both may have an insidious or abrupt onset. The child may have fever and a productive or nonproductive cough, as well as malaise.

Prognosis is good, although respiratory viral infections make the child susceptible to secondary infection. Treatment is usually symptomatic and provided at home. Measures include oral fluids, antipyretics, a humidified environment, and rest.

Bacterial Pneumonia Symptoms are usually more severe than those of viral pneumonia. There is usually a sudden onset and children appear ill. Early signs include fever, malaise, headache, and abdominal and chest pain. There may be a hacking, nonproductive cough, decreased breath sounds, and fine crackles. Later, the child may exhibit a productive cough, coarse crackles, and rhonchi. If it is a severe case of pneumonia, signs of respiratory distress such as tachypnea, dyspnea, retractions, and **hypoxia** may be present.

Hypoxia. Lower than normal amounts of oxygen in the blood.

Older children can be treated at home if the illness is recognized and treatment initiated early. Home management includes antipyretics, antitussives, fluids, oral antibiotics, and a cool mist vaporizer. Hospitalization is indicated for infants with pneumonia and children with respiratory distress and hypoxia. Inpatient treatment includes antipyretics, intravenous fluids and antibiotics, chest physiotherapy, oxygen if necessary, and bed rest.

Mycoplasma Pneumonia The onset of mycoplasma pneumonia may be insidious or sudden. Early symptoms are vague, such as fever, chills, headache, and malaise. Later, the child has signs of upper airway congestion, sore throat, nonproductive cough (it later becomes productive), and fine crackles. Children with mycoplasma pneumonia usually require home management that includes antibiotics and symptom relief.

Diagnosis

Diagnosis of pneumonia is made largely by the history, the child's age, the physical examination, radiography, and laboratory findings.

Nursing Management

Nursing management for the child with pneumonia includes ensuring adequate hydration, promoting airway clearance and gas exchange, easing the work of breathing, managing fever, and controlling the cough.

Care for the child is primarily to relieve symptoms and to be supportive. Thorough respiratory assessment, administration of antibiotics, and oxygen are provided. The child is disturbed as little as possible and activities are clustered so as not to disturb sleep.

Children may be placed in a mist tent with oxygen. A cool mist environment moistens the airways and aids in temperature reduction. Children require frequent changes of clothing and linen to prevent becoming chilled in the damp atmosphere. They are comfortable with the head of the bed elevated, but should be allowed to be in their position of comfort. If the pneumonia is unilateral, lying on the affected side splints the chest and promotes airway exchange in the unaffected lung.

Postural drainage and chest physiotherapy are usually prescribed every 4 hours. Infants should have their nose and nasopharynx suctioned with a bulb syringe.

The child and family need support. Hospitalization and many of the treatments and tests are frightening. Reducing stress and anxiety allows the child to relax and decreases respiratory effort. The presence of the parent or caregiver provides the child comfort and support. Caregivers are also in need of the nurse's support. Most children have been ill for several days before hospitalization, and in many cases the dry, hacking cough has disturbed the family's sleep.

Acute Laryngotracheobronchitis

Laryngotracheobronchitis (LTB) is the most common cause of croup and typically affects children younger than 5 years old, mainly in the winter. It is an inflammation of the larynx, trachea, and bronchi. Common causative agents are parainfluenza, RSV, *Haemophilus influenzae* type B, and *Mycoplasma pneumoniae*.

Pathophysiology

Acute LTB is usually preceded by an upper respiratory infection, which slowly descends to adjacent anatomical structures. The acute infection causes inflammation of the mucosal lining of the larynx and trachea and subsequent narrowing of the airway. With significant airway narrowing, the child has difficulty inspiring air past the obstruction and into the lungs, producing inspiratory stridor (a high-pitched whistling) and a barking or hoarse cough. When the child is unable to inspire an adequate volume of air, hypoxia occurs, and the child may progress to respiratory failure.

Therapeutic Management

The child with mild signs and symptoms of acute LTB usually receives care at home. High humidity and cool mist provide relief for most children. A steamy bathroom or cool-air vaporizer can be used. Parents are instructed to recognize and report symptoms of respiratory distress.

Children who have continuous inspiratory stridor or who progress to serious respiratory symptoms are hospitalized. Mist tents for toddlers and hoods for infants are sometimes used to provide mist. Aerosolized racemic epinephrine is often prescribed for the child with significant airway obstruction. This is a bronchodilator whose effects decrease subglottic edema. The child must be observed for several hours after receiving the racemic epinephrine because of the possibility of a rebound effect. The use of corticosteroids is beneficial because the anti-inflammatory effects decrease airway edema.

It is essential for the child with mild croup to drink fluids. Parents are encouraged to offer liquids that their child likes to drink and to provide comfort measures. If the child is unable to take fluids by mouth or has severe respiratory symptoms, intravenous fluids should be administered.

Nursing Management

Nursing care focuses on maintaining a patent airway, easing the work of breathing, and maintaining hydration. The most important nursing function is to carefully and accurately assess the child's respiratory status. Changes in treatment are usually based on the nurse's observations and documentation. Signs and symptoms of increased respiratory distress are immediately reported.

The mist tent system is maintained to ensure a patent airway. Children often do not want to stay in the mist tent. This stress, along with crying, cough, and laryngeal spasm, may cause symptoms to worsen. A child who will not stay in the mist tent may be more cooperative if held in the parent's lap with the cool mist directed toward his/her face.

The family should be encouraged to stay with the child as much as possible to help allay fears and reduce stress. Procedures that induce crying should be kept to a minimum and the child's ability to tolerate them assessed. To allow the child to conserve energy, nursing care activities are alternated with frequent rest periods. Sufficient fluids should be offered and if intravenous fluids are necessary, the fluids and IV site are maintained.

Parents need reassurance that as the child responds to therapy, recovery will be prompt. Teaching includes how to make their child comfortable during the acute phase of the illness. Home care after discharge from the hospital includes continued humidity, adequate hydration, and nourishment.

$\mathcal{A}$CUTE EPIGLOTTITIS

Acute epiglottitis is a potentially life-threatening inflammation of the epiglottis. It is a condition that requires immediate medical attention. Most common in children 2 to 8 years old, it can occur from infancy to adulthood, especially during the winter. The causative agent is usually *H. influenzae*.

Pathophysiology

The acute bacterial infection causes inflammation and potentially fatal obstruction of the epiglottis. With significant airway narrowing, the child has difficulty inspiring air.

Clinical Manifestations

Acute epiglottitis has a sudden onset. Typically, the child goes to bed asymptomatic and awakens later with complaints of sore throat, dysphagia (difficulty swallowing), inspiratory stridor, drooling, and high fever. The child automatically assumes a sitting position, looks toxic, is irritable, is extremely restless, and has a fearful expression. If the child is able to talk, his/her voice is muffled and sounds froglike. There is an absence of cough. The throat is red and inflamed, and the epiglottis appears large and cherry-red on inspection.

Therapeutic Management

A suspected diagnosis of acute epiglottitis constitutes an emergency. Throat inspection is performed only when emergency equipment is available for intubation or tracheotomy and only by experienced personnel. If a lateral neck x-ray is indicated and a portable film is not done, the child is accompanied to the radiology department by a physician or someone able to perform emergency intubation or tracheotomy. Usually the child remains on the parent's lap during the examination or procedures.

Endotracheal intubation or tracheotomy is usually considered for the child with severe respiratory distress. Whether or not the child has an artificial airway, he/she requires intensive care and observation by experienced personnel. The swelling of the epiglottis usually improves after 24 hours of antibiotic therapy and should be near normal size by the third day. Intubated children are usually extubated at this time.

Intravenous antibiotics are administered to children with acute epiglottitis and followed by oral antibiotics for 7 to 10 days. Corticosteroids are used to reduce edema in the course of treatment.

Prevention

The American Academy of Pediatrics recommends that all children receive the *H. influenzae* type B conjugate vaccine beginning at 2 months of age.

Since administration of the vaccine has become part of routine immunizations, there has been a decline in the incidence of epiglottitis.

Nursing Management

Because epiglottitis can be fatal and is frightening to the child and family, the nurse must be sure to provide support to ease anxiety and allay their fears. Actions must be quick without increasing anxiety. The child should be allowed to remain in the position that provides the most comfort and security.

Asthma

Asthma (reactive airway disease) is a chronic respiratory disorder characterized by hypersensitivity of the bronchi after exposure to a stimulus, which is reversible either spontaneously or with treatment. Asthma can be intermittent, in which the child can be symptom-free for long periods without medication, or chronic, in which the child requires frequent or continuous therapy. Chronic asthma affects the child's school performance and activities and may contribute to poor self-confidence. Asthma is the leading cause of chronic illness in children, typically appearing between age 2 and 8, affecting more boys than girls until puberty. Asthma is a common cause of school absence and is responsible for a major portion of pediatric admissions to the emergency department and hospital.

Etiology

Asthma is an extremely complex disorder involving biochemical, immunologic, infectious, endocrine, and psychological factors.

Both heredity and allergic factors are suspected causes of asthma. The family or child may have a history of atopic conditions, such as allergic rhinitis, eczema, or asthma. Although allergy does provide an explanation for triggering asthma, there are instances when allergic factors are not present. A strong relationship exists between viral infections and asthma, especially in infants.

Asthma triggers may include the following:

Allergens: *outdoors:* trees, shrubs, grass, molds, spores, pollen, air pollution; *indoors:* dust, dust mites, cockroach antigen, mold; *irritants:* household cleaners, strong odors, wood-burning stove smoke, tobacco smoke, fumes
Medications

Foods: shellfish, eggs, milk, nuts, chocolate, food additives, food dyes, sulfites
Animals: dogs, cats, birds
Viral infections
Cold air
Changes in weather
Exercise
Strong emotions: fear, anxiety

Pathophysiology

Most theories do not explain all types and causes of asthma. Spasms of the smooth muscle cause the lumina of the bronchi and bronchioles to narrow. Edema of the mucous membranes lining these bronchial branches, increased production of thick mucus within them, and bronchial spasm cause airway constriction. Gas trapping occurs in areas obstructed by thick bronchial obstruction.

Clinical Manifestations

The onset of an attack may be abrupt, or it may progress over several days. Asthma attacks frequently occur at night, waking the child from sleep. Clinical findings in the child with asthma occur in early and late stages.

Early Signs

Cough—dry, hacking, nonproductive
Wheezing—audible on expiration
Prolonged expiration—the child has the most difficulty during the expiratory phase of respiration
Retractions—the child may be using accessory muscles for respiration
Dyspnea
Apprehension
Restlessness
Shortened speech

Late Signs

Wheeze—audible on inspiration and expiration
Rhonchi and crackles
Cough—rattling, productive; sputum is clear and frothy
Decreased breath sounds
Tachypnea
Tachycardia
Difficulty speaking
Anxiety and restlessness
Hypoxia

Diagnosis

The diagnosis of asthma depends on a family history of atopic conditions, the physical examination, clinical manifestations, and abnormal pulmonary function test results indicating decreased peak expiratory flow rates. When a child has a chronic cough without infection or has diffuse wheezing in the expiratory phase of respiration, it is suggestive of asthma. A definitive diagnosis is made when obstruction of the airways is reversed with bronchodilators.

Therapeutic Management

Prevention is the most important aspect in the treatment of asthma. Children and their families must be taught to recognize the symptoms that lead to an acute attack so treatment can start quickly. Use of a peak flowmeter is a way to objectively measure airway obstruction and response to treatment. Children as young as 4 years old can be taught to use a peak flowmeter. A peak flow diary should be maintained, which also can include symptoms, exacerbations (worsening of symptoms), actions taken, and outcomes. Compliance with prescribed regimens is essential to successful management.

Allergen Control Families must make an effort to eliminate any possible allergens from the home. House dust mites and dust are the agents most often identified in children allergic to inhalants. Skin testing identifies specific allergens, so steps can be taken to eliminate them. Often the removal of an animal from the home decreases the frequency of asthma attacks. Parents must not allow smoking in the house or near the child. Air conditioning and dehumidifiers help control temperature changes.

Drug Therapy Medications usually do not have to be administered continuously. Bronchodilators are the drugs of choice to reverse bronchospasm. Several drugs, often in combination, are prescribed. Many of the drugs are given by inhalation by nebulizer or metered-dose inhaler (MDI). The MDI may have a spacing unit or reservoir attached to make it easier to use and so the child will receive an adequate amount of bronchodilator. Children who are unable to use an MDI obtain relief with nebulization or aerosol.

Corticosteroids are the most effective anti-inflammatory drugs for treatment to reverse airflow obstruction, control symptoms, and reduce hyperactivity of the bronchioles in chronic asthma. Corticosteroids can be administered parenterally, orally, or by aerosol. Onset of action is 3 to 6 hours with peak effectiveness within 6 to 12 hours. Usually short-term therapy that begins with high doses is prescribed for 5 to 10 days.

Cromolyn sodium prevents mast cells from releasing chemical mediators that cause bronchospasms and mucous membrane inflammation. It is used to decrease allergen-induced daily wheeze and exercise-induced asthma.

The ß-adrenergic or sympathomimetic drugs are first-choice medications for the treatment of acute exacerbations of asthma and the prevention of exercise-induced asthma. They can be given by inhaler, oral, or parenteral preparations. The inhaled drug has a more rapid onset of action, but is more costly.

Methylxanthines, specifically theophylline, have been used for decades to relieve symptoms and prevent asthma attacks. Theophylline preparations are available in short-acting and long-acting forms. Short-term forms are most effective when used for intermittent episodes of asthma because they enter the bloodstream quickly. Side effects are nervousness, insomnia, muscle spasms, irritability, palpitations, upset stomach, anorexia, perspiration, and frequent urination. Long-acting preparations are helpful in patients who need medication continuously because these drugs sustain more consistent theophylline levels in blood than do short-acting forms. When theophylline is used, it is available in intravenous, intramuscular, oral, and rectal preparations.

Monitoring serum concentrations of theophylline is important in both acute care and long-term management. A therapeutic theophylline level is 10 to 20 mcg/mL, and the dosage of theophylline is adjusted to maintain that level. Signs and symptoms of theophylline toxicity involve many systems. The earliest symptoms are nausea and vomiting. Cardiopulmonary effects include tachycardia, dysrhythmias, tachypnea, diuresis, irritability, and possibly seizures.

Exercise Exercise-induced asthma (EIA) is an acute, reversible airway obstruction that develops 5 to 15 minutes after strenuous exercise and lasts 30 to 60 minutes after onset. Children with asthma are often excluded from physical exercise and activities by their parents and teachers. This can hamper peer relationships. If the asthma is under control, children can participate in activities at school and in sports with minimum difficulty. Prophylactic treatment with ß-adrenergic drugs or cromolyn sodium before exercise will usually allow strenuous exercise to be tolerated. Swimming is a sport that is well tolerated by children with EIA because they are breathing moisturized air and exhale under water.

Chest Physiotherapy Chest physiotherapy (CPT) includes breathing exercises, physical training, and inhalation therapy. Breathing exercises improve respiratory function and help control asthma attacks. These exercises teach children how to control their own symptoms and build self-confidence.

Status Asthmaticus Children who continue to have respiratory distress despite vigorous therapy are considered to be in status asthmaticus. These children are very ill and require hospitalization for careful monitoring and observation. Therapeutic management is directed toward improvement of ventilation, correction of dehydration and **acidosis,** and treatment of infection, if present.

Acidosis. Condition caused by too much acid in the blood.

Nursing Management

Nursing management focuses on relieving the child's respiratory distress and reassuring the child and family. Continuous teaching of the child and family is important throughout the child's hospitalization.

During an acute asthma attack, the child should be continuously monitored with pulse oximetry. Observations include respiratory rate, effort, and presence of nasal flaring, retractions, and color changes. The head of the bed should be elevated, and an older child may be more comfortable leaning forward. The child is monitored for response to medications and possible side effects, such as gastrointestinal upset, restlessness, and seizures. Supplemental oxygen may be necessary during an acute attack. Nursing activities are coordinated to allow the child long periods of rest.

During an acute attack children lose fluids through the respiratory tract and diaphoresis, and may have poor oral intake because of coughing and vomiting. Strict monitoring of fluid intake and output is necessary. Offer oral fluids that the child prefers. Administer intravenous fluids if necessary.

The child's fear may be intensified by the behavior of the parent. The child's and the caregiver's fear and anxiety can be reduced by teaching them the signs and symptoms and treatment of an impending asthma attack. Child and family teaching is essential in the care of asthmatic children. Acute asthma attacks can be prevented or decreased by prompt attention and adequate intervention. Aspects that must be taught to the parents and the child (according to the child's ability to understand) are the disease processes, recognition of symptoms of an acute attack, environmental control, avoidance of infection, exercise, drug therapy, and chest physiotherapy. The child and parent must be taught how to use the metered-dose inhaler or nebulizer, the peak flowmeter, and peak flow diary.

$\mathcal{C}$YSTIC FIBROSIS

Electrolytes. Substances that are charged particles when they are dissolved.

Cystic fibrosis (CF) is a hereditary disorder transmitted by an autosomal recessive inheritance pattern. The mutated gene responsible is located on the long arm of chromosome 7, along with its abnormal protein product, cystic fibrosis transmembrane regulator (CFTR). The affected child inherits the defective gene from both parents. With each pregnancy, the chance is 1 in 4 that the child will have the disease. Cystic fibrosis occurs predominantly in Caucasians and affects both sexes equally.

Several features characterize cystic fibrosis: increased viscosity of mucous gland secretion, elevation of sweat **electrolytes,** and excessive electrolytes excreted from the salivary glands. The basic defect of CF is related to abnormal secretions of the exocrine (mucus-producing) glands, which produce thick, tenacious mucus rather than the thin, free-flowing secretions normally produced. This thick mucus leads to obstruction of the secretory ducts of the pancreas, liver, and reproductive system. Thick mucus obstructs the respiratory passages, trapping air and overinflating the lungs. The thick secretions also cause abnormalities in autonomic nervous system functioning.

Clinical Manifestations

Symptoms of cystic fibrosis may occur during infancy, childhood, or adolescence. A harsh, nonproductive cough may be the first sign. Bronchial infections become frequent. Development of a barrel chest and clubbing of the fingers indicates lack of oxygen. Despite a hearty appetite, malnutrition is apparent and becomes severe. The abdomen becomes distended, and body muscles become flabby.

Meconium ileus is the earliest symptom of cystic fibrosis in the newborn. Depletion or absence of pancreatic enzymes before birth results in impaired digestive activity, and the meconium becomes viscid (glutinous) and mucilaginous (sticky). The inspissated (thickened) meconium fills the small intestine, causing complete obstruction. Symptoms of meconium ileus are bile-stained emesis, distended abdomen, and absence of stool. Intestinal perforation may occur.

Pancreatic Involvement Malabsorbed fats cause frequent steatorrhea (frothy, bulky, greasy stools with a foul odor). In the pancreas, the thick secretions block the pancreatic ducts, eventually causing pancreatic fibrosis. This blockage prevents the pancreatic enzymes lipase, trypsin, and amylase from reaching the duodenum, causing impaired digestion. The islands of Langerhans may decrease in number as pancreatic fibrosis progresses. The incidence of diabetes in children with CF is higher than in the general population. In the liver, localized biliary obstruction and fibrosis are common. Anemia or rectal prolapse frequently occurs if the pancreatic condition remains untreated.

Pulmonary Involvement Lung involvement is present in almost all children with cystic fibrosis and is the most serious threat to life. The degree of lung involvement determines the prognosis of survival. Severity of pulmonary involvement differs in individual children, a few showing only minor involvement.

Abnormal amounts of thick, viscid mucus clog the bronchioles. The child is unable to expectorate the thick secretions; this provides an ideal growth medium for bacteria. Repeated respiratory infections cause bronchial fibrosis. If bronchial obstruction leads to atelectasis, the patient exhibits decreased breath sounds, hypoxia, and hypercapnia. Small pulmonary blebs may rupture spontaneously, causing pneumothorax. Rupture of small capillaries leads to hemoptysis (blood-tinged sputum). In advanced disease, increased pulmonary vascular resistance results in **pulmonary hypertension** and right-sided heart failure (cor pulmonale). Long-term use of accessory muscles causes barrel chest. Chronic hypoxia results in finger clubbing.

Pulmonary hypertension.
Condition resulting from chronic body volume overload through the pulmonary arteries.

Diagnosis

Diagnosis is based on family history, elevated sodium chloride levels in the sweat, absence of pancreatic enzymes, chronic pulmonary involvement, and failure to thrive. Cystic fibrosis is assumed in any infant born with meconium ileus.

The consistent finding of abnormally high sodium and chloride concentrations in the sweat is characteristic of cystic fibrosis. Parents often report that their infant tastes salty to them. The sweat chloride test, using the pilocarpine method, confirms the diagnosis of cystic fibrosis. This method induces sweating by using a small electric current that carries topically applied pilocarpine into a localized area of skin. Elevations of 60 mEq/L or above are diagnostic. False positive results do occur and the test is done only in infants older than 6 months because younger infants do not produce enough sweat for the test to be valid. Genetic testing may identify asymptomatic carriers of the disease. Prenatal diagnosis of cystic fibrosis is possible through genetic testing of the parents and the fetus.

Therapeutic Management

Goals of therapy include preventing or minimizing pulmonary complications, ensuring adequate nutrition, and supporting the child and family in coping with a chronic and fatal disorder.

Pulmonary Complications Management of pulmonary problems is directed toward the prevention and treatment of pulmonary infection by promoting airway clearance, improving gas exchange, and giving antibiotics. Prevention of infection involves a daily routine of chest physiotherapy (CPT) to maintain pulmonary hygiene. CPT is a combination of postural drainage and chest percussion. It is performed routinely at least every morning and evening, even if little drainage is present. Chest percussion, which is clapping and vibrating of the affected areas, if performed correctly, helps loosen and remove the secretions from the lungs. Aerosolized bronchodilators help open bronchi for easier expectoration and are administered before CPT when the child has wheezing.

Physical exercise is essential because it provides a sense of well-being and self-esteem. The child is encouraged to participate in any aerobic activity that he/she enjoys. Activity should be limited only by the child's endurance.

Antibiotics for the treatment of infection are necessary as soon as infection is recognized. A culture and sensitivity of sputum determine the choice of drug. Some children are prescribed prophylactic antibiotic therapy when diagnosis is confirmed. Antibiotics may be administered orally or parenterally, even in the home. Most children have central venous catheters for home administration of IV antibiotics.

Immunizations against childhood communicable diseases are important for these children. The immunization schedule should be maintained at the proper intervals.

Ensure proper nutrition. Pancreatic enzymes given during meals and snacks aid digestion and absorption of fat and protein. Because pancreatic enzymes become inactivated in the acidic environment of the stomach, enteric-coated products that deliver the enzymes to the alkaline environment of the duodenum are preferred. These enzymes are administered as capsules to be swallowed or opened and sprinkled on food or mixed into cereal or fruit. The amount of enzyme administered is adjusted to achieve normal growth and decrease the number of stools to 2 to 3 a day.

Children with cystic fibrosis require a diet high in calories and high in protein without restriction of fat. The child may need up to 150 to 200% of the normal caloric intake to promote growth. If the infant is breast-fed, nursing is continued with pancreatic enzyme. Commercial infant formula is usually adequate. Absorption of fat-soluble vitamins is decreased; a water-soluble form of vitamins (A, D, E, K) is given along with multivitamins. When high-fat foods are eaten the child takes extra enzymes. Total parenteral nutrition or tube feedings may be given during sleep hours, if necessary to promote growth and maintain weight.

Nursing Considerations

Nursing management focuses on promoting airway clearance, improving respiratory function, preventing infection, and ensuring adequate nutrition, teaching, and support of family and child.

Mucus causes obstruction of the airways and decreases gas exchange. The nurse assesses the child's respiratory status with special attention to any dyspnea, tachypnea, nasal flaring, or other signs of respiratory distress. Aerosols and CPT are carried out as ordered and kept on a schedule. CPT should not be performed before or immediately after meals. Coordination of CPT and meals is usually difficult in the hospital setting, so the nurse should plan these interventions. Deep breathing and coughing are encouraged. The child's position is changed every 2 hours. The nurse notes the color, amount, and consistency of pulmonary secretions. Cultures are obtained if necessary. Supplemental oxygen is delivered to maintain oxygen saturation above 90%. Pulse oximetry is monitored.

The child with CF is at risk for respiratory infections. As a first defense, the nurse practices good handwashing techniques and the family is instructed to do the same. People with an infectious process, including health care workers, family members, and visitors, should be restricted from visiting. Intravenous antibiotics are administered in the hospital on schedule.

The diet is maintained for the hospitalized child and instituted for the newly diagnosed child. Children should be assisted in choosing meals and snacks that are high in calories and nutritious. Newly diagnosed children have hearty appetites. Hospitalized children with pulmonary infection or increased lung involvement lose their appetites. Encouraging a sick child to eat and to accept extra fluids can be a challenge for the nurse, especially if that child has extra nutritional needs. Caloric intake should be increased and adequate salt provided. Pancreatic enzyme is given with every meal and snack. If the child has constipation or bouts of diarrhea, it is reported so the enzyme dosage can be adjusted. Daily weights allow for assessment of any weight loss or gain.

Supporting the child and family is crucial to nursing care of the child with cystic fibrosis. The nurse is the person who best provides overall support and families are encouraged to remain in contact with health care workers. Families are faced with a long-term, fatal illness. They may have already seen deterioration in their child's health and the possibility of death. The need for treatment several times a day puts a strain on the entire family. Children often become uncooperative and refuse treatment—putting parents in the position of insisting on compliance. Cystic fibrosis restricts the activities of the child, who has no choice but to live with an inflexible schedule of treatment, medications, and diet. This may make the child resentful and unwilling to socialize for fear of being "different." These children should be encouraged to join groups with children their own age and to attend school.

Adolescent males with the disorder eventually need to be informed that they will have normal sexual function, but most likely will be sterile and unable to produce children. Adolescent females may become pregnant, but should be aware that the pregnancy will affect their respiratory function and that their children will be carriers of cystic fibrosis.

The nurse should evaluate the family's knowledge of the disease process because it will help in determining their needs. The family and child need opportunities to voice their fears and anxieties. The family may need referrals for counseling and genetic testing. The cost of a chronic illness and the time necessary to provide the home care the child requires place a tremendous strain on the family emotionally as well economically.

Preparation for Home Care   A treatment plan for home care is planned when diagnosis is confirmed and the child's and family's needs are assessed. Parents will need assistance to acquire medical equipment. They must learn to give aerosol treatments and operate the nebulizer. The child may require administration of intravenous antibiotics and tube feedings at home.

One of the most important aspects of home care teaching is educating parents to perform breathing exercises and chest physiotherapy. These exercises must be done exactly as prescribed. Postural drainage can be made fun for the child when a parent raises the child's feet in the air and walks the child "wheelbarrow" style, or allows the older child to hang from monkey bars.

Hot weather activity should be closely monitored, with attention on increasing fluid and salt intake during exercise.

SUMMARY

This chapter examines disease that involves the airway, affected by age-related differences in structure and function, as transient conditions that can be managed at home. Systemic disorders are closely examined in order to diagnose and develop nursing interventions aimed at relieving the symptoms as well as bringing resolution to the condition. Emotional and physical stress are the biggest contributors to the development of respiratory conditions in children. This chapter also emphasizes the history and objective assessment of these conditions. As the nurse learns about the conditions and the treatment that is needed to resolve their pathology, he/she learns about nursing interventions such as positioning for lung expansion, maintenance of effective airways, general support measures, promotion of parent and child competence in the management of the disease, and anticipatory guidance.

CRITICAL POINTS IN THE CARE OF RESPIRATORY DISORDERS

Pulmonary conditions in children are reportedly the most common causes of hospitalizations in the United States. It is reported that 48% of infant deaths are related to pulmonary diseases and that 7% of the children in our country suffer from some kind of chronic condition related to pulmonary disease. Breathing difficulties are more frequent in children and infants because of the developmental differences in structures at these ages. The biggest challenge that the nurse faces is the fear that parents experience when their child is ill, and the seriousness of an acute respiratory episode if it is not treated efficiently.

Parents' observations are valuable for the formulation of a correct diagnosis. Their perceptions of the course of the disease and of its onset become as important as the knowledge of the pathophysiology of the disease. More important than the report of the progression of the illness is the knowledge of the precipitating factors. Often the precipitating factors can be food intake, exercise, or plain irritation from insertion of a foreign object, as well as exposure to an infected person, or a chemical or environmental irritant. Only the parent can give this information. The second component of this evaluation for the nurse is the assessment of the family stress level in response to the child's illness. Many young families—and unfortunately most families with young children are very young—have poor skills in coping with stress. If the nurse does not use his/her best interviewing skills or is rushed, he/she will not realize the family's strength or absence of coping capabilities.

In considering all the above factors the nurse uses subjective assessment as the cornerstone on which to base objective assessment. The objective assessment consists of a thorough physical examination. The most important element of this exam is a clear explanation to the child and the parent of all the procedures that are going to be performed, before starting the examination. A clear explanation ahead of time ensures that the child's heart will not react in fear, and also that the child will not cry, making it impossible to assess how patent the upper respiratory tract is. The lung field will also be better assessed.

The important points to remember while doing the physical exams are: Evaluate the heart and lungs before the child gets agitated or scared. Clarify what kind of language the parents are using (an example is the confusion by the parents of the terms *stridor* and *wheezing*, or the confusion between *inspiration* and *expiration*). Most important, always remember that upper respiratory problems interfere with air entry, and stridor is always associated with air entry. This will lead the nurse to consider common disorders such as croup, epiglottitis, laryngitis, and bacterial tracheitis. Expiratory wheezing is commonly associated with disorders of the lower respiratory tract that cause inflammation, infection, or bronchoconstriction. The child may also have fever, while fear may cause the child to hyperventilate. This adds to the difficulty of the determining the real illness.

In teaching the parents, remember that education should be geared first to alleviate their anxiety. It is important to acknowledge to parents that respiratory illness can be very frightening. Second, the nurse should teach the parent and the child about the etiology and normal course of the conditions along with the use of humidification and hydration. Giving the child some responsibility for his/her own care will prevent overprotection of the child, which often translates into feelings of anxiety for the child, sending the message that the child's illness is very serious. When instructing parents on how to administer medication, remember that often parents treat the child with over-the-counter medications. It is important to educate them that such medications cause irritability, stimulation, insomnia, sedation, and sometimes gastrointestinal upsets. Teaching should be done when the parent is calm and may often need to be repeated two to three times.

Another phase of the complexity of respiratory conditions is that these conditions also are chronic. Taking care of a child with chronic conditions also means taking care of the family. Parents often blame themselves for a child's chronic illness. Families with children with chronic conditions have needs that extend further than the help that the health care system can give them. It is pivotal that the nurse empower the family with the ability to function independently on a daily basis and understand that chronic conditions are irreversible and require comprehensive care.

$\mathcal{Q}$UESTIONS

1. A 10-year-old girl with asthma is allergic to birds. She went to a playmate's house after school where there was a pet canary. Several hours later, on arriving home, she starts to wheeze. Which of the following drugs should have been administered in the afternoon to prevent her wheezing?
   A. Serevent
   B. Albuterol
   C. Cromolyn sodium
   D. Theophylline

2. A 10-month-old infant boy will undergo an evaluation to rule out cystic fibrosis. For which test should the nurse prepare the infant to confirm the diagnosis?

   A. Complete blood count
   B. Bronchoscopy
   C. Pulmonary function studies
   D. Sweat test for sweat electrolytes

3. Clinical manifestations of laryngotracheobronchitis (croup) in a child include:

   A. Absence of cough
   B. Inspiratory stridor
   C. Expiratory wheeze
   D. Clear, frothy sputum

4. The priority nursing action when caring for a child with suspected acute epiglottitis is:

   A. Start an IV immediately and infuse fluids.
   B. Place the child in an isolation room.
   C. Complete the nursing history.
   D. Obtain an intubation tray and notify the physician.

5. The nurse is explaining home care to the parents of a child newly diagnosed with cystic fibrosis. Which of the following statements indicates the need for further teaching?

   A. "I will give the enzymes with breakfast and dinner when I am at home."
   B. "I understand that the enzymes will help food digestion."
   C. "I can expect my child to have a good appetite."
   D. "I do not have to limit my child's salt and fat intake."

6. A 3-month-old infant is admitted to the pediatric unit from the emergency department with diagnosis of RSV bronchiolitis. What equipment should the nurse have in the room?

   A. Intubation tray, IV pump, cardiorespiratory monitor
   B. IV pump, oxygen, cardiorespiratory monitor
   C. Tracheotomy tray, oxygen, infant formula
   D. Cardiorespiratory monitor, pacifier to suck, tracheotomy tray

7. The mother of two school-age children who have asthma asks the nurse to suggest a sport her children can play without triggering an exacerbation. The best response is:

   A. Football
   B. Wrestling
   C. Baseball
   D. Swimming

8. The failure of a newborn to pass meconium within the first 24 hours after birth is suggestive of which of the following?
   A. Hypoglycemia
   B. Cystic fibrosis
   C. Dehydration
   D. Celiac disease

9. A 7-year-old child is admitted to the pediatric unit with suspected right-sided lobar pneumonia. The appropriate position for this child would be:
   A. Head of bed elevated 10°
   B. Turned on right side
   C. In a prone position
   D. In a supine position

10. A toddler is admitted to the hospital with the diagnosis of viral croup. She has fever, inspiratory stridor, and a barking cough. A mist tent has been ordered for her because:
    A. The mist has antitussive effects.
    B. It prevents the spread of infection.
    C. The mist thins mucus, allowing for a productive cough.
    D. It allows for delivery of supplemental oxygen.

$\mathcal{A}$NSWERS

1. *C.* Corticosteroids and cromolyn sodium are useful in the treatment of allergy-induced asthma. Theophylline, albuterol, and Serevent are useful for their bronchodilator effect, but not late-phase allergic response.

2. *D.* Definitive diagnosis for cystic fibrosis is made after two sweat electrolyte tests with chloride level 60 mEq/L or above. Complete blood counts assess a patient's hematological states. Pulmonary function studies and bronchoscopy assist with evaluation of respiratory function, but do not confirm the diagnosis of cystic fibrosis.

3. *B.* Inspiratory stridor is a symptom of croup. The child with acute epiglottitis has an absent cough. An expiratory wheeze is an early symptom of an asthma attack. Expectoration of clear, frothy sputum is a late sign in an asthma attack.

4. *D.* A child with suspected acute epiglottitis is in danger of complete airway obstruction by the edematous epiglottis. Intubation or tracheotomy equipment must be immediately available. Eventually the child will need an IV started for fluids. Antibiotics, respiratory isolation, and the nursing history should be completed, but are not the immediate priority.

5. *A.* Digestive enzymes must be given with every meal and snack. Children with cystic fibrosis have voracious appetites and usually need nutritional supplements. Because sodium chloride is excreted through the skin, salt is not restricted, but encouraged.

6. *B.* Infants that are tachypneic with a respiratory rate of 60 breaths per minute or higher and have symptoms of respiratory distress should be NPO. They receive fluids intravenously. Oxygen should be available. This infant should be placed on cardiorespiratory monitoring.

7. *D.* Swimming is a sport well tolerated by patients with respiratory conditions. Patients inspire moisturized air. Football, wrestling, and baseball require strenuous activity that may trigger an attack.

8. *B.* A diagnosis of cystic fibrosis is suspected when the newborn does not pass meconium within the first 24 hours after birth. The meconium mixes with tenacious mucus and forms a plug, causing a bowel obstruction. Hypoglycemia and dehydration usually do not cause intestinal symptoms. Recurrent diarrhea and steatorrhea characterize celiac disease. Symptoms of celiac disease do not develop until gluten is introduced into the diet.

9. *B.* Lying on the affected side allows splinting and aeration of the unaffected lung. Elevating the bed 10° is not high enough. A prone or supine position will not allow for maximum aeration of the lungs.

10. *C.* The mist in the tent provides humidified air to thin and liquefy mucous secretions. The patient is then able to cough and expectorate easier. The spread of infection is not a concern for the patient with acute laryngotracheobronchitis. The mist tent does not deliver oxygen.

Glossary

acidosis condition caused by too much acid in the blood.

apnea cessation of respiration lasting longer than 20 seconds.

electrolytes substances that are charged particles when they are dissolved.

hypercapnia greater than normal amounts of carbon dioxide in the blood.

hypoxemia abnormally decreased arterial blood oxygen in the blood.

hypoxia lower than normal amounts of oxygen in the blood.

pulmonary hypertension condition resulting from chronic body volume overload through the pulmonary arteries.

retractions a visible drawing in of the skin of the neck and chest, which occurs on inhalation in children and young infants.

tachypnea an abnormally rapid rate of respirations.

$\mathcal{B}$IBLIOGRAPHY

AMERICAN ACADEMY OF PEDIATRICS COMMITTEE ON INFECTIOUS DISEASES. *1994 Red Book: Report of the Committee on Infectious Diseases.* 23rd ed. Elk Grove Village, IL: Author, 1994.

AMERICAN ACADEMY OF PEDIATRICS TASK FORCE ON INFANT SLEEP POSITION AND SIDS: Joint commentary from the American Academy of Pediatrics and selected agencies of the federal government. *Pediatrics* 93:820, 1994.

BARKIN, R. M., AND ROSEN P., ed. *Emergency Pediatrics: A Guide to Ambulatory Care.* 4th ed. Philadelphia: Mosby, 1994.

BEHRMAN, R., KLEIGMAN, R., NELSON, W., AND VAUGHAN, V., eds. *Nelson Textbook of Pediatrics.* 14th ed. Philadelphia: W. B. Saunders, 1992.

BERMAN, S. *Pediatric Decision Making.* Philadelphia: B. C. Decker, 1991.

CAMPBELL, P. W., AND HAZINSKI, T. A. Acute pneumonia. In Hoekelman, R. A., Friedman, S. B., Nelson, N. M., and Seidel, H.M., eds. *Primary Care.* 2nd ed. (Pp. 1457–1459). St. Louis: Mosby Year Book, 1992.

CARLSON, K. L. Assessing a child's chest. *RN* 11:26–32, 1989.

CUNNINGHAM, J. C., AND TAUSSIG, L. M. An introduction to cystic fibrosis for patients and families (Publication No. N8554A-4). Bethesda, MD: Cystic Fibrosis Foundation, 1991.

DENNY, F. W. Tonsillopharyngitis. *Pediatrics in Review* 15:185–191, 1994.

DERSHEWITZ, R. A., ed. *Ambulatory Pediatric Care.* Philadelphia: Lippincott, 1993.

FLEISHER, G. R., AND LUDWIG, S., eds. *Synopsis of Pediatric Emergency Medicine.* Baltimore: Williams & Wilkins, 1996.

FRANKEL, L. R., et al. Bronchoalveolar lavage for diagnosis of pneumonia in the immunocompromised child. *Pediatrics* 81:785, 1988.

HATHAWAY, W. E., HAY, W. W., GROOTHUIS, J. R., AND PAISLEY, J. W. (eds.), *Current Pediatric Diagnosis and Treatment.* 11th ed. Norwalk, CT: Appleton & Lange, 1993.

HAY, W. W. et al., eds. *Current Pediatric Diagnosis and Treatment.* Altos, CA: Lange, 1994.

HOEKELMAN, R.A. et al., eds. *Pediatric Primary Care.* 3rd ed. St. Louis: Mosby, 1996.

KATCHER, M. S. Cold, cough, and allergy medications: Uses and abuses. *Pediatrics in Review* 17:12–18, 1996.

LARSEN, G. L., ABMAN, S. H., FAN, L. L., WHITE, C.W., AND ACCURSO, F. J. Respiratory tract and mediastinum. In W. W. Hay, J. R. Groothuis, A. R. Hayward, and M. J. Levin (eds.), *Current Pediatric Diagnosis and Treatment.* 12th ed. (Pp. 493–543). Norwalk, CT: Appleton and Lange, 1995.

LYBARGER, P. M. Inhalation injury in children: Nursing care. *Issues in Comprehensive Pediatric Nursing* 10:33–50, 1987.

MARTIN, W. J., II. Diagnostic bronchoalveolar lavage in immuno-suppressed patients with new pulmonary infiltrates. *Mayo Clin Proc* 67:296, 1992.

NATIONAL ASTHMA EDUCATION PROGRAM, EXPERT PANEL ON THE MANAGE-
MENT OF ASTHMA. *Guidelines for the Diagnosis and Management of
Asthma* (DHHS Publication No 91-3042A). Washington, D.C.: U.S.
Government Printing Office, 1991.

OSKI, F. A., ed. *Principles and Practice of Pediatrics.* 2nd ed. Philadelphia:
Lippincott, 1994.

RACHELEFSKY, G. S. Asthma update: New approaches and partnerships.
Journal of Pediatric Health Care 9:12–21, 1995.

RUDOLPH, A. M., HOFFMAN, J. I. E., AND RUDOLPH, C. *Rudolph's Pediatrics.* 20th ed. Stamford, CT: Appleton & Lange, 1996.

RUUSKANEN, O. AND OGRA, P. L. Respiratory syncytial virus. *Current
Problems in Pediatrics* 23:50–79, 1993.

TUNNESSEN, W. W. *Signs and Symptoms in Pediatrics.* 2nd ed. Philadelphia: Lippincott, 1988.

WALD, E. R. Sinusitis. *Pediatrics in Review* 14:345–351, 1994.

$\mathcal{H}$ELPFUL INTERNET SITES

PEDINFO: An Index of the Pediatric Internet at http://www.pedinfo.
org   This is an excellent site that covers nearly all topics within this
review. It has a wealth of information and is worth a visit. It is written
for health care professionals but others could also use the information.

The Allergy and Asthma Network/Mothers of Asthmatics at http://
www.aanma.org   Good site about allergies and asthma for both lay
persons and health care professionals. The AAN/MA's mission is to
help all people affected by allergies and asthma.

The American Lung Association at http://www.lungusa.org/asthma/
merck_fact.html   A link to the American Lung Association "fact
sheet" on asthma for a quick check list about asthma.

The American Lung Association at http://www.lungusa.org   This
is the official site for the American Lung Association. It has a great
deal of information and links for both lay persons and health care
professionals.

Virtual Naval Hospital Information for Providers at http://www.
vnh.org/Providers.html   This site is part of the University of Iowa's
health care site and is linked to a very large set of databases that can
be used by health care providers. The site covers a larger number of
links to other sources on health care issues and problems. This is an
excellent starting place to discover information on various common
diseases and their treatments.

ElectricAirway: Upper Airway Problems in Children at http://www.
vh.org/Providers/Textbooks/ElectricAirway/ElectricAirway.html   This
is part of the "Virtual Hospital" site that is maintained by the
University of Iowa. It is a comprehensive overview of upper airway
problems in children and their treatments.

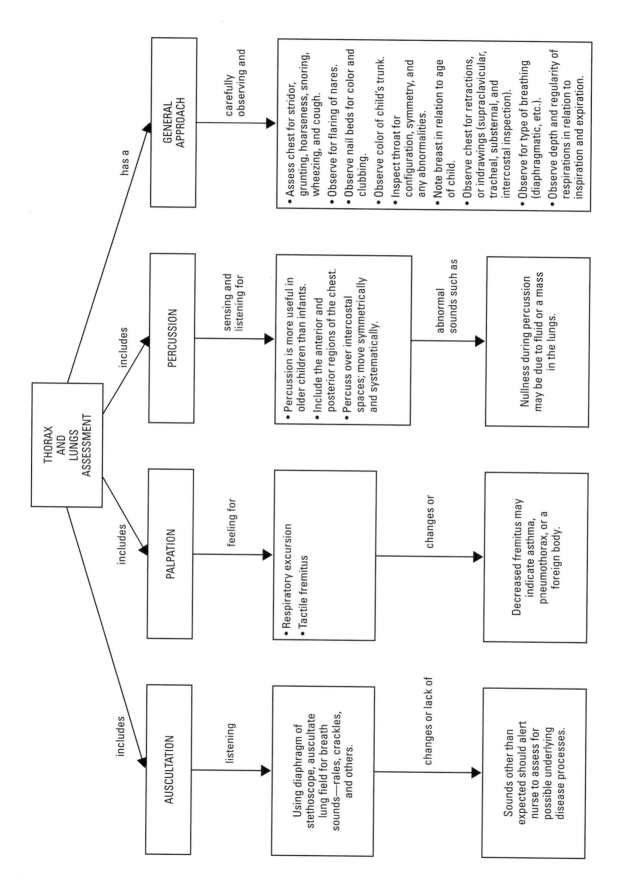

THORAX AND LUNGS ASSESSMENT

has a → GENERAL APPROACH

carefully observing and →

- Assess chest for stridor, grunting, hoarseness, snoring, wheezing, and cough.
- Observe for flaring of nares.
- Observe nail beds for color and clubbing.
- Observe color of child's trunk.
- Inspect throat for configuration, symmetry, and any abnormalities.
- Note breast in relation to age of child.
- Observe chest for retractions, or indrawings (supraclavicular, tracheal, substernal, and intercostal inspection).
- Observe for type of breathing (diaphragmatic, etc.).
- Observe depth and regularity of respirations in relation to inspiration and expiration.

includes → PERCUSSION

sensing and listening for →

- Percussion is more useful in older children than infants.
- Include the anterior and posterior regions of the chest.
- Percuss over intercostal spaces; move symmetrically and systematically.

abnormal sounds such as →

Nullness during percussion may be due to fluid or a mass in the lungs.

includes → PALPATION

feeling for →

- Respiratory excursion
- Tactile fremitus

changes or →

Decreased fremitus may indicate asthma, pneumothorax, or a foreign body.

includes → AUSCULTATION

listening →

Using diaphragm of stethoscope, auscultate lung field for breath sounds—rales, crackles, and others.

changes or lack of →

Sounds other than expected should alert nurse to assess for possible underlying disease processes.

Concept Map 9-1

288

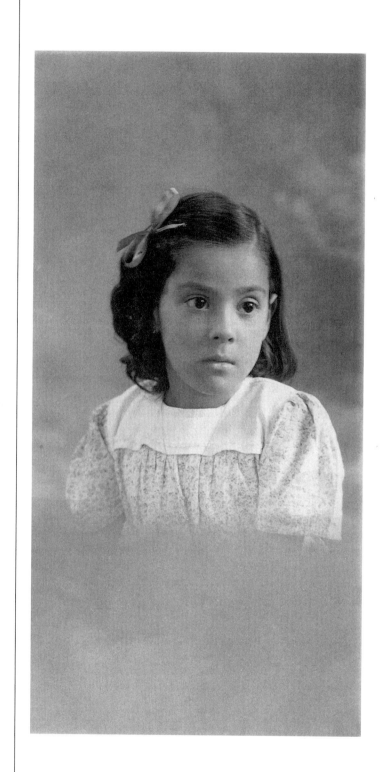

GASTROINTESTINAL DISORDERS

INTRODUCTION

The gastrointestinal system begins to develop during the third week of gestation. The gut is initially formed as a tube and then divides into the foregut, midgut, and hindgut. As the fetus grows, these structures develop into a complex system that becomes the gastrointestinal (GI) tract. The GI tract extends from the mouth to the anus. It is comprised of organs that aid the digestion and accessory organs that include the liver, pancreas, and gallbladder. The functions of the GI tract are ingestion of food, movement of food from the mouth to the rectum, mechanical and chemical changes to the food, absorption of the nutrients, and elimination of the waste products. Digestion begins in the mouth, where the food is mixed with saliva, which aids with the release of the gastric juices. Immediately the esophagus transports the food from the mouth to the stomach by **peristalsis**. Afterwards the stomach becomes the reservoir for the food, where digestion continues, aided by the digestive juices; once the process is completed, the food turns into liquid material, which is propelled to the small intestine. The major function of the small intestine is to absorb the nutrients into the systemic circulation. Carbohydrates are converted into monosaccharides before they are absorbed. Fat absorption occurs mainly in the jejunum, accomplished with the aid of the pancreatic enzymes, which also convert protein into amino acids. After this process is completed, the liquid is sent to the large intestine, where water is removed from the stool, and it becomes the fecal mass that is expelled from the rectum. The functions of the GI tract are essential for normal growth and conservation of the whole body.

Peristalsis. Progressive wavelike movement that occurs involuntarily in hollow tubes of the body.

Even though the GI system is new in children, it can be affected by illness, trauma, or malformation that can prevent its normal functioning.

The chapter discusses upper gastrointestinal tract and lower gastrointestinal tract disorders. The dysfunctions include infection, metabolic disorders, malabsorption, motility disorders, congenital malformations, genetics, injuries, and behavioral disorders.

*L*OWER GASTROINTESTINAL TRACT DISORDERS

Colic

Infantile colic is characterized by episodes of intense crying lasting 3 to 4 hours a day in infants younger than 3 months old. Colic usually starts at 3 weeks of age and resolves itself by 3 months. There is no specific cause of colic. However, several theories attribute colic to sensitivity to certain formulas, swallowing air when nursing, immaturity of the GI tract, food allergies, and to psychological factors such as family tensions. Colic is estimated to occur in one-third of all infants. Babies with colic usually outgrow the disorder and their prognosis is good.

The sequelae to this condition, however, can be detrimental to bonding and to the development of a close relationship between parent and infant. Mothers can feel desperate and become very tense and nervous, which in turn affects their perception of motherhood and their relationship with their infant.

On objective examination of the infant, the nurse finds that the infant displays excessive gas in the stomach, is tense, keeps the lower extremities tense, and demands frequent feedings. Since there is no cure for colic, the nurse's goal should be to calm the infant, decrease stimulation from the child's environment, ensure proper feeding techniques, support the parents, reinforce what they are doing well, and allow the parents to express their feelings.

Recurrent Abdominal Pain

Pain. Sensory or emotional experience associated with actual or potential tissue damage.

Epigastric. Region over the pit of the stomach.

Periumbilical. Region around the umbilicus.

Acute **pain** is the onset of severe abdominal pain. The subjective diagnosis of recurrent abdominal pain is based on the occurrence of three or more episodes of abdominal pain over a period of 3 months. The objective diagnosis is based on the physical examination of the child's abdomen. The location of the abdominal pain is helpful in identifying its cause, which can be related to preexisting illness, appetite, food intake, fever, history of recent illness, nausea, vomiting, diarrhea, hematuria, or dysuria. **Epigastric** pain usually indicates pain from the liver, stomach, pancreas, and upper small bowel. **Periumbilical** pain is usually from the distal small intestine, appendix, and ascending colon. **Suprapubic** pain could be caused by urinary tract infection, pelvic organs, and distal intestines. **Referred pain** is usually the result of localized pain felt in adjacent areas of the abdomen. The most common cause of referred pain, in all age groups, is gastroenteritis. In children younger than 2 years, it could be the result of trauma, intussusception, incarcerated hernias, or intestinal malrotation. In children 2 to 5 years of age, the pain can be the result of sickle cell anemia or right-lobe pneumonia; in children older than 5 years, appendicitis; in adolescents, ovulary pain, ectopic pregnancy, ovarian torsion, or testicular pain. The most uncommon causes of abdominal pain in all ages are pancreatitis, cholecystitis, renal stones, and peptic ulcer disease. Other causes of recurrent pain include stool retention, lactose intolerance, parasitic infection, inflammatory bowel disease, and psychogenic pain.

Physical examination should encompass rectal examination along with vital signs, and pelvic examination if indicated. The laboratory tests should include a complete blood count (CBC) with differential, SMA 15, stool test for **occult blood**, abdominal x-rays, and if needed, ultrasound examination. Parents should be told that it may be necessary to reexamine the child during acute episodes. The management of abdominal pain varies. If it is suspected that the disease is a **functional disorder**, the family and the child should be assured that the symptoms are real and they will be treated. The family needs to be told that there is no organic cause in order to relieve their anxiety about the possibility of physical danger. If the cause is due to **organic disease**, the treatment is directed to correcting the underlying cause of the pain.

Appendicitis

Appendicitis is the most common surgical condition that produces abdominal pain in school-age children. Frequency increases with age and the peak of incidence is around 15 to 25 years of age. Appendicitis is an inflammation of the appendix, initiated by obstruction of the appendical lumen. The appendix becomes distended, causing ischemia and necrosis. A complete physical examination is required. The most prevalent findings are periumbilical pain concentrated in the right to the lower quadrant, rebound tenderness over McBurney's point, and low-grade fever. Tenderness may be noted on rectal examination. There is anorexia, vomiting, and diarrhea. The most comfortable position for the child is on the side with legs flexed. A CBC with differential shows an increase in neutrophils and leukocytes over 15,000/μL. A urinalysis (UA) shows pyuria. A chest x-ray is needed in order to rule out pneumonia, which sometimes mimics appendicitis. The only treatment is the surgical removal of the appendix in order to prevent perforation, necrosis, peritonitis, sepsis, shock, or death. If treated early, the prognosis is very good.

Constipation

Constipation is the diminished passage of fecal material. Fecal continence is the ability to control defecation voluntarily; it requires normal contractions

Suprapubic. Region above the pubic arch.

Referred pain. Felt in a part removed from its point of origin; may be the result of visceral pain or from proximal organ.

Occult blood. Blood in such minute quantity that it can be recognized only by microscopic examination or by chemical means.

Functional disorder. Changes or disturbances of any organ's functions.

Organic disease. A disease associated with observable or detectable changes in the organs of the body.

Constipation. Difficulty in defecation; infrequent passage of hard, dry fecal material.

of the anal sphincter. Usually, the movement of fecal material into the rectum stimulates automatic coordinated reflexes. The lower colon, including the rectum, contracts, and the external sphincter relaxes. Then the external sphincter contracts, and a total inhibition of the external and internal sphincter occurs, leading to defecation. At the time of defecation, intra-abdominal pressure increases voluntarily, the pelvic floor descends, and the stool is expelled. Retention of stool for prolonged periods of time can lead to stretching of the rectal wall and the development of megarectum. The most common causes of constipation include ignoring the urge to defecate, a sedentary life-style, medications, neurologic diseases, anorectal disorders, and endocrine disorders. Familial, cultural, and social factors also influence its genesis, development, and course. Psychological factors such as toilet training techniques and diet (excessive milk intake and low fiber intake) may also influence bowel habits. Subjective findings such as nervousness, school failure, and bad breath have been attributed to constipation. Normal infants often appear to have problems with constipation, and parents should be taught that this is a normal developmental pattern. The use of laxatives should be discouraged because it can lead to rectal retention of stool. Fecal retention can lead to impaction of the rectum with involuntary leakage. Constipation is prevalent among mentally retarded children. Diagnostic tests include abdominal x-rays, barium enema, and rectal biopsy if Hirschsprung disease is suspected. The treatment of constipation in children encompasses reduced milk intake and increased intake of fluids; if the condition does not improve, the use of dioctyl sodium sulfosuccinate, 5 to 10 mg/kg/d, is recommended.

Diarrhea

Diarrhea. Frequent passage of unformed watery bowel movements. A frequent symptom of gastrointestinal disturbance.

Electrolytes. Substances that, in solution, conduct an electric current and are decomposed by the passage of an electric current.

Infectious disease. The invasion of a pathogenic agent into the body.

Diarrhea is abnormally frequent and liquid fecal discharge, with excessive loss of fluids and **electrolytes** in the stool. It is classified as acute (lasts less than 2 weeks) or persistent (lasts 2 to 3 weeks or more). Diarrhea or acute gastroenteritis is one of the most common pediatric illnesses. Although bacteria and parasites can be the cause of these conditions, diarrhea is hard to define because there is a wide variation of normal bowel habits. Diarrhea can be caused by: (a) interruption of normal cell transport processes, (b) decrease in the surface area available for absorption, (c) increase in bowel motility, (d) increase in absorbable active molecules in the intestinal lumen, or (e) increase in intestinal permeability (Nurko, 1993).

Most symptoms of viral enteritis derive from dehydration. The cause of viral diarrhea can be rotavirus or calicivirus. Bacterial diarrhea can be caused by *Salmonella, Shigella,* or *Escherichia coli.* Other viral and bacterial agents include *Campylobacter jejuni, Clostridium difficile, Yercinia enterocolitica,* and viruses that invade the intestinal mucosa. Parasites can also cause diarrhea, as can *Staphylococcus.*

The causes of acute diarrhea are usually **infections,** inflammatory bowel disease, or medications such as antibiotics, antacids, or laxatives. Inflammatory bowel disease, malabsorption, hyperthyroidism, HIV, functional bowel disease, irritable bowel syndrome, or fecal impaction cause chronic diarrhea.

Osmotic diarrhea is the result of osmotically active particles in the intestine, a condition seen in dumping syndrome and overfeeding. Secretory diarrhea is the result of inhibition of ion absorption, as seen in the presence of bacteria. Bile salt and pancreatic enzyme deficiency cause diarrhea by inhibiting the normal absorption process. Inflammatory processes due to bacterial infection that cause abnormal peristalsis can become acute diarrhea.

In pediatrics, diarrhea is most common in children age 6 months to 2 years. Other than the diarrhea associated with antibiotic therapy, viruses are the most common cause of diarrhea all over the world. And the most common viral cause of diarrhea, worldwide, is rotavirus. The incidence depends on many factors, the most prevalent being geographical location, living conditions, climate or season, socioeconomic status, and hygiene practiced in daily activities.

Treatment is aimed at restoring fluid and electrolyte balance, including oral rehydration. When stooling has diminished, half-strength formula is offered to infants; 24 to 48 hours after the diarrhea has subsided, the child should be offered full-strength formula. Constipation-producing solids such as rice, applesauce, cereal, and bananas may be given to older children when feeding resumes. The use of antidiarrheal agents to decrease bowel motility is not recommended if the diarrhea is caused by a germ; the underlying cause should be treated. Parents should be instructed not to feed an infant nonsterile food, and that good hygiene reduces fecal-oral spread of the germs.

Hepatitis

Hepatitis is an inflammation of the liver that occurs as a response to exposure to a drug or an infection. It tends to occur both epidemically and sporadically. Viruses are the most common cause of hepatitis in children; they can result in hepatitis A or B. Approximately 60,000 cases of viral hepatitis are reported each year in the United States. Autoimmune chronic active hepatitis is most common in teenage girls, yet it also occurs in all ages and in both sexes. Chronic active hepatitis may also follow hepatitis B.

Children with hepatitis present with diffuse abdominal pain, decreased appetite, nausea and vomiting, and sometimes fever and malaise. Children with hepatitis do not present with jaundice, but a nonspecific macular rash and arthralgia occur sometimes early in the course of hepatitis B. There are five types of hepatitis: A, B, C, D, and E.

Hepatitis A Hepatitis A (HAV), also called infectious hepatitis, is caused by a picornavirus composed of single-stranded RNA. It is transmitted through close personal contact and contaminated food and water. In children, the infection can be spread by fecal contamination; it is also seen in food handlers with poor hygiene habits. Other sources are shellfish: oysters, clams, and mussels.

The average incubation period is 28–30 days. The virus is shed in the stool for 2 to 3 weeks. Because the children are anorectic, their infection goes unnoticed during the most highly contagious period. Children that have had hepatitis A have lifelong immunity. There are no specific measures for treatment, but the child should not be given corticosteroids or sedatives. Diet should be light, especially at the beginning of the disease process, and foods ought to be low in fat. Ninety percent of children recover without any sequelae.

Hepatitis B Hepatitis B (HBV) or serum hepatitis is spread by contact. The disease is spread by contact with infected blood or blood products. Hepatitis B is transmitted through percutaneous inoculation (tattooing, dirty needles) and cuts exposed to dirty objects such as razors. Sexual transmission occurs via semen, vaginal secretions, and saliva. The average incubation period is 3 to 4 months. In contrast to hepatitis A, hepatitis B has a delayed onset with an incubation period of 21 to 160 days.

The disease is caused by a DNA virus that is usually acquired perinatally from the mother. The symptoms are nonspecific, consisting of a slight fever and mild gastrointestinal upset. Visible jaundice is the first symptom, accompanied by pale stools and darkened urine. Hepatomegaly is present. Infants display a yellow pigmentation of the skin; older infants, children, and adolescents also display jaundice and arthralgia or rashes can be the first sign. The diagnosis is made via the HBsAg, HBcAg (core), HBeAg, and antibodies to these antigens.. The treatment consists of supportive measures such as bed rest and a nutritious diet during the active phase of the disease.

Hepatitis C Hepatitis C (HCV) is caused by illicit use of intravenous drugs. Children with hemophilia or in chronic hemodialysis are at risk. The risk from transfused blood products has diminished since the advent of blood testing for serum aminotransferase (ALT) and anti-HCV. The incubation period is 1 to 5 months, and the onset of symptoms is insidious. Most childhood causes are asymptomatic despite the development of chronic hepatitis. The treatment is supportive and relapses are common. The prognosis for children is not well defined, though cirrhosis may develop rapidly or after decades. Infants infected at birth tend to develop HIV infection.

Hepatitis D Hepatitis D (HDV) can only occur in the presence of HBV infection. In developing countries, transmission is by intimate contact; in Western countries, by parental infection. In children, there is a strong association between chronic HDV co-infection with HBV and chronic, active hepatitis and cirrhosis. The diagnosis is made by the anti-HDV IgM test. Treatment is directed at therapy for HBV infection.

Hepatitis E Hepatitis E (HEV) is the cause of enterically transmitted, epidemic non-A, non-B hepatitis. It is rare in the United States. The agent is transmitted via the fecal-oral route. It occurs predominantly in developing countries, is associated with waterborne epidemics, and has only a

3% secondary attack in household contacts. Its clinical manifestations are similar to those of HAV except that it is rare in children and more common in adolescents. Hepatitis E is also associated with a high mortality rate.

Hernias

A **hernia** is a protrusion of abdominal viscus through the abdominal wall. Incarcerated hernias cannot be reduced and the contents of the hernia sac cannot be returned to the peritoneal cavity. Strangulated hernias occur when blood supply to the viscera lying within the hernia sac is cut off. Hernias can be congenital, from obesity, chronic airway disease, chronic coughing, or ascites. Chronic constipation with straining and hard physical labor are conditions that increase intraabdominal pressure and may contribute to the appearance of a hernia.

Physical exam determines the type of the hernia and whether it is reducible, incarcerated, or strangulated. In doing the initial exam for a suspected hernia, the nurse should examine the patient in standing and supine positions. Inspect the abdomen and groin and ask the patient to do a Valsalva maneuver. Inspect the hernia for discoloration, edema, tenderness, and signs of bowel obstruction. If it is suspected that the hernia is strangulated, it should not be reduced because of the danger of causing a gangrenous bowel.

Inguinal Hernia The presence of a scrotal or inguinal swelling or both is known as an inguinal hernia. In females, inguinal hernias present with swelling in the inguinal area and labia majora (Figure 10-1). In males, inguinal hernia is the incomplete closure of the processus vaginalis through which the testes descend into the scrotum. An inguinal hernia allows the presence of abdominal contents in the inguinal canal or scrotum in males, and in the labia majora in females. They occur in 2% of boys and are more common in males than in females.

Diagnosis is done during the first year of life. Bilateral hernias are the most common. Unilateral hernias are more likely to occur on the right side. The parent reports that the swelling in the scrotal area or labia majora comes and goes, and is more prominent when the infant cries. An inguinal hernia does not resolve by itself, so it ought to be referred to a surgeon for repair. Parents usually become very upset when they realize that their infant has to undergo surgery. They need to be educated in the dangers of postponing surgery and in recognizing the symptoms of incarcerations, and the action that they must take if this occurs.

Umbilical Hernia Umbilical hernias are more common in premature infants than in full-term infants. This condition is also more common in black infants. Most umbilical hernias regress spontaneously if the diameter of the fascial defect is less than 1 cm. Larger umbilical hernias should be treated surgically.

Hernia. Protrusion or projection of an organ through the wall of the cavity that normally contains it.

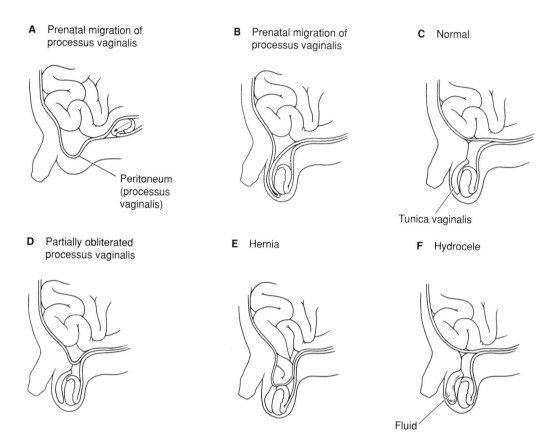

A   Prenatal migration of processus vaginalis

Peritoneum (processus vaginalis)

B   Prenatal migration of processus vaginalis

C   Normal

Tunica vaginalis

D   Partially obliterated processus vaginalis

E   Hernia

F   Hydrocele

Fluid

FIGURE 10-1 The development of an inguinal hernia. (A, B) Prenatal migration of processus vaginalis. (C) Normal. (D) Partially obstructed processus vaginalis. (E) Hernia. (F) Hydrocele.

Intussusception

Intussusception is the most common cause of intestinal obstruction in the first 2 years of life, with a peak incidence at 3 months to 1 year. The bowel begins proximal to the ileocecal valve and is usually ileocolic, but it can be ileoileal or colocolic. The parents usually report that the child has episodic abdominal pain with vomiting and screaming with drawing up of the legs. Once the pain has subsided, they report, the child is lethargic, and there is diarrhea, which can have a small amount of bleeding. Objective physical examination reveals a mass like a thick cord in the right upper quadrant of the abdomen. The abdomen is tender when **palpated** and is distended. A flat plate x-ray of the abdomen is taken to confirm the diagnosis; 40% of the time the x-ray can appear normal. If this occurs a barium enema is given and sometimes this procedure is therapeutic.

The treatment is geared to resolving the condition. The child is treated in the hospital where intravenous fluids are started. If the condition is not resolved with the barium enema and if the pediatrician suspects perforation, immediate surgery is performed. The prognosis is good but there is a possibility that if perforation occurs the child can develop sepsis.

Palpation. Process of examining by application of the hands or fingers to the external surface of the body to detect evidence of disease or abnormalities in the various organs.

*U*PPER GASTROINTESTINAL TRACT DISORDERS

Gastroesophageal Reflux

Gastrointestinal esophageal reflux (GER) is the effortless passage of gastric contents into the esophagus from the stomach through the lower esophageal sphincter. There are three classifications of GER (Boyle, 1989):

1. Physiological: the child has infrequent episodic vomiting.
2. Functional: the child has effortless vomiting, does not complain of pain or discomfort, and has no subsequent physical problems.
3. Pathological: the child has frequent vomiting, which causes alteration in physical functioning. This kind of GER is usually seen in infants with failure to thrive.

The three main physiological barriers that prevent reflux of gastric content into the esophagus are functional esophageal sphincter, normal distal esophageal motility, and efficient gastric emptying. Therefore, physiological reflux occurs when there is a delay in the maturation of one or more of the three barriers. This condition is the result of many factors. While taking the initial history, the nurse should give extra consideration to the historical information about the birth, complaints of feeding difficulties, type of feeding, amount and frequency of feeding, and amount of reflux when the child was an infant. Also, it is important to determine if the infant was bottle- or breast-fed. In assessing the family history, it is important to verify if the child has choking spells during feedings and if the vomiting has bilious content or blood, which should alert the nurse to the possibility of chronic gastritis. Headache, fever, and abdominal pain are also indications that the child could be developing an infection secondary to bleeding. Obtaining a 24-hour diet history of the child from the parents gives the nurse a clear picture of the attainment of developmental milestones. Besides the history and the physical exam, the following tests are performed: CBC with differential, stool for occult blood, UA with culture, upper GI series, endoscopy to rule out esophagitis, and esophageal pH monitoring.

The complexity of this condition obliges the nurse and the doctor to suspect its presence as secondary to anatomic anomalies such as malrotation of the bowel, esophageal webs, gastroenteritis, formula intolerance, Reye's syndrome, pancreatitis, and hepatobiliary problems. In 80% of patients, GER is self-limiting, disappearing between 6 and 12 months. The treatment is geared to preventing reflux and to maintaining nutrition. The role of the nurse is important in teaching parents the importance of giving the child small, frequent feedings and the correct technique in burping the infant, encouraging breast-feeding, and incorporating solid food into the diet. Infants are usually introduced to rice early; 1 tablespoon per 1 ounce of milk is given in the beginning. If tolerated, the quantity is increased. It is also important to stress that after feedings the infant should be propped up with his/her head elevated.

Parents of older children should be educated about the problems that foods rich in caffeine, fat, and spices can cause to children with this condition. The major problem that the nurse faces with children with this condition is the follow-up over time, since poor nutrition contributes to delays in growth and development.

If the condition does not improve and if the medical treatment is not successful, surgery is necessary in order to prevent aspiration pneumonia, apnea, or severe esophagitis. The major complications of GER are bleeding and formation of strictures in the esophagus.

Diaphragmatic Hernia

Diaphragmatic hernia is a malformation that consists of a herniation of abdominal organs into the hemothorax, usually on the left side. This is due to a posterolateral defect in the diaphragm. Infants with this condition usually present in the delivery room with signs of respiratory distress, cyanosis, decreased breath sounds on the side of the hernia, and shift of the mediastinum to the side opposite the hernia. This condition is critical and the infants are usually hard to resuscitate, requiring immediate intubation. The treatment is surgery, performed immediately after the infant is stabilized. The mortality rate is 50% with survival depending on the degree of pulmonary hypoplasia in the contralateral lung.

Tracheoesophageal Fistula and Esophageal Atresia

Tracheoesophageal fistula and esophageal atresia are associated conditions that are characterized by a blind esophageal pouch and a fistulous connection between either the proximal or distal esophagus and the airway (Figure 10-2). In 80% of infants with this condition, the fistula is between the distal esophagus and the airway. Infants with this condition have copious secretions, cyanosis, and choking during the first hours after birth. Diagnosis is confirmed with chest x-ray after careful placement of a nasogastric tube to the point at which resistance is met.

The treatment consists of elevating the head of the bed immediately to prevent reflux of gastric contents, and aspirating the lungs. Intravenous fluids are started immediately and oxygen is started. Surgery depends on the distance between the segments of the esophagus. If the distance is not too great, the fistula can be ligated and the ends of the esophagus anastomosed. The prognosis depends on the presence or absence of associated anomalies.

Nausea and Vomiting

Nausea is an unpleasant feeling of impending vomiting, and vomiting is the forceful expulsion of gastric contents. Nausea and vomiting are pro-

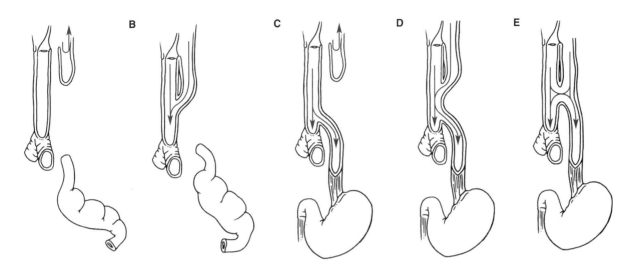

FIGURE 10-2 The most common types of esophageal atresia and tracheo-esophageal fistula.

tective mechanisms activated by numerous gastrointestinal and nongastrointestinal causes. Among the most common gastrointestinal causes are peptic ulcer disease or gastritis and motility disorders. Among the central nervous system causes are motion sickness and migraine headaches. Systemic causes include pregnancy, infections, and food poisoning, and iatrogenic causes may be medications or bulimia.

The diagnosis is based on the duration, quantity, and quality of the vomitus. It is also important to assess the timing, whether it occurs before or after meals, and if it is associated with abdominal pain, diarrhea, dizziness, headache, or systematic symptoms of fever and malaise. In infants, it is important to assess feedings, activity level, irritability, lethargy, and the number of wet diapers. The physical exam should pay more attention to fever, abdominal tenderness, rigidity, bowel sounds, and liver and spleen sizes. Children should be examined rectally to rule out occult blood.

Pyloric Stenosis

Pyloric stenosis is characterized by a hypertrophied pyloric muscle, causing a narrowing of the pyloric sphincter (Figure 10-3). The disease occurs in 1 out of 500 births, and males are more affected than females. Infants with this condition develop vomiting after the first 2 weeks of life, which becomes **projectile** after every feeding. The vomitus does not contain bile but may be bloodstreaked. The infant usually is hungry and presents a picture of weight loss and dehydration. On physical examination the baby presents a mass like an olive in the epigastrum, and there

Projectile vomiting. Forceful ejection through the mouth of gastric contents, in cases of obstruction.

A   B

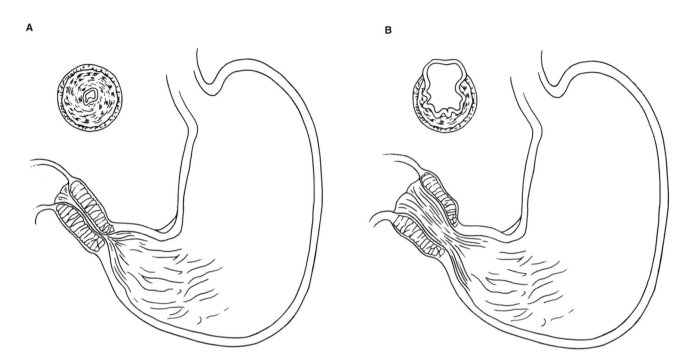

FIGURE 10-3 Hypertrophic pyloric stenosis. (A) Muscular tumor nearly
annihilates the pyloric channel. (B) Pyloric channel after longitudinal
surgical division of muscle down to the mucosa.

is an obvious peristaltic wave across the abdomen (see Figure 10-4;
Color Insert 9). Diagnosis is made by gastrointestinal series and the
treatment is a surgical intervention called pyloromyotomy. In postoperative care, feedings should be introduced in small amounts, and the nurse
must be aware that vomiting can continue for few weeks postsurgery.
The prognosis is very good.

Celiac Disease

Celiac disease is the result of intestinal sensitivity to the gliadin fraction of
the gluten from wheat, rye, barley, and oats. The disease appears to be
more prevalent in persons of European descent and almost nonexistent in
blacks and Asians. The causal factor for the sensitivity is not known; however, the intestinal lesion is hypothesized to be the result of a cell-mediated
immune response to gliadin. Affected children present with a history of
gastric problems during early infancy. Initially, diarrhea is intermittent,
but later it becomes continuous, with bulky, pale, frothy, greasy, foul-
smelling stools. The clinical picture of the infant is one of anorexia, dehydration, and muscle weakness, with very thick fatty stools.

The management of this disease is very complicated because not only are there physical sequelae, but also psychological problems, such as failure to bond, retardation of growth, and parents' feelings of guilt and pain. Treatment consists of dietary gluten restriction for life. Dietary supervision is essential, and the diet should be tailored to the child's appetite and capacity to absorb nutrients. The prognosis is determined according to the rate of clinical recovery, which is usually slow.

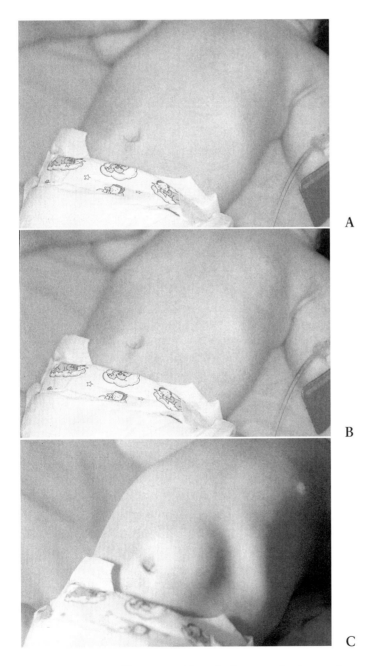

A

B

C

FIGURE 10-4 Gastric wave of hypertrophic pyloric stenosis. A gastric wave can be seen traversing the abdomen in this series of photographs of a patient with HPS. (Courtesy of Kevin J. Knoop, MD, MS.) (See also Color Insert 9.)

*L*OWER GASTROINTESTINAL TRACT INFECTIONS

Intestinal Parasites

Multiple organisms can cause parasitic infestation in the gastrointestinal tract. The following are among the most common.

Ascariasis Ascariasis is defined as an intestinal parasitic infection caused by *Ascaris lumbricoides*, a large roundworm. It is considered the most common parasitic worm, is found globally in humans, and affects both children and adults. The child ingests the eggs of the worm, which are found in the soil, by eating dirt (pica) or food that was grown where the eggs are found (unwashed vegetables), or drinking water contaminated by human feces.

Diagnosis of ascariasis is based on a comprehensive history and physical examination. The presenting signs and symptoms include anorexia, nausea, vomiting, weight loss, fever, irritability, and cough. The child will normally give a history of pica ingestion and stool examination will reveal adult worms. The visualization of adult worms in the stool is considered the most conclusive diagnostic test. Normally, three stool specimens are collected and analyzed for ova and parasites (O & P). Upon physical examination, the child demonstrates progressive weight loss with abdominal tenderness and masses. Included in the physical examination is a check for occult blood. The nurse must include a differential diagnosis of asthma, pneumonia, poor nutrition, and giardiasis.

Management of a child with ascariasis includes using pyrantel pamoate 11 mg/kg in a single dose or mebendazole 100 mg bid for 3 days. A pregnant woman must consult a physician before beginning any medication that could affect her unborn child. The nurse should stress the importance of a clean play area, the elimination of pica ingestion, and the sanitary disposal of feces. Follow-up is not considered essential.

Enterobiasis Enterobiasis is defined as an intestinal parasitic infection caused by *Enterobius vermicularis*, a white pinworm. Humans are the only known host for this worm. The pathogenesis follows a chronological series of events. An adult gravid female worm deposits eggs on the child's perianal skin. The child scratches the perianal area and then places his/her hands in or near the mouth, so the eggs are able to enter the child's body. The pathogenesis is therefore related to poor handwashing, which permits autoinfection by ingestion of the eggs. A comprehensive history will reveal the time and circumstances surrounding the onset of symptoms. The physical examination of the child will reveal anal pruritus, and genital irritation in females. Often, similar histories and physicals of others in the household will reveal a similar pattern of pruritus and genital irritation. Differential diagnosis considerations include poor hygiene and chemical irritants such as bubble bath as causes of the signs and symptoms. The primary diagnostic examination technique is to place Scotch tape on the anus area just before the child goes to bed and then to remove the tape just before the child normally rises. The tape is then evaluated for the presence of ova. The management of enterobiasis is the same as for ascariasis.

Visceral Larva Migrans Visceral larva migrans is defined as an intestinal parasitic infection caused by *Ancylostoma duodenale* and *Necator americanus*. The eggs of the adult worm are normally found in the stool of the host, who then passes the eggs in feces left in the soil. In the soil, the eggs hatch into larvae. A person is infected by the larvae by walking barefoot in areas where feces are left. Contact with contaminated soil for 5 to 10 minutes will result in skin penetration through the soles of the feet or the palms of the hands. The larvae are carried throughout the circulatory system and normally enter the lungs and eventually the small intestine, where they move down the intestinal tract and leave the host in feces.

A comprehensive history and physical will reveal episodes of intense pruritus of the feet, palms of the hands, and even buttocks of the child. Physical examination will demonstrate the pruritus as well as chest symptoms of the infection such as cough and wheezing. Further examination will show abdominal pain, a history of diarrhea, and weight loss. Physical examination of the skin, especially the palms of the hands and soles of the feet, will reveal erythematous papular vesicular lesions that may be excoriated from scratching. Such lesions can be found on the buttocks and thighs as well. The abdomen will have masses and tenderness. The nurse should also consider the differential diagnoses of asthma, pneumonia, poor nutrition, and giardiasis as possible causes for the patient's presenting signs and symptoms. The diagnostic test of choice is the collection of a stool specimen for examination for O & P. The management of visceral larva migrans is the same as for ascariasis.

Giardiasis Giardiasis is defined as an infection of the small intestine and/or biliary tract by *Giardia lamblia*, a flagellate protozoan considered one of the most common intestinal parasites in the United States. The pathogenesis of giardiasis is from the ingestion of contaminated drinking water where the protozoa are found. Humans are the principal reservoir of infection. The main route by which the protozoa spread is by fecal materials, or the oral transfer of cysts from the feces of an infected individual to a noninfected person. The incubation period is normally 7 to 14 days. The disease is considered **communicable** as long as the cysts are being excreted in the stool.

Diagnosis is made through a comprehensive history and physical examination. The patient normally demonstrates abdominal pain and bulky, malodorous stools with eructation and flatulence. There is a history of weight loss and the patient's family members will demonstrate similar signs and symptoms. The nurse needs to question the family as to possible water sources that could be considered contaminated and stress the need to use only a clean water source for drinking and bathing. The history and physical examination should include a determination if weight loss has occurred and whether abdominal masses, tenderness, and bowel sounds are present.

Communicable disease. A disease that is directly or indirectly transmitted from one person to another.

Salmonellosis Salmonellosis is an infection caused by *Salmonella*, a gram-negative rod bacteria belonging to the family *Enterobacteriaceae*. The primary reservoir for *Salmonella* are such animals as poultry, livestock, and pets. *Salmonella* can be found in contaminated and improperly cooked foods such as poultry, eggs, dairy products, and sausage. The pathogenesis, or mode of transmission, is by ingestion of infected food or water, and direct contact with infected animals or persons. The diagnosis of salmonellosis is made through a comprehensive history and physical.

If salmonellosis is suspected, the nurse should assess for the onset, duration, and systemic symptoms, which include mucoid and/or bloody stools. Ask about the possibility of exposure to infected animals or persons, and ingestion of contaminated food or water. The patient's family normally will present with similar signs and symptoms, so the nurse should ask about their general health as well. The physical examination will reveal a febrile child, abdominal tenderness, rigidity, and abnormal tympani with liver and spleen enlargement. Included in the assessment should be bowel sounds, rectal examination for tenderness and mass, and stool for occult blood.

Management is similar to that for other intestinal infections and includes restoring and maintaining hydration. Once the infant or child is able to take and retain fluids, he/she should be returned to full-strength formula as quickly as possible. For those children who are taking solid foods, give bland, soft foods within the first 24 to 48 hours of rehydration. Bananas, rice, applesauce, toast, and carrots are generally tolerated and assist in firming up the stool.

Salmonella diarrhea normally resolves spontaneously in most cases. Antibiotic therapy can prolong the carrier state, and therefore is indicated only for neonates and children younger than 1 year who are considered at risk for bacteremia. Other patients at risk are patients with lymphoproliferative diseases, hemolytic anemias, or hemoglobinopathies, immunosuppressed individuals, and those who have cardiac or valvular disease.

Shigellosis Shigellosis is defined as an acute infection of the bowel by *Shigella* organisms, gram-negative rods belonging to the family *Enterobacteriaceae*. Shigellosis is most common in children 6 months to 3 years of age. The pathogenesis is ingestion of contaminated food or water, and homosexual transmission. The source of infection is human feces. There is no known animal reservoir.

The diagnosis of shigellosis is made through a comprehensive history and physical. Included in the assessment is the onset, duration, systemic symptoms, and if there are mucoid or bloody stools. Ask whether the person has been exposed to infected persons, ingested contaminated food or water, or had homosexual contacts. The child's family will have similar signs and symptoms of the illness, and the family members' general health status should also be assessed. If the child attends day care, ask about the children's health at the day care. In the physical examination, the nurse should include the child's hydration and cardiovascular status, and determine if there is any abdominal tenderness, masses, abnormal tympani, bowel sounds, or liver and spleen enlargement. A rectal examination should be done to determine tenderness, masses, and stool for occult blood.

Preventing Parasitic Infestations Simply ensuring that the patient and family use good handwashing techniques and have good sanitation practices can prevent most parasitic infestations. Many parasites can be avoided or eliminated through various means. *G. lamblia:* Reduce or eliminate by treating questionable water with iodine or boiling it for 20 minutes. Have children who are symptomatic stay home from day care or school until they are asymptomatic. *E. vermicularis* (pinworm): Reduce by having the child avoid scratching. Have the parent wash the child's sheets and clothing in hot water and detergent. *N. americanus* (hookworm): Practice sanitary disposal of feces. Wear shoes in high-risk areas. *A. lumbricoides* (roundworm): Eliminate by using appropriate food preparation techniques. *Strongyloides* (threadworm): Avoid by simply wearing shoes. *Taenia* (tapeworm): Eliminate by avoiding raw or undercooked beef or pork.

Complications of Parasitic Infections A number of complications can occur with various parasitic infections, but they can be avoided with early detection and treatment of the underlying cause. *G. lamblia* can lead to malabsorption, weight loss, and failure to thrive. *E. vermicularis,* even untreated, is self-limiting, but reinfections should be eliminated. *N. americanus* can cause anemia and malnutrition. *A. lumbricoides* can lead to Loeffler syndrome (fever, respiratory symptoms, pulmonary complications such as infiltrates, and excessive serum eosinophilia), produced as an allergic response to the larvae.

$\mathcal{S}$UMMARY

In this chapter, common gastrointestinal abnormalities involving the digestive tract were discussed. Various gastrointestinal defects and/or infections may be described according to anatomical abnormalities or influences that defects or infection might have upon ingestion, digestion, absorption, or elimination processes. Understanding the normal organization and function of the digestive tract is important, since changes in a structure or a functional process of the digestive system will have profound influences on other systems. The major signs and symptoms associated with various infectious agents that attack the digestive system are often manifested in similar complaints. Therefore, the nurse must be comprehensive while doing a history and physical assessment in order to differentiate between various causes. Chronic diarrhea and/or dehydration can lead to acidosis, which can then lead to cardiovascular collapse and ultimately death.

In the case of the child with congenital gastric malformations, the nurse has to be aware that the anomalies can happen anywhere in the GI tract. Any infant who has excessive drooling and cyanosis should be suspected as having malformation problems. The nurse needs to prepare the infant for measures that will maximally alleviate the condition, and also prepare the infant for immediate or imminent surgery. Special care and support should be given to the parents through this difficult time. Although educating parents is important, at this time teaching should be postponed in order to allow the parents to express their fear and anxiety. The nurse has to be aware that this is a time when families need support and care from the health team in order to deal with their situation.

CRITICAL POINTS IN THE MANAGEMENT OF GASTROINTESTINAL DISORDERS

Appropriate functioning of the gastrointestinal system is essential for children's growth and development. A clear understanding of its anatomy and physiology allows the nurse not only to manage the health problems, but also to guide parents and children in order to prevent further deterioration and complications. The emphasis in the care of these conditions is an anticipatory guidance for the parents, since they are the ones who will be managing the condition at home. In order to provide the necessary guidance, the nurse must create a longitudinal plan of care, taking into consideration not only the disease process but also the main milestones in the development of the child. In this context, the appropriate nutritional status must be achieved as quickly as possible.

Growth and development of the child is the number one goal of the treatment, and planning for the incidentals of the disease becomes second. Recognizing early signs of interruptions in the development of the child allows the nurse to treat the child as a whole, and not merely the disease process.

In the case of malabsorption syndromes, it is important to assess the child and the family, but most important to understand the social structure within the family. A clear understanding of the society in which the child lives allows the health care team to provide a more comprehensive plan of care. Simultaneously, this approach challenges families to leave their circle of familiar beliefs in order to successfully treat their children.

Often parents do not understand the disease process or misinterpret explanations in order to deal with their guilt or with their societal rules. Families of children with malabsorption syndromes many times do not want to hear that the condition will not go away, and that it is a slow process. For example, in the case of the child with chronic diarrhea, the most valuable tool that the nurse must teach the parent is the ongoing assessment of the infant's nutritional balance and the danger of dehydration. Special attention should be given to educating the parents in how to rehydrate the child and how to reintroduce milk and solid food. In addition, parents must learn how to avoid placing the infant in danger of reinfection and also how to relieve skin deterioration due to diarrhea.

QUESTIONS

Diagnosis: Diarrhea Due to Shigellosis

History: 1-year-old Johnny is taken to the pediatrician's office because he has had loose bowel movements for 2 days. His mother states that Johnny was okay before this episode, that no one in the family is sick, and that no one has diarrhea. Johnny has been eating the same food that they all had. The only difference in the household is a new dog. The little dog is healthy, but not housebroken yet, so sometimes he defecates in the house. Johnny is just starting to walk, but he still crawls a lot and he loves the little dog.

Nursing problems: Fluid and electrolyte imbalance, dehydration, fever, malaise, excessive diarrhea.

Symptoms: Dehydration, low-grade fever, vomiting during the first 12 hours of illness, and abdominal pain. The vomiting was not bilious and did not have blood. The stools had some blood streaks.

Physical exam: Johnny is dehydrated, pale, with poor skin turgor, tenderness in his abdomen, and clear lungs. He looks as though he was well developed before this illness.

Laboratory findings: Stool testing: *Shigella* present. Electrolytes reflect the degree of dehydration and bicarbonate loss in the stools. Temperature: 101.8°F (axillary). Urinalysis: concentrated with some WBC. Weight: 19 pounds; normal weight, 20 pounds.

1. Considering all the lab reports, which pharmacological treatment should Johnny receive?

   A. Ampicillin
   B. Erythromycin
   C. None
   D. Furazolidone

2. Which of the following assessment data is most clinically diagnostic of dehydration?

   A. Skin turgor
   B. Moisture of mucous membranes
   C. Weight
   D. Urinary output

3. Johnny is placed on NPO status and intravenous fluids have been started. Johnny is very upset because he is thirsty. His mother asks the nurse when she will be able to feed Johnny again.

   A. In one week.
   B. When stooling diminishes.
   C. When the fever subsides.
   D. In 24 hours.

4. Johnny has had only two stools in the last 24 hours. The nurse tells his mother that now she will be able to feed Johnny
   A. Ginger ale
   B. Rice
   C. Milk
   D. Applesauce

5. Johnny's condition has improved and the doctor's orders include feeding him with half-strength milk. His mother asks when she will be able to feed Johnny whole milk.
   A. After two feedings of half-strength milk.
   B. After assessment of how he tolerates the half-strength milk.
   C. After 24–48 hours of tolerating the half-strength milk.
   D. After 1 week, to make sure he is all right.

6. Johnny is being discharged from the hospital. What is the most important information that the nurse must impart to Johnny's mother?
   A. Do not wait so long the next time before you take Johnny to the doctor.
   B. As soon as Johnny has diarrhea place him on NPO for 8 hours.
   C. Good hygiene reduces fecal-oral spread.
   D. Start with antidiarrheal medication before bringing Johnny to the doctor.

Diagnosis: Peritonitis after Appendicitis

Nursing problems: Impaired physical motility. Risk of alteration in thermoregulation. Risk of further infection. Altered nutrition.

History: 13-year-old Mary Williams just came back from a weekend at her grandmother's home. While she was visiting, she felt diffuse cramping in her abdomen, with right lower quadrant tenderness. Her grandmother thought that she might be having her first period, so she took care of Mary by keeping her in bed and giving her some warm fluids and soup. Mary got worse and when she arrived at home she was anorexic, had low-grade fever, and had more acute pain. Mrs. Williams took Mary to the doctor's office. After examining Mary, the doctor decided that Mary had to have surgery right away.

1. What symptoms are suggestive of appendicitis?
   A. Anorexia, vomiting, pain in the abdomen
   B. Persistent lower quadrant pain, abdominal tenderness, low-grade fever
   C. Diarrhea, vomiting, low-grade fever
   D. Persistent lower quadrant pain, diarrhea, vomiting

2. After surgery, the doctor tells the Williams that Mary has peritonitis, and that the reason is because Mary's appendix has perforated. In preparing the Williams to see Mary after the surgery, the most important nursing intervention is to tell them that Mary:

A. Will have oxygen when she comes to her room.
B. Will have intravenous fluids for at least 48 hours.
C. Will have a drainage of the localized abscess.
D. Will only have an small incision.

3. In peritonitis, the leukocyte count is initially high, greater than $20,000/mm^3$, and later may fall to neutropenic levels. Supportive therapy is aimed at correcting which of the following?

A. Dehydration and acidosis
B. Infection
C. Pain
D. Healing

4. CBC and differential was one of the tests that were done in order to confirm the diagnosis. Which of the following would be increased in this condition?

A. Platelets
B. Red blood cells
C. Neutrophils
D. Erythrocytes

Diagnosis: Celiac Disease

Nursing problems: Altered family process. Altered nutrition. Altered fluid volume.

History: Mr. and Mrs. Leon suspect that their small baby, Clara, is not well. Six months after her birth, Clara developed diarrhea, but it was not continuous, so the parents did not worry. At Clara's 7-month checkup, Mrs. Leon told the nurse that Clara had stomach problems and that her stools were foul smelling.

1. The nurse immediately suspects that Clara may have celiac disease. Her judgment is based on her knowledge that the most important symptom of celiac disease is:

A. Presence of foul-smelling stools
B. Persistent diarrhea
C. Intermittent diarrhea
D. Intolerance of milk

2. The treatment of celiac disease is aimed at the prevention of which of the following:

    A. Celiac crisis
    B. Fat reabsorption
    C. Protein depletion
    D. Muscle wasting

3. Children with celiac disease often fail to thrive. This condition is due to which of the following?

    A. Loss of appetite
    B. Increased irritability
    C. Increased hunger
    D. Decreased peristalsis

4. The main part of the treatment is diet. Treatment consists of:

    A. Introduction of gluten slowly
    B. Restriction of gluten for life
    C. Replacement of proteins slowly
    D. Restriction of proteins for life

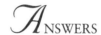

ANSWERS

Shigellosis

1. *A.* Diarrhea accompanies antibiotic therapy. Children develop fever, abdominal pain, and tenesmus, and may pass feces that contain leukocytes and sometimes blood for up to 8 weeks. Treatment with ampicillin is recommended.

2. *C.* When doing a physical exam of the child with dehydration, many factors should be taken into consideration. One of the most important determinants of the degree of dehydration is the child's weight, since this can assist in determining the percentage of total body fluids lost.

3. *B.* When stooling has diminished, rehydration by mouth should be started. Half-strength milk is offered as tolerated for 24–48 hours.

4. *A.* Clear fluids such as ginger ale and fruit-flavored gelatin are first introduced after the child has been on NPO.

5. *C.* Whole milk is introduced after 24–48 hours of tolerating half-strength milk.

6. *C.* Parents and children should be educated in the importance of washing their hands after going to the bathroom and, in the case of Johnny, after handling the urine or feces of the little dog.

Peritonitis

1. *B.* The triad of persistent localized right lower quadrant pain, localized abdominal tenderness, and slight fever strongly suggests appendicitis.

2. *C.* After the removal of the appendix, the peritoneal cavity sometimes has residual fluid and leukocytes. Often it is necessary to drain the abscess.

3. *A.* Along with antibiotic therapy, supportive treatment with intravenous therapy will correct dehydration and acidosis.

4. *C.* Neutrophils are always elevated in the presence of inflammation.

Celiac Disease

1. *A.* The hallmark of celiac disease is the presence of pale, watery stools with foul odor.

2. *A.* The nursing consideration is aimed at helping children and their parents adhere to dietary restrictions, which will prevent the celiac crisis, characterized by dehydration, shock, and acidosis.

3. *A.* The onset of diarrhea is usually accompanied by loss of appetite, failure to gain weight, and increased irritability.

4. *B.* Gluten needs to be eliminated from the child's diet. This is very simple when the child is an infant but more difficult when the child goes to school. The nurse's role, in teaching the parents and children about the dietary needs, is to stress the long-range consequences of not adhering to the diet.

 GLOSSARY

communicable disease   a disease that is directly or indirectly transmitted from one person to another.

constipation   difficulty in defecation; infrequent passage of hard, dry fecal material.

diarrhea   frequent passage of unformed watery bowel movements. A frequent symptom of gastrointestinal disturbance.

electrolytes   substances that, in solution, conduct an electric current and are decomposed by the passage of an electric current.

epigastric   region over the pit of the stomach.

functional disorder   changes or disturbances of any organ's functions.

hernia   protrusion or projection of an organ through the wall of the cavity that normally contains it.

infectious disease   the invasion of a pathogenic agent into the body.

occult blood   blood in such minute quantity that it can be recognized only by microscopic examination or by chemical means.

organic disease   a disease associated with observable or detectable changes in the organs of the body.

pain   sensory or emotional experience associated with actual or potential tissue damage.

palpation   process of examining by application of the hands or fingers to the external surface of the body to detect evidence of disease or abnormalities in the various organs.

peristalsis   progressive wavelike movement that occurs involuntarily in hollow tubes of the body.

periumbilical   region around the umbilicus.

projectile vomiting   forceful ejection through the mouth of gastric contents, in cases of obstruction.

referred pain   felt in a part removed from its point of origin; may be the result of visceral pain or from proximal organ.

suprapubic   region above the pubic arch.

$\mathcal{B}$IBLIOGRAPHY

AMERICAN ACADEMY OF PEDIATRICS. Workgroup on cow's milk protein and diabetes mellitus: Infant feeding practices and their relationship to the etiology of diabetes mellitus. *Pediatrics* 94:752–753, 1994.

BARKIN, R. M., AND ROSEN, P. *Emergency Pediatrics: A Guide to Ambulatory Care*. 4th ed. St. Louis: Mosby, 1994, pp. 276–282.

BARNESS, L. A. *Manual of Pediatric Physical Diagnosis*. 6th ed. St. Louis: Mosby, 1981.

BEHRMAN, R. E., AND KLIEGMAN, R. M. *Essentials of Pediatrics*. Philadelphia: W. B. Saunders, 1994.

BEHRMAN, R. E., et al., eds. *Nelson Textbook of Pediatrics*. 14th ed. Philadelphia: W. B. Saunders, 1992.

BOYLE, J. Gastrointestinal reflux in the pediatric patient. *Gastroenterology Clinics of North America* 18:315–337, 1989.

CASTEEL, H., AND FREDOREK, S. Oral rehydration therapy. *Pediatric Clinics of North America* 37(2):295–311, 1990.

CERVISI, J., CHAPMAN, M., NIKLAS, B., AND YAMAOKA, C. Office management of the infant with colic. *Journal of Pediatric Health Care* 5:184–190, 1991.

CHANG, T., AND WINTER, H. Gastroesophageal reflux. In R. A. Dershewitz (ed.), *Ambulatory Pediatric Care*. 2nd ed. Philadelphia: Lippincott, 1993, pp. 393–396.

CONNER, G. Foreign bodies of the ear, nose, airway, and esophagus. In R. A. Hockelman, S. Blatman, S. B. Friedman, N. M. Nelson, and H. M. Seidel (eds.), *Primary Pediatric Care*. St. Louis: Mosby, 1987, pp. 1245–1247.

HYAMS, J. A simple explanation of chronic abdominal distress. *Contemporary Pediatrics* 8(3):88–104, 1991.

KIRSCHNER, B. Inflammatory bowel disease in children. *Pediatric Clinics of North America* 35(1):189–208, 1988.

LEHTONEN, L., AND KORVENRANTA, H. Infantile colic: Seasonal incidence and crying profiles. *Archives of Pediatrics and Adolescent Medicine* 149:533–536, 1995.

LENCER, W. Malabsorption syndromes and chronic diarrhea. In R. A. Dershewitz, ed., *Ambulatory Pediatric Care.* 2nd ed. Philadelphia: Lippincott, 1993, pp. 411–415.

LERMAN, S. Common intestinal parasites. In R. A. Dershewitz (ed.), *Ambulatory Pediatric Care.* 2nd ed. Philadelphia: Lippincott, 1993, pp. 761–765.

NURKO, S. Acute diarrheas. In R. A. Dershewitz (ed.), *Ambulatory Pediatric Care.* 2nd ed. Philadelphia: Lippincott, 1993a, pp. 404–411.

NURKO, S. Recurrent abdominal pain. In R. A. Dershewitz (ed.), *Ambulatory Pediatric Care.* 2nd ed. Philadelphia: Lippincott, 1993b, pp. 400–404.

PETER, G., LEPOW, M., MCCRACKEN, G., AND PHILLIPS, C. (eds.), *Report of the Committee on Infectious Diseases.* Elk Grove Village, IL: American Academy of Pediatrics, 1991.

SONDHEIMER, J. Gastroesophageal reflux in infants and children. Personal communication, 1992.

SONDHEIMER, J., AND SILVERMAN, A. Gastrointestinal tract. In W. E. Hathaway, J. R. Groothuis, W. W. Hay, and J. W. Paisley (eds.), *Current Pediatric Diagnosis and Treatment.* Norwalk, CT: Appleton & Lange, 1991, pp. 538–573.

*H*ELPFUL INTERNET SITES

PEDINFO: An Index of the Pediatric Internet at http://www.pedinfo. org   This is an excellent site that covers nearly all topics within this review. It has a wealth of information and is worth a visit. It is written for health care professionals but others could also use the information.

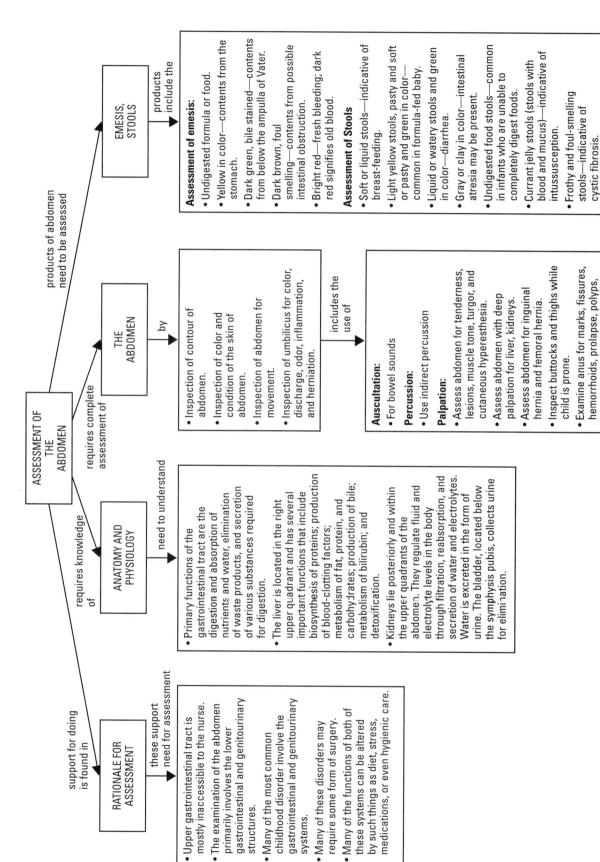

ASSESSMENT OF THE ABDOMEN

products of abdomen need to be assessed → **EMESIS, STOOLS**

requires complete assessment of → **THE ABDOMEN**

requires knowledge of → **ANATOMY AND PHYSIOLOGY**

support for doing is found in → **RATIONALE FOR ASSESSMENT**

EMESIS, STOOLS — products include the

Assessment of emesis:
- Undigested formula or food.
- Yellow in color—contents from the stomach.
- Dark green, bile stained—contents from below the ampulla of Vater.
- Dark brown, foul smelling—contents from possible intestinal obstruction.
- Bright red—fresh bleeding; dark red signifies old blood.

Assessment of Stools
- Soft or liquid stools—indicative of breast-feeding.
- Light yellow stools, pasty and soft or pasty and green in color—common in formula-fed baby.
- Liquid or watery stools and green in color—diarrhea.
- Gray or clay in color—intestinal atresia may be present.
- Undigested food stools—common in infants who are unable to completely digest foods.
- Currant jelly stools (stools with blood and mucus)—indicative of intussusception.
- Frothy and foul-smelling stools—indicative of cystic fibrosis.

THE ABDOMEN — by
- Inspection of contour of abdomen.
- Inspection of color and condition of the skin of abdomen.
- Inspection of abdomen for movement.
- Inspection of umbilicus for color, discharge, odor, inflammation, and herniation.

includes the use of

Auscultation:
- For bowel sounds

Percussion:
- Use indirect percussion

Palpation:
- Assess abdomen for tenderness, lesions, muscle tone, turgor, and cutaneous hyperesthesia.
- Assess abdomen with deep palpation for liver, kidneys.
- Assess abdomen for inguinal hernia and femoral hernia.
- Inspect buttocks and thighs while child is prone.
- Examine anus for marks, fissures, hemorrhoids, prolapse, polyps, and skin tags.

ANATOMY AND PHYSIOLOGY — need to understand
- Primary functions of the gastrointestinal tract are the digestion and absorption of nutrients and water, elimination of waste products, and secretion of various substances required for digestion.
- The liver is located in the right upper quadrant and has several important functions that include biosynthesis of proteins; production of blood-clotting factors; metabolism of fat, protein, and carbohydrates; production of bile; metabolism of bilirubin; and detoxification.
- Kidneys lie posteriorly and within the upper quadrants of the abdomen. They regulate fluid and electrolyte levels in the body through filtration, reabsorption, and secretion of water and electrolytes. Water is excreted in the form of urine. The bladder, located below the symphysis pubis, collects urine for elimination.

RATIONALE FOR ASSESSMENT — these support need for assessment
- Upper gastrointestinal tract is mostly inaccessible to the nurse.
- The examination of the abdomen primarily involves the lower gastrointestinal and genitourinary structures.
- Many of the most common childhood disorder involve the gastrointestinal and genitourinary systems.
- Many of these disorders may require some form of surgery.
- Many of the functions of both of these systems can be altered by such things as diet, stress, medications, or even hygienic care.

Concept Map 10-1

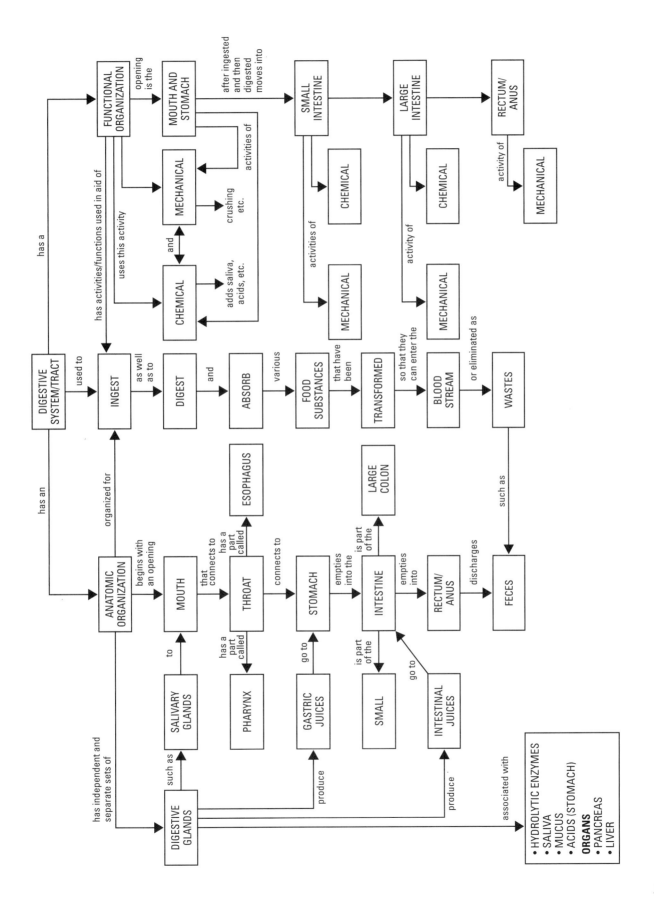

Concept Map 10-2

317

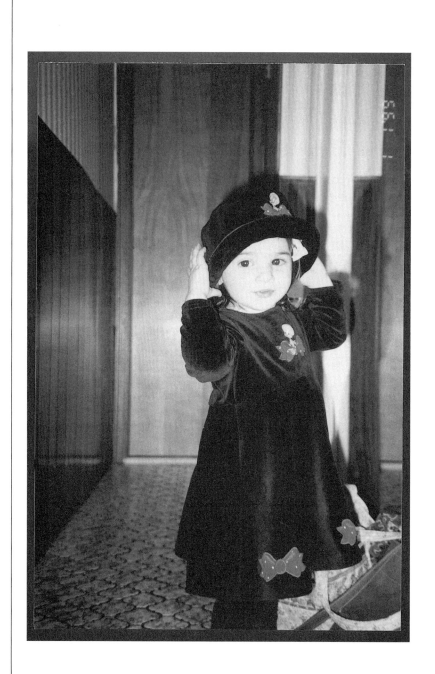

MUSCULOSKELETAL DISORDERS

INTRODUCTION

The musculoskeletal system is one of the major structural systems of the body. Any abnormality in this system signifies a major disruption in a child's life. A variety of congenital and structural disorders can present serious problems, not only in the child's physical development, but also because of the emotional scarring that these conditions may cause. The nurse plays a significant role in the outcome of these conditions by predicting problems before they occur, thereby preventing them. The nurse also assists the family in coping with any stigma they may harbor because of a disability of one of their members.

CONGENITAL HIP DYSPLASIA

Congenital hip dysplasia (congenital hip dislocation) results from defective development of the acetabulum with or without dislocation. The head of the femur does not sit correctly in the acetabulum and becomes displaced upward and backward. This disorder is more common in females than males. Usually only one hip is involved, the left more often than the right.

Congenital hip dysplasia. Hip disorder resulting from defective development of the acetabulum.

Etiology

The cause of congenital hip dysplasia is unknown. There is evidence of hereditary factors (increased incidence in twins). It is more common in infants with a frank breech delivery.

Three forms of congenital hip dysplasia exist. The degree of deformity can be mild (acetabular dysplasia), in which the femoral head remains in the acetabulum; intermediate (subluxation) (Figure 11-1), in which the femoral head remains in contact with the acetabulum, but is displaced; and the most severe, complete dislocation, in which the femoral head does not touch the acetabulum.

Ideally, diagnosis should be made in the first 2 months of the infant's life. The nurse plays an important role in the detection of this disorder. The newborn is observed during routine nursing activities and any deviations from normal are reported. Assessment of the hips should be part of the overall newborn assessment and continue until the child walks with a satisfactory gait. An older child's gait is observed at well-child checkups. The practitioner may detect an audible click using the Barlow (Figure 11-2) or Ortolani (Figure 11-3) maneuvers. These maneuvers are done one hip at a

FIGURE 11-1

⌘

Nine-year-old with developmental dislocation of left hip.

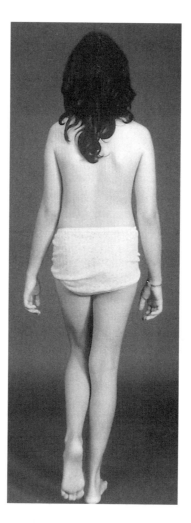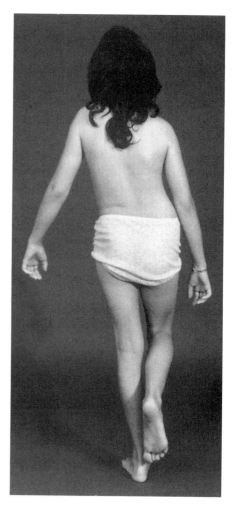

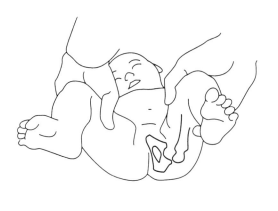

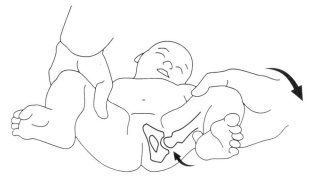

FIGURE 11-2

The Barlow test for dislocation of a located hip.

FIGURE 11-3

The Ortolani maneuver reduces a posteriorly dislocated hip.

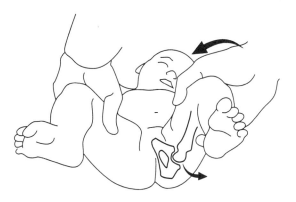

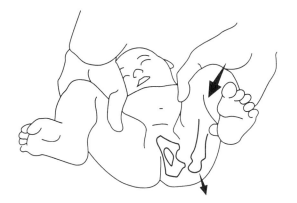

Lordosis. Lumbar curvature of the spine.

time, dislocating and relocating the acetabulum in adduction and abduction; however, these techniques are effective only for the first month. Signs used for diagnosis once the child is more than a month old include: asymmetry of the gluteal folds, which includes limited abduction of the affected hip, and obvious shortening of the femur. After the child starts walking, diagnostic signs include **lordosis,** protruding abdomen, swayback, duck waddle gait, and a positive Trendelenburg sign. Radiographic studies will confirm the diagnosis in the older infant and child.

Clinical Manifestations of Congenital Hip Dysplasia

In the Infant:

Positive Ortolani test—first 4 weeks
Positive Barlow test—first 4 weeks
Asymmetry of gluteal folds—higher on affected side
Limited hip abduction of affected hip—tested by placing infant in supine position with the knees flexed; both knees are passively abducted until they reach the examination table; if dislocation is present, the affected side cannot be abducted past 45°
Shortening of the femur on the affected side

In the Older Infant and Child:

Shortened lower extremity
Lordosis
Swayback
Protruding abdomen
Positive Trendelenburg sign—child stands on the affected leg holding on to a chair, rail, door, etc., and raises the normal leg; the pelvis tilts downward instead of upward as it would under normal circumstances (Figure 11-4)

Treatment is initiated as soon as the condition is detected. Early management allows for a more favorable prognosis, because the longer treatment is delayed, the more severe the deformity becomes, and the more difficult treatment becomes. Treatment depends on the age of the child and the severity of the dysplasia.

When dislocation is detected during the first few months of life, treatment is the manipulation of the femur into place and the application of a brace. The most frequently used brace is the **Pavlik harness** (Figure 11-5). The infant wears this harness continuously for 3 to 6 months until the hip is stable. Often, no further treatment is necessary.

After diagnosis, parents are given instructions concerning the Pavlik harness. The nurse should stress that the harness must be worn continuously. Sometimes, the harness may be removed for an occasional tub bath; however, the parents must be instructed on how to give a tub bath while

Pavlik harness. Frequently used to maintain flexion and stability of the hips in infants with congenital hip dysplasia.

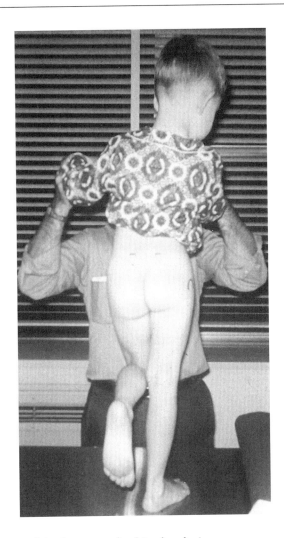

FIGURE 11-4 Trendelenburg test for hip dysplasia.

maintaining flexion and stability of the hips, which requires two people. Parents should also be instructed on how to reapply the harness properly.

If the child is placed in a cast, the parents must be taught cast care as well as techniques to keep the child and cast clean, especially in the diaper area. Parents also need to be instructed on how to feed their infant in a spica cast.

Children 6 to 18 months old may develop hip contractures if hip dysplasia goes unrecognized. These children require reduction by Bryant's traction and hospitalization. A spica cast is applied after the hip dislocation has been reduced. The child wears the cast until the hip is stable. If early treatment is unsuccessful or detection has been delayed until after the child walks, open reduction followed by a spica cast is necessary.

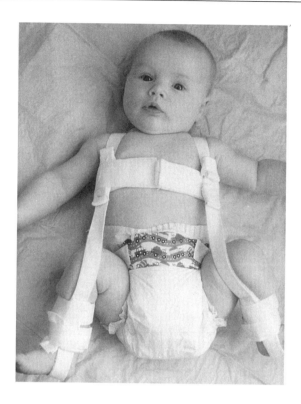

FIGURE 11-5

⌘

A 5-month-old infant being treated for bilateral right dislocation of hip in a Pavlik harness.

CONGENITAL CLUBFOOT

Clubfoot. Describes a condition in which the foot appears twisted out of shape.

The term **clubfoot** describes a condition in which the foot appears twisted out of shape. Deformities or talipes (from the Latin *talus,* meaning ankle, and *pes,* meaning foot) of the foot and ankle are named according to the position of the foot and ankle (Figure 11-6). The most frequently occurring type (95%) is talipes equinovarus, in which the foot is pointed downward and inward.

Congenital talipes equinovarus is the most common congenital foot deformity, appearing as a single anomaly or in combination with other defects. More males are affected than females and the clubfoot may be unilateral (one foot) or bilateral (both feet).

The exact cause of clubfoot is unknown. A hereditary factor is demonstrated by a higher incidence in identical twins. Some experts propose that arrested embryonic growth of the foot during the first trimester of pregnancy may be a cause. Abnormal positioning in utero may also be an explanation.

Clubfoot is apparent at birth. It is easily detected prenatally on ultrasound. The true clubfoot must be differentiated from a persistent fetal position of comfort. The positional deformity may be corrected by passive exercise; the deformity of clubfoot is fixed. Radiographic studies confirm the diagnosis.

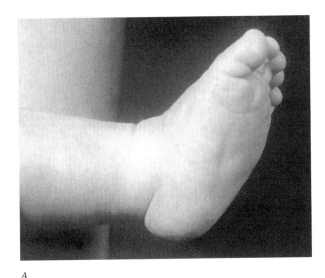
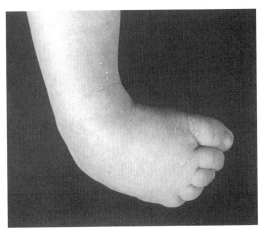

A

B

FIGURE 11-6 Clubfoot.

Manipulation and serial casting are used to correct the deformity and maintain correct positioning of the foot. The first cast is often applied in the newborn nursery. While the cast is being applied, the foot is gently moved into as close to normal positioning as possible. Force is not used. Manipulation and casting are repeated frequently, every few days for several weeks, then every week or two. The foot remains casted until complete correction is achieved. Following correction, a splint such as a **Denis-Browne splint** with corrective shoes is used to maintain the correction for 6 months or longer. A special clubfoot shoe is worn after overcorrection is attained. If these techniques fail, open reduction is necessary.

Nursing care of the child with nonsurgical correction is similar to that required by any child in a cast. Parents are instructed to observe for complications. Parents need a detailed explanation of the entire treatment and plan of care. They need to understand that frequent cast changes are necessary and they must protect against the cast becoming damaged.

Denis-Browne splint. A splint with corrective shoes used in the treatment of clubfoot.

OSTEOMYELITIS

Osteomyelitis is an infection of the bone that occurs frequently between 5 and 16 years of age. It is more common in boys than girls. Most often it is the tibia and femur that are affected.

Bacteria, which cause the infection, can enter the bone in one of two ways: by direct invasion (exogenous osteomyelitis), such as from a penetrating wound, open fracture, or surgical contamination, or, more commonly, by indirect invasion by blood-borne pathogens (hematogenous

Osteomyelitis. An infection of the bone.

osteomyelitis) originating from a preexisting infection. Sources of infection may be otitis media, tooth abscess, impetigo, and burns. *Staphylococcus aureus* is the most common causal organism in older children; *Haemophilus influenzae* is more common in younger children.

Bacterial invasion begins in the bloodstream and is carried to the metaphysis of the bone. An abscess forms. Bony tissue within the abscessed area becomes necrotic. If infection is not treated promptly, pressure from the accumulated pus causes the periosteum to rupture, spreading infection along the bone, under the periosteum, and allows bacterial invasion into the closest joint space.

Diagnosis is based on clinical observations, laboratory findings of significant leukocytosis, increased erythrocyte sedimentation rate, and positive blood cultures. Radiographic findings do not reveal the process until 5 to 10 days after the onset or show only soft tissue swelling.

The signs and symptoms of acute hematogenous osteomyelitis have an abrupt onset and intensify over several days. The child may have a high fever, malaise, irritability, tachycardia, and tachypnea. There is often pain and local tenderness over the metaphysis of the affected bone (hematogenous osteomyelitis usually involves a single bone). There may be tenderness, warmth, and swelling of the skin over the affected bone. The child may refuse to use or put weight on the involved bone.

Treatment must be immediate. Once blood cultures have been drawn a 3 to 4 week course of high-dose intravenous antibiotic therapy is started. Hospitalization is necessary for 5 to 7 days to evaluate the child's response to therapy. With a good response and compliance, the child may continue with intravenous antibiotics at home or be switched to oral antibiotics.

The child is placed on complete bed rest in the hospital and at home until the infection is gone. The affected extremity is immobilized with a splint. Bed rest and immobilization help prevent the spread of infection to other joints. Surgical drainage of the involved metaphysis may be performed to prevent the rupture of the periosteum; tubes are placed in the wound for drainage of pus and for irrigation. If the abcess has ruptured into the subperiosteal space, chronic osteomyelitis follows, requiring further antibiotic therapy. Weight bearing on the affected bone is not permitted because of a high risk of fracture.

Nursing management focuses on controlling the infection, enhancing bone healing, and promoting comfort.

Antibiotics are administered as ordered and the IV site is carefully observed and maintained. Frequently, the child will have a peripherally inserted central catheter (PICC) for long-term antibiotic therapy. Response to antibiotic therapy is evaluated by measuring temperature and reviewing laboratory values. Blood drug levels are monitored. The child is observed closely for adverse systemic effects of high-dose antibiotic therapy (many of the drugs are renal and ototoxic). Parents are instructed on the importance of compliance with antibiotic therapy.

Adequate nutrition is essential to aid healing and the formation of new bone. The child should have a diet high in calories, protein, and calcium. In the beginning, the child will probably have a poor appetite, so high-calorie food supplements are encouraged until the appetite returns.

The nurse should stress the need to maintain bed rest and be certain that the child and the parents know the purpose of the immobilization device, that this protects the bone from further injury. Techniques to avoid weight-bearing on the affected extremity should be demonstrated.

Usually the child has significant pain during the acute phase of illness. The nurse positions the child comfortably with the affected extremity elevated. Movement and turning of the patient must be done carefully and gently. Pain medication is administered on schedule. Diversional activities that are age appropriate are also important nursing interventions to lessen pain and provide comfort.

$\mathcal{L}$EGG-CALVÉ-PERTHES DISEASE

Legg-Calvé-Perthes disease (coxa plana) is an aseptic necrosis of the head of the femur. The disease typically affects children 4 to 8 years old. Boys are affected 4 to 5 times more than girls and the disorder is seen 10 times more often in whites than blacks.

The exact cause of the disorder is unknown. There is an interruption of blood circulation to the proximal femoral epiphysis, possibly due to trauma or inflammation, causing necrosis of the femoral head. Normal physical activity causes microfractures of the necrotic bone tissue. **Synovitis** (inflammation of a joint) of the hip may follow.

There are four stages of the disease. In the first stage, radiographic studies show opacity of the epiphysis. In the second stage, the epiphysis becomes mottled and fragmented. The third stage shows new bone formation and increased density, and during the fourth stage gradual reformation of the head of the femur, hopefully in a spherical form. This process may take 18 to 36 months.

The diagnosis is suspected from the clinical signs and symptoms and confirmed by radiography showing characteristic bone changes.

Legg-Calvé-Perthes disease has an insidious onset. Initial symptoms include intermittent or constant hip soreness or stiffness or a limp on the affected side. The child may complain of more pain after physical exertion, upon rising, and at the end of the day. Range of motion (ROM) is limited.

The goal of medical therapy is to prevent deformity of the femoral head by containing it in the acetabulum. Containment allows the femoral head to preserve its spherical shape during bone regeneration.

Most children do not require hospitalization and receive conservative treatment at home. They are prescribed a period of bed rest to reduce inflammation and non-weight-bearing devices, such as braces, casts, or harnesses. The child must continue to wear braces for 2 to 4 years until the disease process is complete. Surgical correction and containment is another option that allows the child to return to full physical activity within 3 to 6 months.

The disease is self-limiting. Successful outcome of therapy depends on early and compliant treatment, as well as the age of the child at onset of

Legg-Calvé-Perthes disease. Disorder in which there is an aseptic necrosis of the femoral head.

Synovitis. Inflammation of a joint.

the disorder. With the cooperation of the child and family the prognosis is excellent.

Nursing management focuses on promoting normal hip and femur function and providing diversional activities. The nurses, especially the school nurse, may be the first health care professional to identify the symptoms of Legg-Calvé-Perthes disease.

Since most of the care for this child is in an outpatient setting, nursing care involves teaching the child and family the purpose and expected outcomes of therapy. Instructions are also given on the care, application, and management of the corrective devices along with the importance of compliance with treatment. Parents should be advised that a child can easily remove a brace, so monitoring the child is important.

Probably the most challenging aspect of nursing care is finding suitable activities for this child, whose physical activity is severely limited, but at the same time feels well. It is difficult for a child to adjust to inactivity while watching other children playing outdoors, riding bicycles, and running. The nurse should suggest activities that will keep the child occupied as well as foster developmental growth. This is an opportune time to encourage a hobby such as crafts, card or stamp collecting, or model building.

$\mathcal{S}$COLIOSIS

Scoliosis. Lateral curvature of the spine.

Kyphosis. Thoracic curvature of the spine.

Scoliosis is a lateral curvature of the spine, and is the most common spinal deformity, appearing most frequently in preadolescent girls. The curvature may occur in the thoracic (**kyphosis**), lumbar (lordosis), or thoracolumbar spine.

Scoliosis occurs in two forms, structural and functional (most common). Structural scoliosis is caused by malformed and rotated vertebrae. It may be idiopathic (most common and having no known cause), congenital, or associated with some other disorder. Structural scoliosis may progress rapidly during the adolescent growth spurt. Functional scoliosis may be caused by poor posture, muscle spasms, or unequal leg lengths.

Scoliosis is diagnosed by observation and radiography, which reveals the degree of spinal curvature. A school nurse may identify children with scoliosis during routine screenings. During the screening the child is undressed except for underpants and faces forward so the nurse has a posterior view. The nurse observes and notes any lateral curve. The nurse then has the child bend forward at the hips and observes for the presence of a rib hump, flank asymmetry, or prominence of the scapula on one side.

The treatment for structural scoliosis depends on the severity of the spinal curvature (see Figures 11-7, 11-8, and 11-9). Curvatures of less than 20° are considered mild and, if the curve does not progress, require no treatment. Curvatures between 25° and 40° are usually corrected with a brace or electrical stimulation, and those of more than 40° are usually corrected surgically.

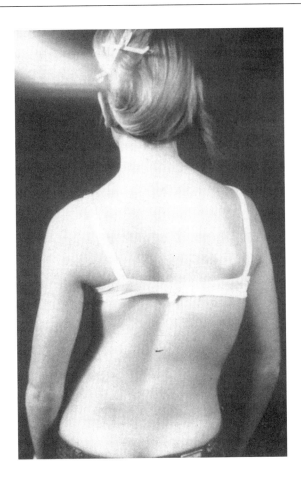

FIGURE 11-7

⚬

Inspection of an adolescent girl with right thoracic scoliosis.

Functional scoliosis is treated by eliminating the primary problem. Exercises to strengthen back and abdominal muscles may be prescribed.

External bracing is required for a child with mild to moderate structural scoliosis. Bracing does not correct the curvature, but prevents further progression of the curve. The **Milwaukee brace** (Figure 11-10) is the one most often prescribed. It is a plastic and metal appliance that extends from the neck to the pelvis and exerts lateral pressure in a longitudinal traction, achieving vertical alignment. The Milwaukee brace is worn 16 to 23 hours a day and adjusted as the child grows. It should be worn over a T-shirt to protect the child's skin from irritation. The brace does not interfere with routine activities. The child wears the brace until the spinal bones reach maturity (approximately 18 to 21 years of age); then only at night for 1 to 2 years.

Adolescence is a time when body image concerns are very important. Acceptance of the brace and possible limitation of some activities may cause anger, a grief reaction, or noncompliance with the treatment. The understanding support of the nurse, family, and peers is required to successfully work through these feelings.

An alternative to bracing for the child with mild to moderate structural scoliosis is electrical stimulation to the muscles on the outward (convex) side of the curvature. This causes the muscles to contract, halting the progression of the curvature and possibly straightening the spine. The electrodes are

Milwaukee brace. Most often prescribed brace; prevents progression of curvature.

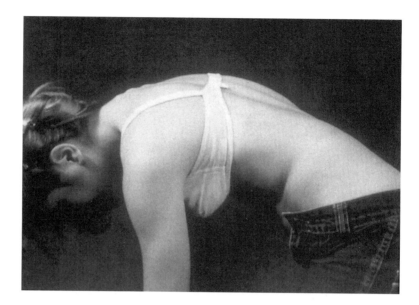

FIGURE 11-8

⬟

Inspection of a patient from the lateral aspect during Adams forward bend test.

applied to the skin or surgically implanted. If the electrodes are placed externally on the skin, maintaining and assessing skin integrity is important. This therapy takes place at night while the child is asleep.

Surgical correction may be necessary for children with moderate to severe scoliosis, and sometimes for certain children with mild scoliosis. Indications for surgery include diminished pulmonary function, back pain (which is not usual), and noncompliance with a brace. Surgical techniques consist of realigning and straightening the spine by inserting an internal fixation device (often a Harrington rod) and fusing the realigned vertebrae.

Preoperatively, some children with a severe curvature may require traction for a time before spinal fusion is performed to begin the correction process. Traction can either be manual or skeletal. Frequently, **halo traction**

FIGURE 11-9

⬟

Posterior inspection of a patient during Adams forward bend test.

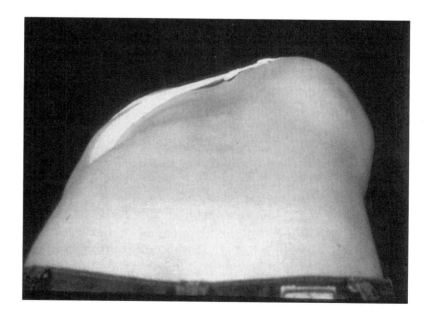

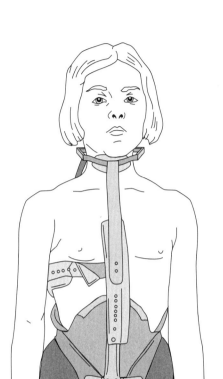
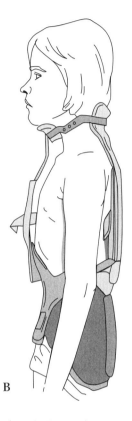
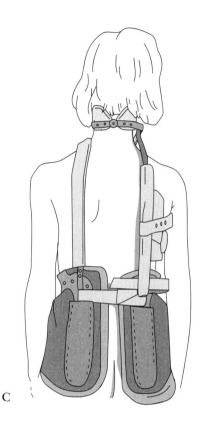

FIGURE 11-10 Milwaukee brace. (A) Front. (B) Side. (C) Rear view.

is added: a metal ring attached to the skull using stainless steel pins, pulleys, and weights.

Treatment of scoliosis extends over a long period of time in an adolescent's life. This is the time in which their identity is formed. For some young people, it means treatment that may limit activities and wearing appliances that make them look different. Developing a sense of identity and positive self-worth is crucial during the preadolescent period when the scoliosis develops, and during adolescence as treatment continues. The child may feel unattractive because of the brace or the deformities. In the hospital setting, these children are often immobilized and cut off from social interaction with their peers.

If a brace is necessary, the course of treatment, expected outcomes, how the correction takes place, limitation of activities, and how to remove and replace the device should be thoroughly explained to the child and the parents prior to the onset of treatment. Compliance should be stressed as the most critical responsibility of the child for the treatment to be successful. Management of the therapy should include the expertise of a multidisciplinary team, including the orthopedic physician, nurse, physical therapist, **orthotist** (specialist in fitting braces), and possibly a social worker and pulmonologist. The nurse can suggests ways to perform activities of daily living: dressing, bathing, getting out of bed. Suggest oversized

Halo traction. Metal ring attached to the skull by stainless steel pins.

Orthotist. Specialist in fitting braces.

clothing to camouflage the brace and encourage socialization with peers as well as participation in social activities. Always stress the positive outcome of the therapy.

The child who must undergo major surgery will require a long postoperative course. Preoperative teaching is of great importance. The child should have a full explanation concerning the procedure, the necessity of the procedure, and everything that will happen postoperatively.

After the surgery is completed, the surgical site must be protected. Most children prefer to have the head of the bed flat. Proper body alignment is maintained with the spine kept straight. Log-rolling techniques are used to turn the child from side to side. Twisting movements are avoided. The surgical dressing is observed frequently and kept dry and intact.

The child usually has significant pain, especially in the first 3 postoperative days. Narcotic analgesia is administered regularly around the clock. For many, patient-controlled analgesia (PCA) is the most effective pain relief modality.

Included in the usual postoperative observations and vital signs are assessments of circulation, movement, and sensation of the lower extremities. There is usually some degree of paralytic ileus following surgery. The nurse assesses the abdomen for the return of bowel function. Urine output is closely monitored because of the large blood loss during the surgery, and many patients experience urinary retention.

Physiotherapy is begun as soon as it is tolerated by the patient. Range of motion to the extremities is provided by the nurse or family member at first; then the patient is taught how to get out of bed without twisting and ambulate.

The family is encouraged to remain with the child to offer emotional support and participate in the child's care while he/she is in the hospital. Family members are taught wound care, how to apply the postoperative brace, and/or cast care if necessary.

Fractures

Fractures are common injuries that can occur at any age. A fracture is defined as a broken or crushed bone, when injurious forces exceed the strength of the normal bone. In infants, the major causes of fractures are often the result of injury, birth trauma, motor vehicle accidents, or child abuse. Children's bones are easily injured and minor falls or twists may result in fractures. A fracture may be incomplete or complete, with the latter involving separated fragments of the bone. All fractures affect the cross section of the bone. A fracture can be transverse, perpendicular to the long axis of the bone, oblique, slanting but straight, or spiral, circular, and twisting around the bone shaft. There are four major types of fractures: (1) closed fracture—skin integrity is intact, (2) open fracture—skin and tissue involvement, (3) epiphyseal injury, involving a growth plate and cartilage, and (4) articular fracture, involving the entrance of an articular surface. The types of fractures are illustrated in Figure 11-11.

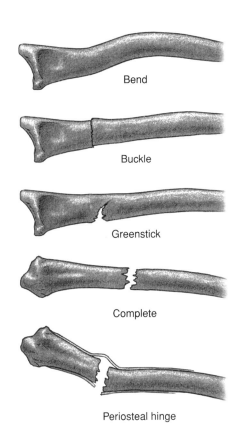

Bend

Buckle

Greenstick

Complete

Periosteal hinge

FIGURE 11-11A

⌖

Types of fractures in children. Fractures are the result of the resistance of the bone against the stress force. Fractures are common in children.

FIGURE 11-11B Epiphyseal injuries from minor to complex.

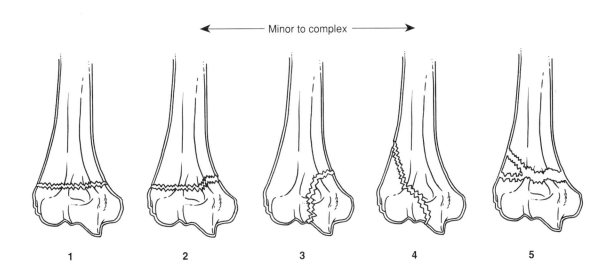

Minor to complex

1   2   3   4   5

Children with fractures often report generalized pain, swelling, tenderness, and inability to move the injured part. When a child refuses to walk, a fracture should be suspected. In assessing the extent of an injury, the nurse should key in on the 5 Ps: pain, pulse, pallor, paresthesia, and paralysis. The mechanism of injury should be investigated, and should correlate with the type of fracture; otherwise physical abuse may be involved. Radiographic examination, x-ray, is the most effective diagnostic tool. When soft tissue, bone, or muscle injury is severe, a complete blood count (CBC) should be done to determine hematocrit and hemoglobin levels. SGOT (serum glutamic-oxaloacetic transaminase), LDH (lactate dehydrogenase), creatinine, and alkaline phosphatase levels should also be obtained to determine the extent of muscle damage.

Reduction of the bony fragments, immobilization, and restoration of function to regain alignment of the injured bone are the main goals in fracture management. Traction and casting are the management treatments for realigning and immobilizing the injured part, until adequate callus is formed. Fractures of the supracondylar area of the distal humerus, the femur, and complex maligned fractures require hospitalization. Sometimes, when a fracture is severely maligned, surgical intervention is warranted and the most common complication is infection.

Nurses are responsible for initial assessment. Observation of the injured extremities for cuts, bruises, and swelling, and neurovascular and circulatory checks should be done. The injured part should be handled as little as possible and the involved bone or joint should be promptly immobilized by application of splints, elevated, and ice applied to reduce the swelling.

The cast is made of gauze strips and bandages with fiberglass and polyurethane resin. The cast dries in approximately 30 minutes. Turning the child every 2 hours will help the cast dry evenly, and aiming a regular fan at the site may be helpful during humid weather. The nurse is responsible for checking the neurovascular status of the extremity involved. If neurovascular integrity is compromised, permanent muscle and tissue damage may occur in 6 to 8 hours. The most common observations that should alert the nurse to complications include pain, swelling, pallor or cyanosis, coldness, faint or absent pulses, increased capillary refill time, and inability to move the extremities distal to the fracture.

The parents and the child should also be educated on home cast care, use of crutches, and symptoms that warrant immediate medical help. Home cast care includes keeping the cast clean and dry; avoiding putting objects, powders, or lotions inside the cast; elevating the injured extremity with pillows; checking for circulation, movement, color, and sensation of the distal visible extremities; and properly using crutches to avoid further injuries.

When simple traction or casting is not enough to realign the bone fragments, an extended pulling force is needed, and continuous traction may be administered. There are three types of traction: manual, skin, and skeletal. Manual traction is used for immediate cast application on uncomplicated arm or leg fractures. Nurses provide the manual traction by applying a pull to the distal bone fragment. Applying the pull directly to the skin surface and indirectly to the skeletal structures is skin traction. Direct pull to the skeletal structure by pins, wires, or tongs inserted through the diameter of the bone distal to the fracture is called skeletal traction.

Upper extremity traction is the treatment of fractures of the humerus. It is done by overhead suspension in which the arm is bent at the elbow and vertically suspended with the traction applied to the distal end of the humerus. The Dunlop traction may also be utilized. In this traction the arm is suspended horizontally.

Lower extremity fractures usually have significant overriding and minimum displacement. The types of lower extremity traction are illustrated in Figure 11-12 (also see Table 11-1).

FIGURE 11-12 Different types of traction. The use of traction in the management of fractures is the direct application of forces to produce equilibrium at the fracture site.

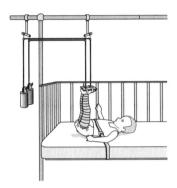

A Bryant traction

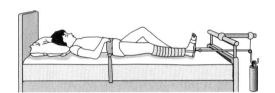

B Buck extension traction

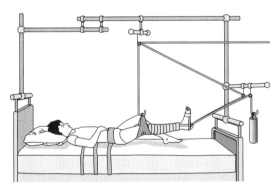

C Russell traction

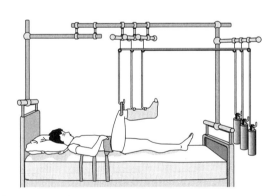

D "90-90" traction

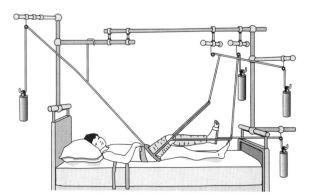

E Balance suspension with Thomas ring splint and Pearson attachment

◙

TABLE 11-1
GUIDELINES FOR ASSESSMENT OF TRACTION

Check desired line of pull and relationship of distal fragment to proximal fragment	Check whether fragment is being directed upward, adducted, or abducted.
Check function of each component	• Position of bandages, frames, splints • Ropes—in center tract of pulley, taut, no fraying, knots tied securely • Pulleys—in original position on attachment bar; have not slid from original site; weights freely moveable • Weights—correct amount of weight; hanging freely; in safe location
Check bed position	Head or foot elevated as directed for desired amount of pull and counter-traction.
Assess child's behavior	To determine if traction causes pain or discomfort.
Skin traction	• Replace nonadhesive straps and/or Ace bandage on skin traction when permitted and/or absolutely necessary, but make certain that traction on limb is maintained by someone during procedure. • Assess bandages to ascertain if they are correctly applied (diagonal or spiral), not too loose or too tight, which could cause slippage and malalignment of traction.
Skeletal traction	• Check pin sites frequently for signs of bleeding, inflammation, or infection. • Check pin screws to be certain that screws are tight in metal clamp that attaches traction apparatus to pin. • Note pull of traction on pin; pull should be even.
Observe for correct body alignment	• Emphasis should be on alignment of shoulders, hip(s), and leg(s). • Check again after child moves.
Assess any circular dressing	Assess for excessive tightness.
Assess restraining devices, if prescribed	• Make certain that they are neither too loose nor too tight. • Remove periodically and check for pressure areas. • Note if any tightness, weakness, or contractures are developing in uninvolved joints and muscles.
Note any neurovascular changes	• Color in skin and nail beds • Alterations in sensation • Alterations in motor ability
Check under child	Check for small objects (e.g., foods, toys, etc.).

Buck traction, also called running traction, pulls only in one direction. Both hips are flexed at 90° and the legs are suspended by pulleys and weights. The weight of the child is the counteraction and the buttocks should be slightly elevated at all times. This type of traction is utilized in children less than 2 years old with a weight limit of 12 to 14 kg because of the risk of postural hypertension. Impairment of circulation is usually the complication and should be frequently checked.

Buck extension is a type of skin traction with the legs in an extended position. The hips are not flexed. This traction is frequently used for short-term immobilization or correcting contracture and in bone deformities such as Legg-Calvé-Perthes disease. This traction allows greater mobility and turning from side to side (with care to maintain alignment) is permitted.

Russell traction is a skin traction on the lower leg with a padded sling under the knee. One pull is along the longitudinal line of the lower leg and the other is perpendicular to the leg. The two lines of pull immobilize the hip and knee in flexed position and allow realignment of the lower extremity. The two ropes are pulling in the same direction of the footplate; therefore the traction pull will be twice the amount of weight at the end of the bed. Five pounds of weight will then produce 10 pounds of pull. Nursing responsibilities include checking the position of the traction to make sure that the correct hip flexion is maintained to prevent footdrop.

A 90-90 traction is the most common skeletal traction. This is the most convenient for nurses because it facilitates toileting, prevention of traction complications, and easy positioning. This is a skeletal traction in which a Steinmann pin or Kirschner wire is placed in the distal fragment of the femur.

Balance suspension traction may be used with or without skeletal or skin traction. The balanced suspension suspends the leg in a flexed position to ease the hip and hamstring muscles. A Thomas splint, which extends from the groin to the midair above the foot, and a Pearson attachment support the lower leg and will stay wherever positioned. A balanced traction is created by the ropes attached. The traction lifts when the child is lifted from the bed with no loss of alignment. The nurse must make sure that the splints and the ropes are intact so that there is no fraying or slippage.

*J*UVENILE RHEUMATOID ARTHRITIS

Juvenile rheumatoid arthritis (JRA) is the most common pediatric connective tissue disease, with arthritis as the major manifestation. It is also the most common chronic disease and the leading cause of disability and blindness in children. The etiology of JRA is unknown. Most likely, it is not caused by one condition but by a conglomerate of diseases of different pathogenesis. It has been common to associate JRA with mumps and rubella. Immunodeficiency is associated with the occurrence of arthritis in children with selective IgA deficiency. Children with JRA may form antibodies to surface membrane antigens on T cells of the suppressor-inducer type. These cells are also low in number in the peripheral white cell population of affected children. The synovial membrane in JRA is characterized by villous hypertrophy and hyperplasia of the synovial lining layer. Edema and hyperemia are present. Infiltrates of inflammatory cells may be seen in parenchymal organs such as the liver. Rheumatoid nodules result from the small blood vessel vasculitis that occurs in JRA. The rash of JRA is characterized by an infiltration of round cells surrounding capillaries and subdermal venules and neutrophilic perivasculitis.

Although the onset of JRA before 6 months of age is unusual, the mean onset is between 1 and 3 years, with many cases having onset anytime throughout childhood and adolescence. Girls are more affected than boys. The JRA child usually begins to complain of fatigue and low-grade fever, anorexia, and failure to grow. In the morning, the child complains of being stiff, and when the disease is advanced the child complains of night pain. Most of the children affected do not complain about the symptoms to their parents; instead, they refuse to walk long distances or run, and they guard their joints from being touched. There are three different modes of onset:

1. Polyarthritis: This classification is given when the disease begins in five or more joints. The onset can be acute or insidious. More than half of the children diagnosed with JRA have this type. The arthritis usually involves large joints such as the knees, wrists, elbows, and ankles. The smaller joints are involved later on as the disease progresses. The pattern of arthritis is usually symmetric. The child may not complain of pain even though the joints are tender and painful in motion. The cervical spine is often involved in this type of onset. The neck may be painful or stiff with an alarming loss of extension over time. Temporomandibular joint disease is relatively common in these children and leads to limitation or asymmetry of bite.

2. Oligoarthritis: This classification is given when the disease involves four or fewer joints. Oligoarthritis is confined to the joints of the knees or ankles, or may involve a single joint at onset and through the course of the disease. The hips are usually spared at onset.

3. Systemic disease: The hallmark of this disease is the presence of high spiking fever with the presence of rheumatoid rash. Temperature elevations occur once or twice a day, often in the late afternoon or at night, with a quick return to baseline temperature or lower. The rash that develops with this fever consists of 2 to 5 mm erythematous macules. It is more commonly seen in the trunk and proximal extremities, and over pressure areas, but can also occur on the face, palms, or soles. The rash is not generally pruritic; the most salient characteristic is that it is transient. Children with this condition have hepatosplenomegaly and lymphadenopathy. Pericarditis, hepatitis, and other visceral diseases may occur. Pulmonary involvement consists of a wide spectrum of abnormalities such as pleuritis and effusion. The central nervous system may be affected.

In arriving at the diagnosis of JRA, the nurse must remember that the diagnosis is a process of exclusion, and therefore other diseases must be considered. The differential diagnosis usually includes other rheumatic and connective tissue diseases, especially rheumatic fever.

Treatment is very conservative and attempts to control clinical manifestations of the disease and prevent and minimize deformity. Because of the nature of the treatment, care is ideally given by a multidisciplinary team, which follows the child through his/her illness. The care is managed by the family and by the community where the child lives. The family and the child have to be helped to accept that the care will be over a long period of time. Prognosis, however, is excellent for most children, and the treatment usually is simple, safe, and conservative. The child usually is treated with nonsteroidal anti-inflammatory drugs such as aspirin. More than half of the children with this disease are treated with aspirin alone, while the rest are treated with a nonsteroid anti-inflammatory drug. If the child does not respond to such therapy, hydroxychloroquine, gold, glucocorticoid, and immunosuppressive drugs can be given, in that order.

Physical therapy and occupational therapy are employed in order to prevent deformities and to maintain preservation and function of the limbs. Orthopedic surgery is sometimes used as a means for prevention and/or reconstruction. The child and the family should be aided via the use of counseling and peer group involvement in the school and community. In addition, the parents and the child should be referred to community agencies that can facilitate coping processes.

In caring for arthritic children, the nurse must realize that every child, regardless of his/her disease or condition, has a tremendous potential for physical and psychological growth. All efforts should be aimed at optimizing the child's normal development.

SUMMARY

This chapter describes disorders that are congenital and acquired, and conditions that are both long- and short-term. Answers to pivotal questions are provided, including: "Why do children develop certain musculoskeletal disorders?" and "What impact do musculoskeletal disorders have on the growth and development of affected children?" By comprehensively understanding the disease process, nurses are able to plan for more efficient nursing interventions.

CRITICAL POINTS IN THE CARE OF MUSCULOSKELETAL DISORDERS

Nurses who care for children with musculoskeletal conditions require a thorough knowledge of orthopedics in order to treat injuries, to recognize skeletal manifestations of systemic diseases, and to provide appropriate nursing care for congenital and developmental abnormalities. Nurses also need a thorough understanding of the environmental factors that contribute to the treatment of these conditions. Nurses are in a unique position to observe the child and the parents, to assess the social environment in which they live, and to determine where support is strongest.

Often, when parents are told that their child has an abnormality, they become anxious and defensive. Assessment of parenting skills and a determination, by the nurse, as to the level of support needed by the parents is of vital importance to the ultimate level of care a child will receive. The management of musculoskeletal conditions implies care over an extended period of time, with different treatments required at different stages of growth and development. Therefore, the nurse must be prepared to change his/her approach as the child matures, and to be sensitive to parents' desire to understand and participate in these changes.

QUESTIONS

Diagnosis: Idiopathic Scoliosis

History: Barbara is a 14-year-old girl who has been followed at the pediatric orthopedic clinic since she was 12 years old, when she was referred there by the school nurse. On a routine screening she was noted to have a lateral curve of less than 20°. One year later, the curve was the same. Now the curve is measured at greater than 20°. There is an obvious rib hump and one hip is higher than the other. Barbara denies any pain. She has just started a new school and is trying to make friends. The orthopedist recommends nonsurgical treatment of her scoliosis.

Nursing problems: Adolescent female with disorder of the musculoskeletal system. Potential noncompliance with prescribed treatment. Altered body image

Chief concern: Patient will not understand potential positive outcome of nonsurgical therapy.

Plan: Encourage compliance with treatment by emphasizing potential positive outcome. Provide emotional support to patient and family.

1. What physical finding is not expected on physical examination?
    A. Pain
    B. Uneven hemline
    C. One shoulder higher than the other
    D. An obvious lateral curve

2. Barbara is to wear a Milwaukee brace. She asks the nurse when she should have it on. The best response is:
    A. Wear the brace only at night.
    B. Take off the brace whenever it is necessary for comfort.
    C. Wear the brace only when there will be physical activity.
    D. Wear the brace 16–23 hours a day and do not remove it unless ordered to.

3. Barbara's mother asks, "Will this brace straighten her spine?" The nurse's best response is:

A. Yes, the brace corrects the spine.
B. The brace is meant to limit physical activity and at the same time correct the curve.
C. You will not be able to tell there was a curvature by the end of treatment.
D. The brace will stop the progression of the curvature, but not straighten the spine.

Diagnosis: Complete Tibial Fracture

History: Arnold is a 7-year-old who was playing in the street when a car hit him. He tried to get up, but could not. Now he complains of right lower leg pain. A visible deformity on that leg is seen. The paramedics transport him to the emergency room.

Plan: Immobilize the leg and take the child to the emergency room for treatment and evaluation. X-ray, cast, admission, and traction.

Nursing problems: Pain management; explanations of procedures; cast care; crutches; prevention of injury; management of traction.

1. To assess the extent of injury, the nurse should focus on the 5 Ps, which are:

A. Pain, pulse, pink, prosthesis, partner
B. Pain, pulse, portion, parameter, pus
C. Position, paralysis, perfusion, palsy, performance
D. Pain, pulse, pallor, paresthesia, paralysis

2. To determine and confirm the extent and diagnosis of a fracture, which of the following tests are usually ordered?

A. CT scan of the legs
B. MRI of the legs
C. X-ray of the right tibia and fibula
D. Chest x-ray

3. Gross deformity is noted and upon inspection, a fracture is suspected. The initial intervention is:

A. Immobilization, ice, elevation, pain medication
B. Casting and traction
C. Orthopedic surgery for insertion
D. Teaching Arnold how to use the crutches

4. Arnold's right leg is put in a cast with his toes exposed. His mother is taught how to check for circulation, movement, and sensation. The nurse should also instruct the mother to call if:
   A. The toes of the right extremities are warm and capillary refill is less than 2 seconds.
   B. Arnold complains of numbness in his right toes and refill is more than 2 seconds.
   C. Arnold's brother starts writing on the cast with a thick black marker.
   D. Arnold can wiggle his toes and the capillary refill is less than 2 seconds.

5. Arnold is to be admitted to the hospital for traction. The nurse explains to his mother that the purpose of the traction is:
   A. To make the bone grow faster
   B. To prepare the area for surgery
   C. To realign bone fragments
   D. To prevent future fractures

6. Arnold is placed on Buck extension traction. This traction is a type of:
   A. Skeletal traction that is 90-90 degree
   B. Skin traction with legs in an extended position
   C. Traction wherein the hips are flexed
   D. Traction that has a Pearson attachment and Thomas splint

7. When a diagnosis of fracture is confirmed in a 6-year-old, but the cause does not correlate with the parent's story and the child's story, what should be suspected?
   A. Physical abuse
   B. Developmental delay
   C. Malnutrition
   D. Pathologic fracture

𝒜NSWERS

Idiopathic scoliosis

1. *A.* Pain is not a common symptom of scoliosis. The rest of the choices are common physical findings in a patient with scoliosis.

2. *D.* Treatment with the Milwaukee brace requires the patient to wear the brace for 16–23 hours a day. It is only removed for bathing and with orders from the orthopedist.

3. *D.* The Milwaukee brace halts the progression of the curvature. Surgical rod instrumentation and fusion of the vertebrae strengthen the spine.

Fractures

1. *D.* The 5 Ps are pain, pulse, pallor, paresthesia, and paralysis.

2. *C.* X-ray of the involved extremity will determine the diagnosis and extent of fracture.

3. *A.* Initial interventions are ice to reduce the swelling, elevation and immobilization, and very little movement to the injured part.

4. *B.* The complaints are significant and may imply that the cast is too tight, compromising circulation to the lower extremities. The cast may have to be opened to prevent further damage.

5. *C.* Traction is for immobilization and to realign bone fragments.

6. *B.* Buck extension traction is a skin traction with legs in an extended position. *C* is Bryant traction and *D* is balance suspension traction.

7. *A.* Abuse is suspected with fractures that do not correlate with the mechanism of injury and the history.

$\mathcal{G}$LOSSARY

clubfoot   describes a condition in which the foot appears twisted out of shape.

congenital hip dysplasia   hip disorder resulting from defective development of the acetabulum.

Denis-Browne splint   a splint with corrective shoes used in the treatment of clubfoot.

halo traction   metal ring attached to the skull by stainless steel pins.

kyphosis   thoracic curvature of the spine.

Legg-Calvé-Perthes disease   disorder in which there is an aseptic necrosis of the femoral head.

lordosis   lumbar curvature of the spine.

Milwaukee brace   most often prescribed brace; prevents progression of curvature.

orthotist   specialist in fitting braces.

osteomyelitis   an infection of the bone.

Pavlik harness   frequently used to maintain flexion and stability of the hips in infants with congenital hip dysplasia.

scoliosis   lateral curvature of the spine.

synovitis   inflammation of a joint.

ℬIBLIOGRAPHY

ARNHEIM, D. D., AND PRENTICE, W. *Principles of Athletic Training*. 8th ed. St. Louis: Mosby-Year Book, 1993.

BEHRMAN, R., KLIEGMAN, R. M., AND ARVIN, A. M. *Nelson Textbook of Pediatrics*. 15th ed. Philadelphia: Saunders, 1995.

BEHRMAN, R., AND VAUGHN, V. C. *Nelson Textbook of Pediatrics*. 13th ed. Philadelphia: Saunders, 1987.

BLECK, E. Adolescent idiopathic scoliosis. *Developmental Medicine and Child Neurology* 33:167–176, 1991.

BUSCH, M., AND MORRISY, R. Slipped capital femoral epiphysis. *Orthopedic Clinics of North America* 18(4):637–647, 1987.

CURRY, L., AND GIBSON, L. Congenital hip dislocation: The importance of early detection and comprehensive treatment. *Nurse Practitioner* 17:49–55, 1992.

HENSINGER, R. Congenital dislocation of the hip. *Orthopedic Clinics of North America* 18:597–616, 1987.

HOLE, J. W. *Human Anatomy and Physiology*. 6th ed. Dubuque, IA: Brown, 1993.

KING, T. Angular deformities of the lower limbs in children. *Orthopedic Clinics of North America* 18(4):513–527, 1987.

KOOP, S. Infantile and juvenile idiopathic scoliosis. *Orthopedic Clinics of North America* 19(2):331–337, 1988.

KYZER, S. P. Congenital idiopathic clubfoot. *Orthopaedic Nursing* 10(4): 11–18, 1992.

MORRISY, R. T., AND SELMAN, S. Slipped capital femoral epiphysis. *Orthopaedic Nursing* 10(1):11–20, 1991.

NELSON, W., BEHRMAN, R. E., KLIEGMAN, R. M, et al. *Nelson's Textbook of Pediatrics*. 15th ed. Philadelphia: Saunders, 1996.

SHOPPEE, K. Developmental dysplasia of the hip. *Orthopaedic Nursing* 11(5):30–36, 1992.

SKINNER, S. Orthopedic problems in children. In A. M. Rudolph, R. Hoffman, and M. Rudolph (eds.), *Rudolph's Pediatrics*. Stamford, CT: Appleton & Lang, 1996.

STAHELI, L. T. *Fundamentals of Pediatric Orthopaedics*. New York: Raven, 1992.

TURCO, V. Surgical correction of the resistant clubfoot. *Journal of Bone and Joint Surgery* 53-A:477–497, 1971.

WENGER, D. R., AND RANG, M. *The Art and Practice of Children's Orthopaedics*. New York: Raven, 1992.

*H*ELPFUL INTERNET SITES

PEDINFO: An Index of the Pediatric Internet at http://www.pedinfo. org   This is an excellent site that covers nearly all topics within this review. It has a wealth of information and is worth a visit. It is written for health care professionals but others could also use the information. Congenital syndromes, congenital malformations, and inborn errors of metabolism are covered.

Virtual Naval Hospital Information for Providers at http://www.vnh. org/Providers.html   This site is part of the University of Iowa's health care site and is linked to a large set of databases that can be used by health care providers. The site covers a large number of links to other sources on health care issues and problems. This is an excellent starting place to discover information on various common diseases and their treatments.

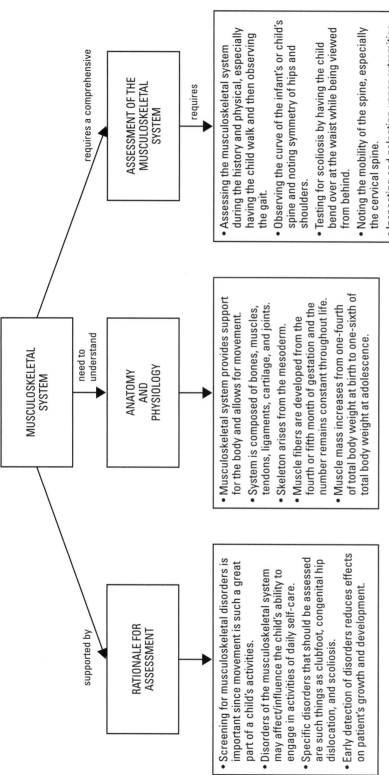

MUSCULOSKELETAL SYSTEM

need to understand → **ANATOMY AND PHYSIOLOGY**

- Musculoskeletal system provides support for the body and allows for movement.
- System is composed of bones, muscles, tendons, ligaments, cartilage, and joints.
- Skeleton arises from the mesoderm.
- Muscle fibers are developed from the fourth or fifth month of gestation and the number remains constant throughout life.
- Muscle mass increases from one-fourth of total body weight at birth to one-sixth of total body weight at adolescence.

supported by → **RATIONALE FOR ASSESSMENT**

- Screening for musculoskeletal disorders is important since movement is such a great part of a child's activities.
- Disorders of the musculoskeletal system may affect/influence the child's ability to engage in activities of daily self-care.
- Specific disorders that should be assessed are such things as clubfoot, congenital hip dislocation, and scoliosis.
- Early detection of disorders reduces effects on patient's growth and development.

requires a comprehensive → **ASSESSMENT OF THE MUSCULOSKELETAL SYSTEM**

requires →

- Assessing the musculoskeletal system during the history and physical, especially having the child walk and then observing the gait.
- Observing the curve of the infant's or child's spine and noting symmetry of hips and shoulders.
- Testing for scoliosis by having the child bend over at the waist while being viewed from behind.
- Noting the mobility of the spine, especially the cervical spine.
- Inspecting and palpating upper extremities, noting size, color, temperature, and mobility of the joints.
- Assessing the strength of the upper extremities.
- Inspecting and palpating the lower extremities and noting abnormalities of mobility, length, shape, and pulses.
- Assessing lower extremities for bowleg (genu varum) by having the child stand with ankles together.
- Assessing for the presence of clubfoot.
- Assessing for meningeal irritation by flexing the child's hips and then straightening each knee (Kernig sign).
- Assessing for congenital hip dislocation.
- Assessing for strength of lower limbs.

Concept Map 11-1

Notes on Parts 1 and 2

OTHER DISEASES

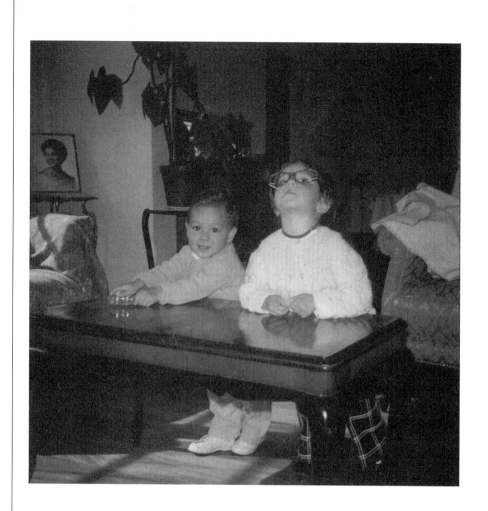

☙
ℋEMATOLOGIC SYSTEM DISORDERS

𝒥NTRODUCTION

Hematologic disorders in children usually result from deficiencies of the formed elements of the blood: red blood cells, white blood cells, and platelets; or deficiencies in coagulation factors. Blood is a major homeostatic force within the body, and essential bodily functions rely upon and are carried out by the blood. These functions include the transfer of respiratory gases, homeostasis, phagocytosis, and the provision of cellular and humoral agents to fight infection. Various abnormalities of blood cells are found in many disease states and result from alterations in the child's nutrition.

Diagnostic hematologic studies (laboratory diagnostic tests) are essential in pediatric health assessment. The types of hematologic disorders the nurse will encounter in clinical practice range from common nutritional deficiencies, whose treatment is rather straightforward, to those rare problems with a genetic or chronic component. Genetic and/or chronic disorders necessitate extensive referral and a multidisciplinary approach to management and treatment. In pediatrics, early detection of blood disorders ensures the best possible prognosis.

Blood is made up of two components: a cellular component with specialized functions; and a fluid component, or plasma. The cellular component consists of red blood cells (erythrocytes), white blood cells (leukocytes), and platelets (thrombocytes). Leukocytes can be further differentiated into granulocytes, monocytes, and lymphocytes. Plasma is a clear yellow fluid in which proteins (mainly albumins, globulins, and fibrinogen) are the major solutes (a substance that is dissolved in a solution). Plasma proteins maintain the intravascular volume, contribute to the coagulation of blood, and are important in maintaining the acid-base balance.

Erythrocytes

Production of red blood cells (RBCs) is regulated by the specific hormone erythropoietin, which is produced primarily from renal glomerular epithelial cells. Erythropoietin stimulates the bone marrow to convert certain stem cells to proerythroblasts. The stimulation to convert these stem cells in RBCs can be from a response to a decrease in the number of circulating RBCs or from a decrease in the partial pressure of oxygen (PaO_2) of arterial blood. Iron, vitamin B_{12}, folic acid, amino acids, and other nutrients are essential substances for RBC formation. RBCs mature through the following stages: proerythroblast, erythroblast, normoblast, reticulocyte, and erythrocyte.

Hemoglobin

Hemoglobin is the oxygen-carrying protein molecule in the RBC. Each of the hemoglobin molecules is composed of two pairs of polypeptide chains (the globin portion) attached to heme groups, which are large disks containing iron and porphyrin (a nitrogen-containing organic compound). Various forms of hemoglobin can be found in the embryo, fetus, child, and adult. The form depends on changes in the globin chain synthesis. By the age of 12 months, 95% of the hemoglobin consists of the normal adult hemoglobin molecules (Hb A). The level of hemoglobin in a newborn ranges from 15 to 22 g/dL. This level drops to its lowest point between 3 and 6 months. This drop indicates a physiologic anemia because of a shortened survival of the fetal RBCs and the rapid expansion of blood volume during this period. However, reduction in hemoglobin can also develop secondary to a decrease in production, blood loss, or an increase in RBC destruction. A reduction in hemoglobin can have clinical significance since the transport of oxygen to the tissues is adversely affected, causing the child to be clinically anemic.

Leukocytes

White blood cells, or leukocytes (WBCs), are larger and fewer in number than erythrocytes. Normally, there are approximately 5000 to 10,000 leukocytes per millimeter of blood. The primary function of leukocytes is to protect the body from the invasion of foreign organisms and to distribute antibodies and other factors of the immune response.

The white blood cells can be divided into five distinctive groups and two general classifications. The two classifications are granulocytes (also called polymorphonuclear leukocytes or "polys") and agranulocytes. Granulocytes contain large granules and are horseshoe-shaped nuclei that become segmented and are connected by thin strands. Granulocytes are further subdivided into neutrophils, eosinophils, and basophils. Agranulocytes include lymphocytes (also called immunocytes) and monocytes.

In children, the granulocytes make up 30 to 60% of all the WBCs. These WBCs mature in the bone marrow through the following stages: stem cell; myeloblast; promyelocyte; myelocyte; metamyelocyte; band forms; and mature, segmented neutrophils. The maturational process takes anywhere from 6 to 11 days. Once the neutrophil is released into the bloodstream, it will stay in circulation for about 6 to 9 hours before it enters the tissue. Within the tissues, the major function of the neutrophils is phagocytosis of harmful substances and cells, particularly bacterial organisms.

Through a differential count (a laboratory test), the frequency distribution of the various types of circulating WBCs can be obtained. The quantitative alterations within the various categories are important diagnostically. A relative increase in the band (or other immature cells) is often called a "shift to the left," a term that comes from how the differential count used to be tabulated on written forms. This "shift to the left" is a phenomenon indicative of the body's immunological response to an infectious process.

Basophils and eosinophils are considered important indicators of the body's inflammatory and allergic responses. Basophils consist of less than 1% of circulating leukocytes. Basophils release heparin and histamine into the bloodstream during systemic allergic reactions. Basophils contain receptor sites for immunoglobulin E (IgE), which becomes elevated in people with allergies, and also prevent clot formation (due to the heparin-releasing ability) in microcirculation. Eosinophils are found in the mucosa of the gastrointestinal tract as well as in the lungs. Eosinophils are considered weakly phagocytic and are also associated with allergic reactions, parasitic infections, and drug reactions.

Monocytes

Monocytes are relatively immature cells that circulate for nearly 8 hours before migrating into the tissues. Once in the tissues they assume their mature form as macrophages. Much like the granulocytes, which are the first line of defense against microbe invasion, the monocytes, as macrophages, have the primary function of phagocytosis of bacteria and cellular debris. Fixed and mobile macrophages are located principally in the liver, spleen, lymph nodes, and gastrointestinal tract.

Lymphocytes

Lymphocytes (or immunocytes) protect the body against specific antigens. They do not have a phagocytic capability. They originate in the bone marrow but differentiate in the lymphoid tissues such as the spleen, liver, thymus, lymph nodes, and intestines. The thymus-dependent lymphocytes, or T cells, are part of the cell-mediated immune response in which cytotoxic agents and macrophages are synthesized. B-cell lymphocytes are precursors of the humoral immune response in which cells are transformed into plasma cells that release immunoglobulins or antibodies into the bloodstream.

Platelet Cells and Coagulation Factors

The platelets are the smallest cellular components in the blood. These thrombocytes are essential to hemostasis and clot formation. Platelets circulating in the blood are fragments of megakaryocytes. Megakaryocytes are precursor cells that are formed in the bone marrow. The normal platelet count ranges from 150,000 to 300,000 cells/mm³. With an injury to a blood vessel or if there is some intrinsic injury to the blood, the platelets will adhere to the inner surface of the vessel and form a homeostatic plug. While the platelet is degraded, a series of at least 13 or more clotting factors or proteolytic enzymes are released into the bloodstream to bring about the clotting process. The basic reaction is as follows: As factor X is activated, prothrombin (factor II) is converted to thrombin, which then catalyzes the conversion of fibrinogen (factor I) to fibrin. The fibrin provides the matrix where the blood cells can aggregate to form a clot. A deficiency in any one of the proteins in the pathway leads to a clotting disorder. For example, if there is a deficiency in factor VIII or an inadequate number of platelets, the activation of factor X is impaired and the result is, in the former, hemophilia, and in the latter, thrombocytopenia.

Pathophysiology

Hematologic disorders and problems generally can be classified as disorders of RBC function, of WBC function, and of platelet and coagulation function. Each of these very broad classifications can be further subdivided into disorders of blood cell production, maturation, or destruction. It is important for the nurse to recognize these distinctions. Knowledge of the pathophysiological classifications provides the nurse with the rationale for routine screening and useful critical pathways as guides for further clinical investigation.

$\mathscr{A}$NEMIA

Anemia. Abnormally low hemoglobin in the blood.

Anemia is a common childhood condition. It is a symptom rather than a disease. **Anemia** is characterized by an abnormally low hemoglobin level in the red blood cells. As a result of this decreased hemoglobin, the capacity of the blood to carry oxygen to the tissues is diminished, resulting in hypoxia.

Anemia may be caused by any one or more of the following processes:

1. Inadequate production of hemoglobin or RBCs, as in iron-deficiency anemia.

2. Excessive blood loss, as in hemorrhage.
3. Increased destruction of RBCs (**hemolysis**), as in sickle cell disease.
4. Hemolysis associated with acquired abnormalities of RBCs from drugs, chemicals, or infectious agents.

Hemolysis. Increased destruction of RBCs.

The different types of anemia are classified by RBC size, shape, and color, or the hemoglobin content. When the anemia has developed slowly, most children adapt to the decreasing hemoglobin. However, if anemia develops suddenly, as in the case of hemorrhage, the effects on the circulatory system are serious. Cardiac workload is increased, resulting in tachycardia and heart murmurs. Congestive heart failure (CHF) may follow.

In blood tests that measure hemoglobin, a level lower than 11 g/dL or a hematocrit lower than 33% means that anemia is suspected. Findings from the history and physical examination, such as fatigue, paleness of the skin and mucous membranes, exercise intolerance, irritability, headache, and decreased attention span may be the first indications that the child is anemic.

Medical management is directed to reversing the anemia by correcting the underlying cause. For example, the child who has suffered from hemorrhage receives blood transfusions. The child who has a nutritional deficiency receives supplements and dietary counseling.

The primary nursing goal for the child with anemia is to reduce tissue oxygen requirements. Physical exertion and stress increase oxygen requirements. The child should avoid strenuous activity and rest frequently. An infant should not be allowed to cry for extended periods and should be given a pacifier, rocked, and comforted by the caretaker during these times. In children with severe anemia, hospitalization may be required with the need for bed rest, oxygen therapy, and intravenous (IV) fluids.

Iron-Deficiency Anemia

Iron-deficiency anemia is a common nutritional deficiency among young children between the ages of 9 and 24 months. It is a hypochromatic, microcytic anemia (RBCs are smaller than normal and deficient in hemoglobin). Premature infants are also at risk because of their reduced fetal iron supply. Adolescents are at risk because of their poor eating habits and rapid growth rate.

Iron-deficiency anemia. Common nutritional deficiency in young children.

Many children with iron-deficiency anemia are undernourished because of the family's economic situation. The Women, Infants and Children (WIC) program provides iron-fortified infant formula for the first year of life in an attempt to decrease the prevalence of iron-deficiency anemia in low-income populations.

Iron-deficiency anemia can be attributed to factors that diminish the supply of iron, impair its absorption, increase the body's need for iron, or affect the synthesis of hemoglobin.

Iron is transferred from the mother to the fetus and stored in the last trimester of pregnancy. The full-term newborn has a high hemoglobin level because of these iron stores. The stored iron diminishes in the first

2 or 3 months of life but is usually adequate until the infant reaches 6 months of age. Premature infants have adequate iron stores for only 2 to 3 months. If dietary iron is not provided to meet the growing infant's needs, iron-deficiency anemia results.

Most infants with iron-deficiency anemia are underweight. However, many are overweight because of excessive milk consumption ("milk babies"). These babies become anemic because milk is a poor source of iron and they have little interest in solid foods. Some infants who are fed fresh cow's milk have an increased loss of blood through feces.

Treatment consists of improved nutrition and the administration of oral iron supplements. In infants who are fed formula, the best sources of dietary iron are iron-fortified commercial formula and iron-fortified infant cereal. Infants younger than 12 months should not be given fresh cow's milk. Dietary addition of iron-rich foods is usually not the sole treatment for iron-deficiency anemia because it is difficult for a child to obtain a large enough quantity of iron from food.

Ferrous sulfate. Oral iron supplement.

Oral **ferrous sulfate** may be prescribed for several months. Ascorbic acid (vitamin C) may also be prescribed along with the ferrous sulfate to enhance its absorption. If the hemoglobin is very low or the level does not rise after 1 month of treatment with the oral iron preparation, an iron dextran mixture for intramuscular (IM) use is administered using the Z-track method.

The family caregivers need instruction on the administration of iron. Ferrous sulfate should be given in 3 divided doses. Iron should not be given with meals. Citrus juice or fruit allows for better absorption. Caregivers should be told that oral iron can cause constipation or turn the child's stools black or dark green in color. Oral iron supplements may stain the teeth. The caregivers should be instructed to administer the medication to the back of the mouth using a syringe or have the child sip the medication through a straw. Brushing the teeth after each dose may help prevent staining of the teeth.

Many caregivers believe that milk is a perfect food. Parents will have to teach their infant to accept foods other than milk. Nutritional counseling is essential. The nurse should discuss the importance of using iron-fortified commercial formulas and cereals. When teaching caregivers, the nurse should keep in mind that attitudes and food choices are often influenced by cultural differences.

Sickle Cell Anemia

Sickle cell anemia. Congenital, chronic disorder characterized by the production of an abnormal hemoglobin that results in a sickle shape under conditions of decreased oxygen tension.

Sickle cell anemia (SCA) is one chronic disorder of a group of autosomal recessive disorders known as hemoglobinopathies. It occurs most commonly in African Americans. Sickle cell diseases (SCD) are characterized by the production of an abnormal hemoglobin that results in the red blood cells taking on a "sickle" shape under conditions of decreased oxygen tension. Normal adult hemoglobin (Hb A) is replaced completely or partially by a different type of hemoglobin (Hb S), fetal hemoglobin (Hb F) or Hb C.

The sickle cell trait occurs when a child inherits one gene for Hb S from one parent and one gene for Hb A from the other parent (heterozygous). Because there is a higher percentage of normal hemoglobin in their RBCs, children with sickle cell trait are usually asymptomatic. When the child inherits two Hb S genes from both parents (homozygous), the child has sickle cell anemia and will be symptomatic. In young infants with sickle cell anemia symptoms will not be apparent until about age 6 months because of the amount of Hb F in their red blood cells. Hb F does not sickle.

The pathological changes from sickle cell anemia are the result of increased blood viscosity and increased red blood cell destruction. Normal, disc-shaped red blood cells move smoothly through the capillaries. The affected red blood cells (Hb S) do the same thing until there is an episode called sickling. When sickling occurs, the abnormal red blood cells become crescent shaped and do not flow smoothly, becoming entangled and enmeshed with one another, causing the blood to be more viscous. The slowing down and sludging of RBCs impair circulation and transport of oxygen, resulting in tissue ischemia and necrosis in multiple organs.

The clinical manifestations of SCA vary in severity and frequency. Children with the disease suffer from periodic sickling episodes called **crises**. There are several forms of crises: vaso-occlusive, splenic sequestration or aplastic crises.

Crises. Episodes of RBC sickling.

Vaso-occlusive crises (painful episodes) occur from the clumping of sickle-shaped RBCs, causing tissue ischemia and the resulting pain. Symptoms of acute tissue ischemia occur mainly in the abdomen, bones, and joints. Splenic sequestration is a pooling of blood in the liver and spleen, resulting in decreased blood volume and shock. Aplastic crises are marked by decreased production of RBCs that causes markedly diminished oxygen transport capacity and a severe anemia. A child may have one or more forms of crises during acute illness.

Vaso-occlusive crises. Clumping of sickle-shaped RBCs causing tissue ischemia and pain.

Tissue ischemia and necrosis result in pathological changes in the following organs:

1. Liver and spleen: Both become enlarged and tender because of the congested blood flow. With repeated blockages (infarcts), liver and spleen cells are destroyed and the organs become scarred and fibrotic. The liver becomes cirrhotic and may fail. The function of the spleen is altered; it can no longer filter bacteria from the blood, leaving the child at risk for infection.
2. Kidneys: Repeated episodes cause congestion of the glomerular capillaries leading to hematuria, inability to concentrate urine, and enuresis.
3. Bones: Joints may become swollen. Children younger than 2 years may have hand-foot syndrome, which is characterized by pain and swelling over the soft tissues of the hands and feet. The child is predisposed to osteomyelitis.
4. Central nervous system: Changes in the central nervous system are attributed to repeated incidences of stasis and thrombosis. Chronic anemia may cause headaches, slowed thought processes, and vision disturbances. Major complications include stroke and cerebral vascular accident, which can result in paralysis and death.

In addition to the effects on various organs, the child with SCA may have complaints of fever, vomiting, abdominal pain, back and joint pain, weakness, and loss of appetite.

Sickledex. Fingerstick screening test that reveals the presence of Hb S.

Hemoglobin electrophoresis. Serum testing used to confirm diagnosis of sickle cell anemia.

Newborn screening is mandatory in most of the United States. Screening for the presence of hemoglobin S may be done with a test called **Sickledex**, a fingerstick screening test that gives results in 3 minutes. This test reveals the presence of Hb S. A positive result does not differentiate between sickle cell trait and sickle cell anemia. **Hemoglobin electrophoresis** ("fingerprinting" of the protein) provides an accurate diagnosis with separation and measurement of the various forms of hemoglobin.

Medical management is aimed at preventing sickling episodes, treating the medical conditions associated with the crisis, and guarding against infection. During a sickle cell crisis, the goal is to prevent further sickling by minimizing oxygen demands and promoting hemodilution. Bed rest is ordered to minimize oxygen requirements. Fluids above normal maintenance requirements by oral and intravenous routes are prescribed. Pain is treated by intravenous (IV) analgesics, acidosis is corrected with bicarbonate administration, and blood transfusions are ordered for severe anemia. Oxygen supplementation may be necessary to treat CHF or if the child has respiratory difficulty.

To prevent infection, pneumococcal and meningococcal vaccines are given to the child at age 2 years. Oral penicillin prophylaxis may be ordered.

The primary goals of the nurse for the child with SCA are to teach the family how to prevent sickling; manage the child's pain during crisis appropriately; increase tissue perfusion and oxygenation during sickle cell crisis; and assist the child and family to adjust to a chronic, life-threatening disease.

Nursing activities and procedures must be planned so the child is disturbed as little as possible. Bed rest is maintained to decrease demands on oxygen supply. Oxygen is administered by mask or nasal cannula to improve tissue perfusion. Vital signs are taken every 4 hours and if fever is present, measures to control it are implemented. Strict measurement of fluid intake and output and daily weights are recorded. The child with sickle cell anemia is prone to dehydration because of the inability of the kidneys to concentrate urine. Signs of dehydration are evaluated by assessment of the mucous membranes or the fontanels of an infant. Parents should be taught that fluid intake must be maintained when the child is not in crisis. Enuresis may be an associated problem and parents should be advised that routine interventions employed to prevent bed-wetting should be avoided.

In any child with anemia, infection is always a concern. Careful hand washing and screening of potentially infectious visitors and staff are essential in caring for this child.

The child in sickle cell crisis usually has severe pain. Enlargement of the spleen causes severe abdominal pain, and joint and muscle pain occur because of poor circulation to the tissues. Accurate assessment of pain, nursing measures to relieve the pain, and prompt administration of analgesics are essential to the child's nursing care. Joints can be supported by pillows, while gentle massage and warm compresses may lessen the pain's intensity. Special consideration is given to the skin. Skin integrity is assessed and documented on every shift. Nursing measures such as extra bed padding, foam protectors, and lotions are helpful.

See Table 12-1 for family teaching to prevent sickling episodes.

◪

TABLE 12-1

FAMILY TEACHING TO PREVENT SICKLING EPISODES

---

1. Be certain the child receives an adequate amount of fluids.
2. Watch for signs and symptoms of dehydration. Observe for dry mucous membranes and skin.
3. Protect the child from all sources of infection.
4. Notify the physician immediately if there are any signs of illness: fever, vomiting, diarrhea, cough.
5. Avoid having the child do strenuous activity.
6. Minimize emotional stress, including prolonged crying.
7. Avoid high altitudes.

$\mathcal{H}$EMOPHILIA

Hemophilia refers to a group of disorders characterized by excessive bleeding and deficiency of one of the factors necessary for coagulation. These disorders are transmitted by an X-linked recessive inheritance pattern. The most common types of hemophilia are hemophilia A (factor VIII deficiency, or classic hemophilia) and hemophilia B (factor IX deficiency, or Christmas disease). Most hemophiliacs have the severe form of hemophilia A.

Clot formation is a complex mechanism that occurs in phases: (1) prothrombin is formed through plasma-platelet interaction, (2) prothrombin is converted to thrombin, and (3) fibrinogen is converted into fibrin by thrombin.

In hemophilia A, **factor VIII** (antihemophiliac factor [AHF]) is present but deficient. AHF is necessary in the first phase of the clotting process. The less AHF present, the more severe the hemophilia. In hemophilia B, factor IX may be present but is deficient or defective. In both disorders, dysfunctional clotting factors prevent normal coagulation and prolonged bleeding.

Bleeding can occur anywhere in the body, but bleeding into joint spaces (**hemarthrosis**) and muscles are the most common sites of internal bleeding.

Diagnosis is usually made from a history of prolonged bleeding episodes. The partial prothrombin time (PTT) is the laboratory test that measures abnormalities of clotting factors I, II, V, VIII, IX, X, and XII.

Medical treatment focuses on replacement of the missing or deficient clotting factor. There are several replacement products available: (1) factor VIII concentrate, (2) cryoprecipitate, a high-potency form of AHF and fibrinogen, and (3) DDAVP, a synthetic form of vasopressin used in children with mild hemophilia and slow response. Purification during manufacture and careful screening of blood products make it unlikely that human immunodeficiency virus (HIV) will be transmitted. However, more than 70% of hemophiliac children who received blood products before 1989 acquired HIV from these products.

Hemophilia. Bleeding disorder characterized by excessive bleeding and deficiency of one of the factors necessary for coagulation.

Factor VIII. Antihemophiliac factor needed in the first phase of clotting.

Hemarthrosis. Bleeding into joint spaces.

Other drugs may also be a part of the medical regimen. Corticosteroids are given to reduce inflammation. Acetaminophen (with or without codeine) may be prescribed for joint pain. Ibuprofen is safe and effective for pain relief. Aspirin and other nonsteroidal anti-inflammatory drugs are avoided.

Aminocaproic acid (Amicar) prevents clot destruction, but use is limited to tongue lacerations and before dental procedures.

For hemarthrosis, ice packs are applied and the affected joint is immobilized and elevated during active bleeding. Once active bleeding ceases, exercise and physical therapy help maintain normal joint function. Treatment is always aggressive and rapid. The faster the bleeding is controlled, the less the likelihood of severe complications.

Nursing goals for the child with hemophilia include prevention of bleeding, recognition and control of bleeding, prevention of joint deformities, support of the family and child dealing with a chronic, potentially crippling disorder, and instruction on preparations for home care.

Prevention of Bleeding

Preventing injury prevents bleeding episodes. During infancy and toddlerhood, acquiring normal motor skills puts the child at risk for injury. The child's hospital and home environment should be made as safe as possible. Outside play should be supervised without inhibiting normal growth and development. The older child may find adjustments to limitations of active sports difficult. Noncontact sports are recommended.

To minimize the risk of hemorrhage the child is encouraged to use a soft bristle toothbrush or a water irrigation device. Adolescents should use an electric razor to shave. Intramuscular injections and venipunctures are contraindicated. Aspirin and aspirin-containing products must be avoided. The earlier a bleeding episode is recognized, the more effective the treatment will be.

The child and family members should be able to recognize signs of occult (hidden) and active bleeding. Early signs of bleeding into the joint spaces are stiffness and mild pain. They should also observe for hematuria, black stools (may indicate gastrointestinal bleeding), and hematemesis (bloody or dark brown emesis). Severe headache, slurred speech, and lethargy may be signs of intracranial hemorrhage. Parents and children 8 years and older are instructed on the preparation and administration of factor replacement therapy, and how to manage active bleeding by applying pressure to the site for 10 to 15 minutes, elevating the injury site above the level of the heart, and applying cold for vasoconstriction.

$\mathcal{I}$DIOPATHIC THROMBOCYTOPENIA PURPURA (ITP)

Idiopathic thrombocytopenia purpura. Blood disorder associated with a deficit of platelets.

Purpura is a blood disorder associated with a deficit of platelets in the circulatory system. **Idiopathic thrombocytopenia** is the most common type of **purpura** occurring in childhood. The exact cause is unknown, but the disorder is often precipitated by an autoimmune response. The condition occurs in one of two forms: an acute disorder that is self-limiting or a chronic condition with intermittent remissions. The onset is frequently acute. Bruising and petechiae (pinpoint subcutaneous hemorrhages) occur. There may be bleeding from the mucous membranes, gums, epistaxis (nosebleed), and hematuria.

In ITP the platelet count may be as low as 20,000/mm³ or lower. The bleeding time is prolonged, and the clot retraction time is abnormal.

Medical management is supportive because of the self-limiting nature of the disorder. Corticosteroids are useful in decreasing the severity and duration of the disease. Intravenous gamma globulin has been effective in increasing the production of platelets until spontaneous recovery takes place.

Nursing care is also supportive. Activity is restricted and the child is protected from falls and trauma. Parents and children should be given explanations concerning the disease and its treatment. Children and parents should be advised to observe for signs of internal bleeding as well as hemarthrosis. Emotional support should be given to the family.

$\mathcal{C}$HILDHOOD LEUKEMIA

Leukemia is the most common type of cancer in children. It is cancer of the blood-forming tissues. The exact cause is unknown. It occurs more frequently in males than females after the age of 1 year; peak onset is between 3 and 5 years. Leukemia is seen more frequently in Caucasian children than African American children.

Leukemia is a general term given to a group of malignant diseases of the bone marrow and lymph system. Leukemia is classified by cell type. In children, two types of leukemia are predominant: acute lymphoid leukemia (ALL), and **acute nonlymphoid** (myelogenous) **leukemia** (ANLL or AML). Alternate terms for ALL include acute lymphatic leukemia, **acute lymphocytic leukemia**, and acute lymphoblastoid leukemia. Alternate terms for ANLL include acute myelogenous leukemia, acute myeloblastic leukemia, and acute nonlymphocytic leukemia. Each form of ALL and ANLL has several subtypes. ALL accounts for about 80% of childhood leukemia cases.

Leukemia is uncontrolled reproduction of immature white blood cells in the blood-forming tissues of the body. These immature WBCs replace normal blood elements (RBCs, WBCs, and platelets) and invade the bone marrow. Leukemic cells then infiltrate the bone marrow and compete with normal, mature WBCs for essential nutrients. Clinical manifestations of bone marrow suppression include: (1) infection from **neutropenia** (decreased WBC count), (2) bleeding tendencies caused by thrombocytopenia (decreased platelet count), and (3) anemia caused by decreased RBC count. Bone marrow infiltration with immature WBCs causes severe bone pain.

Infiltration into the lymph nodes, liver, and spleen causes enlargement and these organs become fibrotic. Not all children develop central nervous

Leukemia. Cancer of the blood-forming tissues.

Acute nonlymphoid leukemia. Type of leukemia that accounts for 20% of childhood cases.

Acute lymphocytic leukemia. Type of leukemia that accounts for 80% of childhood cases.

Neutropenia. Decreased WBC count.

system involvement. However, infiltration of the meninges causes symptoms of intracranial pressure (ICP). Leukemic cells may also infiltrate the gastrointestinal tract, kidneys, ovaries, and testes. Leukemic cells require a tremendous amount of nutrients and energy for reproduction. They eventually deprive all of the body's normal cells of nutrients needed for survival.

Clinical manifestations of leukemia may appear abruptly or have an insidious onset. The exact cause of leukemia is unknown. Children may exhibit few symptoms. It is not unusual for leukemia to be diagnosed on a routine physical examination or after a viral illness or minor infection that does not resolve. The child continues to have low-grade fever, pallor, fatigue, and weight loss. Other symptoms are bone and joint pain caused by the invasion of the periosteum, widespread petechiae, and purpura as a result of a low thrombocyte count. Easy bruising is an ongoing problem. Anorexia, nausea and vomiting, headache, diarrhea, and abdominal pain often occur as the disease progresses. Ulcerations of the mucous membranes (especially the oral mucosa) develop as a result of bacterial infection.

In addition to the history, physical symptoms, and laboratory blood studies, a bone marrow aspiration or biopsy confirms the diagnosis of leukemia. Radiographic studies of the long bones reveal changes caused by infiltration of lymphoblasts.

Regardless of the type of leukemia, treatment is divided into three phases: (1) induction phase, with the goal being to achieve complete remission with no leukemic cells in the bone marrow, (2) prophylactic central nervous system (CNS) therapy or sanctuary, and (3) maintenance.

Induction is begun immediately and lasts for 4 to 6 weeks. A combination of drugs is used during the induction phase. Among the drugs used in ALL are prednisone, L-asparaginase, and vincristine. For children with ANLL, the induction regimen includes prednisone, L-asparaginase, cytosine arabinoside, and doxorubicin or daunorubicin. Most children with ANLL achieve initial remission, but are more likely to suffer a relapse than children with ALL. The child is hospitalized as the induction phase begins for placement of an implantable intravenous device and to monitor response to the chemotherapy. If therapy is tolerated, the child is discharged and treatment continues in an outpatient setting.

Prophylactic CNS therapy or sanctuary begins 6 to 8 weeks after diagnosis. The child receives intrathecal administration (injection into the cerebrospinal fluid by lumbar puncture) of methotrexate, hydrocortisone, and cytosine arabinoside without cranial irradiation or intrathecal methotrexate with cranial irradiation. Because of the concern that cranial irradiation causes late adverse side effects, its use is reserved for high-risk patients.

Maintenance therapy follows successful induction and prophylactic CNS phases and may last for 2 or 3 years for boys (who have a greater relapse rate) and 18 months for girls. The goal of this treatment is to maintain remission and eradicate remaining leukemic cells. For the child with ALL the typical drug regimen is oral doses of prednisone, 6-mercaptopurine, and methotrexate. The child may also receive intravenous vincristine. During maintenance therapy periodic blood counts and bone marrow studies are taken to evaluate therapeutic response and check for possible relapse. After the end of maintenance boys undergo testicular biopsy to detect any possible testicular involvement.

For many children a fourth phase of therapy is necessary when relapse occurs: reinduction phase. Relapse is when the bone marrow studies show the presence of leukemic cells. Relapses usually occur 1 year after therapy is completed. Usually, reinduction for ALL is oral prednisone, intravenous vincristine, and other drugs not previously used. CNS prophylaxis is continued. Second remissions may be achieved, but the prognosis is less favorable with each relapse.

Bone marrow transplant has been used with success for the treatment of children with ALL and ANLL. It is not recommended for children with ALL who are in their first remission because of the excellent results of chemotherapy. It may be a treatment option for the child with ALL who is in a second remission. Since children with ANLL have a less favorable prognosis, bone marrow transplant may be considered after the first remission.

Appropriate nursing management for the child with leukemia is based on the treatment regimen. It includes administration and proper handling of chemotherapeutic agents, managing side effects of chemotherapy and irradiation, managing pain, preventing complications of bone marrow depression, promoting a positive body image, and supporting the child and family.

Precautions must be taken when chemotherapeutic agents are administered. Many of these drugs are vesicants. If the child does not have an implanted IV device established, maintenance of a free-flowing IV is important. If there is any sign of infiltration, the infusion must be discontinued immediately. The child is observed for allergic reaction whenever chemotherapeutic agents are given and an emergency drug box, Ambu bag with mask, and oxygen should be at the bedside. Only experienced nurses should administer chemotherapy. Handling and disposing of these agents may present a health risk to personnel. Protective equipment must be used and special precautions must be taken.

Side effects of chemotherapy and irradiation include:

1. Nausea and vomiting: Managing the side effects of chemotherapy presents challenges in providing nursing care to the child. The nausea and vomiting that occur after administration of chemotherapeutic agents and irradiation can be severe. The child is predisposed to fluid and electrolyte imbalance. An antiemetic should be given before administering these drugs and continued as necessary.

2. Anorexia: Loss of appetite is a result of chemotherapy and irradiation. Nutritional support is an important part of treatment. A child may develop an aversion to foods previously liked and there will be changes in the taste of foods. Allow any food the child desires. Assure the parents that the child's appetite will improve.

3. Mucosal ulceration: The side effect of several drugs is ulceration anywhere in the gastrointestinal tract. Oral ulcers are painful and can become infected, compounding anorexia. Oral hygiene is given with a soft-sponge toothbrush. The child's mouth is rinsed frequently with normal saline and local anesthetics are used. Viscous lidocaine is not

recommended for young children. Provide a bland diet and avoid citrus products. Rectal ulcers are painful and place the child at risk for sepsis. Meticulous, gentle cleaning of the rectal area is needed after each bowel movement. Use sitz baths and a protective skin barrier or an occlusive dressing. Taking temperatures rectally is avoided.

4. Neuropathy: Vincristine can cause neurotoxic effects. Measures to prevent constipation are taken; give stool softeners and laxatives for severe constipation, and ensure adequate fluid intake and a high-fiber diet.

5. Pain: Pain from invasion of lymphoblasts into the periosteum and bleeding into the joints can be excruciating. Gentle handling, foam mattress pads, and frequent positioning can help alleviate discomfort. The child undergoes many painful procedures. The nurse should explain that they are necessary and not meant to be punishment. The child needs to be taught how to communicate pain and its intensity. Analgesics should be appropriate for the pain and administered around the clock.

6. Complications of bone marrow depression: Bone marrow depression may cause anemia, neutropenia, and thrombocytopenia. Administer blood products as prescribed. The child with anemia should have as much uninterrupted rest as possible. To conserve energy the child should be assisted with activities of daily living.

7. Anemia: At the time of diagnosis anemia may be severe from complete replacement of the bone marrow by leukemic cells. During the induction phase of treatment transfusions of packed red blood cells may have to be given to raise the hemoglobin level. Interventions for any child with anemia are provided by the nurse.

8. Neutropenia: The child with neutropenia is at great risk for infection. Infection secondary to neutropenia is the most frequent cause of death from leukemia. Antibiotics are administered and the following precautions are taken: The child is placed in a private room; visitors or personnel with any infections are prohibited; aseptic technique is used for all procedures; and no rectal temperatures are taken (may introduce bacteria into the bloodstream).

9. Thrombocytopenia: Thrombocytopenia places the child at great risk for bleeding and spontaneous hemorrhage. The following measures are included in the child's care: transfuse platelets when prescribed, apply local pressure to bleeding sites, avoid needle sticks, avoid administering products containing aspirin, provide gentle oral hygiene, and restrict any activity that may cause trauma.

10. Poor self-image: The drugs that are administered in chemotherapy cause alopecia (hair loss). The child and family need to be psychologically prepared for this change in appearance. The child may want to choose a wig, cap, or scarf before the hair starts to fall out. Reassure the child and family that the hair will grow back in about 3 to 6 months and may be a different color or texture.

Family members are often devastated when they first learn that their child has leukemia. They need support from the moment of first diagnosis, throughout hospitalization, and during the maintenance phase. Families must cope with the worry that the child will not achieve remission and will relapse. Fear of death causes stress for the child and family. Emotional support is offered to assist the family to cope. Information is provided concerning the disease, treatment, home care, and prognosis.

Summary

This chapter discusses the most common disorders of the blood, which are described according to their pathology and according to how they originate. Understanding the physiological changes of the blood associated with these conditions, including the differences in malignancy and heredity, assists the reader in identifying the appropriate nursing intervention.

Critical Points in the Care of Hematologic System Disorders

Hematologic problems are generally classified as disorders of RBC function, of WBC function, and of platelet and coagulation function. These three very broad classifications can be further subdivided into disorders of blood cell production, maturation, or destruction. Knowledge of RBC function, WBC function, and platelet and coagulation function is essential to understanding the underlying pathogenesis and pathophysiology of hematologic disorders in children.

Anemia is generally defined as a reduction of the blood hemoglobin concentration or of the red cell mass below normal ranges. Anemias that are caused by inadequate production include acquired and constitutional aplastic anemia, red cell aplasia, and transient erythroblastosis of childhood. Maturational anemias are caused by nutritional disturbances such as iron deficiency, lead poisoning, and deficiencies in folic acid and vitamin B_{12}. Other anemias are associated with chronic illnesses where either the bone has a response to the illness or the transport of iron is impaired. Anemias associated with increased cell destruction are hemolytic anemia, which is caused by defects in the red cell membrane, hereditary hemoglobinopathies (like sickle cell anemia), and congenital enzyme defects.

White blood cell dysfunction occurs in pathological conditions such as acute infections, cancer, hemorrhage, hemolysis, tissue necrosis, or toxic exposures. A relative increase in the number of circulating immature band neutrophils is also indicative of an inflammatory process or an acute bacterial infection.

Qualitative abnormalities of granulocytes are felt to be related to defects in the function of phagocytosis. These occur in collagen-vascular disorders and bacterial infections. Certain drugs such as aspirin can lead to dysfunction of the phagocytic process. Granulomatous diseases are considered relatively rare.

Lymphocytosis is produced by viral illnesses such as mumps, measles, rubella, rubeola, varicella, and hepatitis. Pertussis and chronic lymphocytic leukemia also elevate the lymphocyte count. Normally an elevation of atypical lymphocytes indicates an infectious mononucleosis, cytomegalic inclusion disease, or toxoplasmosis.

Leukemia refers to a group of malignant diseases in which there are qualitative and quantitative changes in the circulating leukocytes. Leukemia is characterized by diffuse, abnormal growth of leukocytic precursors in the bone marrow. This uncontrolled increase in immature WBCs will lead eventually to anemia and thrombocytopenia. Life-threatening infections can occur since the immature WBCs are ineffective. Leukemia can be further classified according to the course of the illness and the particular types of cells and tissues involved.

Idiopathic thrombocytopenic purpura is the most common cause of thrombocytopenia in pediatrics. This disorder is associated with the destruction of circulating platelets brought about by an immune-mediated process, whereas disorders of coagulation can be brought about by the deficiencies of any of the clotting factors. Single coagulation factor deficiencies are usually hereditary, the most common being deficiencies in factor VIII (classic hemophilia), factor IX (hemophilia B or Christmas disease), and factor XI (hemophilia C or Rosenthal's disease).

$\mathcal{Q}$UESTIONS

Diagnosis: Iron-Deficiency Anemia

History: John is an 11-month-old infant who had a normal delivery. He has been very healthy, eats well, and is gaining weight. His immunizations are up to date. He eats some table food as well as baby food, including iron-fortified cereals. His mother has been supplementing his commercially prepared infant formula with cow's milk for the past 6 weeks. He is being seen at the pediatric clinic because his mother finds his color "a little pale." A blood count was taken and results indicate a hemoglobin of 10.5 g/dL and hematocrit of 33.0%.

Nursing problems: Infant exhibiting signs of iron deficiency anemia; pale color. Parents' knowledge deficit: Avoid cow's milk in the first year of life. This infant requires oral iron supplement therapy.

Chief concerns: Oxygen-carrying capability of the blood is decreased. Child will experience serious sequelae of iron-deficiency anemia.

Plan: Mother will receive instructions on the purpose, administration, and expected outcomes of oral iron supplement therapy. Mother will understand nutritional needs of infant. Child will have a rise in hemoglobin and hematocrit levels within 1 month.

1. When instructing the parents of an 11-month-old infant in the prevention of anemia, which of the following statements should the nurse include in the discussion?

   A. Anemia can easily occur during infancy. All infants should receive iron supplements.
   B. Cow's milk is an excellent source of iron. All infants should be put on cow's milk as soon as possible.
   C. Anemia during infancy is unusual because infants use fetal iron stores until they are 2 years old.
   D. Anemia can easily occur during infancy. Infants should be given solid foods (meats, vegetables, and cereals) that are good sources of iron.

2. Oral iron therapy may cause all of the following side effects except:

   A. Gastric irritation
   B. Pica
   C. Blackened stools
   D. Darkened teeth

3. To promote absorption of an iron supplement, the nurse should instruct the caregiver to administer the supplement:

   A. During the meal
   B. Two hours after the meal, with orange juice
   C. Two hours after the meal, with milk
   D. Immediately before meals

Diagnosis: Sickle Cell Anemia

History: Michael is a 9-month-old infant who was admitted to the pediatric unit for clinical pneumonia and moderate respiratory distress. He is receiving inhalation therapy, IV antibiotics, supplemental oxygen, and antipyretics. Michael's respiratory symptoms are improving slowly. However, the nurse reports that he is listless, irritable, and difficult for even his mother to comfort. Results from a complete count indicate: white blood cells (WBCs) 12,000; hemoglobin (Hgb) 10.1 g/dL, and hematocrit (Hct) 31%. Based on the clinical symptoms and the latest laboratory findings, a hematology consult is requested. The hematologist confirms a diagnosis of vaso-occlusive crisis of sickle cell anemia.

Nursing problems: Infant in need of appropriate pain management. Infant with reduced oxygen-carrying capability of blood to the tissues. Knowledge deficit: Parents' inability to assess pain in an infant. Parents will need support in dealing with reality of the diagnosis. Knowledge deficit: Parents' knowledge of family history of SCA.

Chief concerns: Infant will receive adequate analgesia. Appropriate care during this crisis.

Plan: Parents will understand teaching of recognition of signs and symptoms of crises and take immediate action. Parents and child will be able to cope adequately with a lifelong, potentially fatal disease. Appropriate referrals for testing for parents and siblings.

1. The nurse should expect which clinical findings in a 9-month-old with sickle cell anemia?
   A. Painful swelling of the hands and feet
   B. Infected leg ulcers
   C. Normal hemoglobin level and hematocrit
   D. Fine macular rash

2. A definitive diagnosis of sickle cell disease is based on which diagnostic results?
   A. Complete blood count (CBC)
   B. Bone marrow aspiration
   C. Blood chemistry tests
   D. Hemoglobin electrophoresis

3. Which of the following nursing actions should the nurse include when developing a care plan for the infant with sickle cell anemia?
   A. Evaluation of acid-base status and administration of sodium bicarbonate as needed
   B. Administration of a high concentration of oxygen to provide adequate oxygenation
   C. Assessment of level of pain and administration of pain medication as needed
   D. Replacement of factor VIII

Diagnosis: Acute Lymphocytic Leukemia

History: Margaret is a 7-year-old girl who was diagnosed with ALL 10 weeks ago. She is currently in the induction phase of chemotherapy. Her treatment regimen includes vincristine, L-asparaginase, and prednisone. She is currently hospitalized in the pediatric oncology unit in a private room. Her latest laboratory findings indicate bone marrow suppression. Her family asks what was significant in the laboratory findings and what interventions need to be taken.

Nursing problems: Child with neutropenia, anemia, and thrombocytopenia; at high risk for infection, especially viral illnesses; with decreased oxygen-carrying capacity of the blood; with a potential for injury and hemorrhage.

Chief concerns: Knowledge deficit: Parents and child, concerning test results and treatment. Protection of child from infectious processes. Protection of child from injury.

Plan: Explain purpose and meaning of results of laboratory findings to parents and child and assess their understanding. Explain expected changes in nursing care due to evidence of bone marrow depression to parents and child if necessary and assess their understanding.

1. Following a course of chemotherapy, a child's WBC count is very low. A specific nursing intervention would include:

   A. No special precautions; a low WBC count is expected
   B. Placing the child in a private room and protecting her from infection
   C. Strict monitoring of intake and output
   D. Administering oxygen and maintaining bed rest

2. A child receiving chemotherapy has a platelet count of 30,000. An appropriate nursing intervention would be:

   A. Keep the child isolated to prevent infection
   B. Encourage a high-fiber diet
   C. Provide frequent rest periods
   D. Discourage active play to avoid getting hurt

3. A child has acute lymphocytic leukemia and is receiving prednisone and vincristine. The child complains of constipation. The most probable cause of the constipation is:

   A. Leukemic mass obstructing the bowel
   B. Enlarged spleen obstructing the bowel
   C. Side effects of vincristine
   D. Toxic effect of prednisone

Diagnosis: Hemophilia

History: Thomas is a 6-year-old who was diagnosed with hemophilia three years ago. He has an implanted IV catheter for home infusion of factor VIII. The last time it was necessary to use it was when he tripped over a toy and fell on his knee, 14 months ago. His parents are well informed about the signs and symptoms of prolonged bleeding and the appropriate action necessary if injury occurs. Today he has been left in the care of his maternal aunt, who has never administered factor VIII, while his parents attend a social event for several hours. Thomas suffers an injury to his left elbow when a softball accidentally hits it. His aunt notices swelling of the elbow and decides to take him to the emergency room. His indwelling IV catheter is accessed by the nurse and factor VIII is administered.

Nursing problems: Knowledge deficit: Caretaker unfamiliar with emergency treatment for a bleeding episode of a child with hemophilia. Hemophiliac with an acute bleeding episode.

Chief concern: Child with a life-threatening bleeding disorder was left in the care of someone with no knowledge of how to take emergency action in the event of active bleeding.

Plan: Emphasize the need for child to be left in the care of an adult who can provide appropriate medical emergency treatment for the child, without criticizing. Referral to an appropriate support group.

1. The most common area for bleeding to occur in a child with hemophilia is:
   A. Brain
   B. Joints
   C. Abdomen
   D. Pericardium

$\mathcal{A}$NSWERS

Iron-Deficiency Anemia

1. *D.* Anemia occurs easily during infancy. Infants have limited iron reserves and must be given foods that are rich in iron. All infants do not require iron supplements because many have adequate dietary iron intake. Cow's milk is a poor source of iron.

2. *B.* Gastric irritation, blackened stools, and stained, darkened teeth are all side effects of the oral administration of iron supplements. A child with pica may be anemic, but this choice is not related to the question.

3. *B.* Iron supplements are absorbed better when the stomach is empty. Citrus products increase absorption of iron. It is best to give the supplement 1 hour before a meal or 2 hours after a meal. Food and milk decrease the absorption of iron.

Sickle Cell Anemia

1. *A.* In sickle cell disease the red blood cells lose their spherical shape and become sickle shaped, slowing blood flow and obstructing small blood vessels. In children age 6 months to 2 years, vessel occlusion in short tubular bones typically causes painful swelling of the hands and feet. Leg ulcers are common in adolescents and adults, not infants. Signs and symptoms in an infant also include pallor and anemia, which result from the shortened life span of the red blood cells. A fine macular rash may occur with skin conditions or drug reactions; it is not specific to sickle cell anemia.

2. *D.* Definitive diagnosis of sickle cell disease depends on hemoglobin electrophoresis, a test in which various types of hemoglobin are separated and identified. The complete blood count helps determine the presence of infection, anemia, or bleeding disorders. Bone marrow aspiration and blood chemistry tests are not used to diagnose sickle cell anemia.

3. *C.* Vaso-occlusive crises are painful experiences. Alterations in acid-base status do not generally occur during a vaso-occlusive crisis. Oxygen may

initially help the child feel better; high concentrations are usually not necessary. Children with hemophilia may require factor VIII replacement; it is not a correct choice because it is not an independent nursing action.

Acute Lymphocytic Leukemia

1. *B.* During chemotherapy a child will become neutropenic because of bone marrow suppression. This causes an inability of the child's immune system to fight infection. The nurse needs to protect the child from possible sources of infection. Placing a child in a private room and restricting visitors assists in protecting the child. Strict intake and output are maintained during chemotherapy, but are not the appropriate answers. Administering oxygen and maintaining bed rest are nursing interventions to be taken when the RBC count is low.

2. *D.* A platelet count of 30,000 is an indication of thrombocytopenia. A normal platelet count is 150,000–500,000. The thrombocytopenic child is at risk for hemorrhage following any kind of injury. Active play is always discouraged. A child who is neutropenic is kept in isolation. A high-fiber diet is indicated to prevent constipation and has nothing to do with a low platelet count. Frequent rest periods are necessary for the child with anemia.

3. *C.* Constipation is a common side effect of vincristine because gastric motility is slowed. A leukemic mass obstructing the bowel is not likely. A different drug would be used. An enlarged spleen would put pressure on the stomach, not the bowel. Constipation is not a toxic effect of prednisone.

Hemophilia

1. *B.* Bleeding can occur anywhere in the body after the child with hemophilia sustains trauma. However, a classic symptom is bleeding into the joints, or hemarthrosis.

𝒢LOSSARY

acute lymphocytic leukemia   type of leukemia that accounts for 80% of childhood cases.

acute nonlymphoid leukemia   type of leukemia that accounts for 20% of childhood cases.

anemia   abnormally low hemoglobin in the blood.

crises   episodes of RBC sickling.

factor VIII   antihemophiliac factor needed in the first phase of clotting.

ferrous sulfate   oral iron supplement.

hemarthrosis   bleeding into joint spaces.

hemoglobin electrophoresis   serum testing used to confirm diagnosis of sickle cell anemia.

hemolysis   increased destruction of RBCs.

hemophilia   bleeding disorder characterized by excessive bleeding and deficiency of one of the factors necessary for coagulation.

idiopathic thrombocytopenia purpura   blood disorder associated with a deficit of platelets.

iron-deficiency anemia   common nutritional deficiency in young children.

leukemia   cancer of the blood-forming tissues.

neutropenia   decreased WBC count.

sickle cell anemia   congenital, chronic disorder characterized by the production of an abnormal hemoglobin that results in a sickle shape under conditions of decreased oxygen tension.

sickledex   fingerstick screening test that reveals the presence of Hb S.

vaso-occlusive crises   clumping of sickle-shaped RBCs causing tissue ischemia and pain.

$\mathcal{B}$IBLIOGRAPHY

AGENCY FOR HEALTH CARE POLICY AND RESEARCH. *Sickle Cell Disease: Screening, Diagnosis, Management and Counseling in Newborns and Infants* (AHCPR Publication No. 93–0562). Silver Spring, MD: U.S. Public Health Service, 1993.

AMERICAN ACADEMY OF PEDIATRICS COMMITTEE ON NUTRITION. *Pediatric Nutrition Handbook.* 3rd ed. Elk Grove Village, IL: Author, 1993.

AMERICAN ACADEMY OF PEDIATRICS COMMITTEE ON PRACTICE AND AMBULATORY MEDICINE. Recommendations for preventative pediatric health care. *AAP News* 19, 1996.

BROWN, R. G. Determining the cause of anemia. *Postgraduate Medicine* 89(6):161–170, 1991.

CENTERS FOR DISEASE CONTROL. *Preventing Lead Poisoning in Young Children.* Washington, D.C.: U.S. Department of Health and Human Services/Public Health Service, 1992.

CORRIGAN, J. Hemorrhagic and thrombotic diseases. In R. Behrman (ed.). *Nelson Textbook of Pediatrics.* 14th ed. Philadelphia: Saunders, 1992, pp. 1272–1287.

DERSHEWITZ, R. A. *Ambulatory Pediatric Care.* 2nd ed. Philadelphia: Lippincott, 1993.

DYMENT, P. G. Pallor. In R. A. Dershewitz (ed.), *Ambulatory Pediatric Care.* 2nd ed. Philadelphia: Lippincott, 1993.

GITHENS, J., AND HATHAWAY, W. Hematologic disorders. In W. Hathaway, J. Groothuis, W. Hay, and J. Paisley (eds.), *Current Pediatric Diagnosis and Treatment.* 10th ed. East Norwalk, CT: Appleton & Lange, 1991, pp. 470–517.

GRIFFIN, J. Interventions for clients with hematologic disorders. In D. Ignatavicus and M. Baynes (eds.), *Medical Surgical Nursing*. Philadelphia: Saunders, 1991.

GUYTON, A. *Textbook of Medical Physiology*. 8th ed. Philadelphia: Saunders, 1990.

HATHAWAY, W. E., WAY, W. W., JR., GROOTHUIS, J. R., AND PAISLEY, J. W. *Current Pediatric Diagnosis & Treatment*. 11th ed. Norwalk, CT: Appleton & Lange, 1993.

LANE, P. A., NUSS, R., AND AMBRUSO, D. R. Hematologic disorders. In W. W. Hay, J. R. Groothuis, A. R. Hayward, et al. (eds.), *Current Pediatric Diagnosis and Treatment*. 12th ed. Norwalk, CT: Appleton & Lange, 1995.

LEVENTHAL, B. Neoplasms and neoplasm-like structures. In R. Behrman (ed.), *Nelson Textbook of Pediatrics*. 14th ed. Philadelphia: Saunders, 1992, pp. 1291–1322.

PARSONS, L. C. Nursing assessment and diagnosis of hematologic function. In D. Jackson and R. Saunders (eds.), *Child Health Nursing: A Comprehensive Approach to the Care of Children and Their Families*. Philadelphia: Lippincott, 1993.

PEARSON, H. The anemia. In F. Oski, C. DeAngelis, R. Feigin, and J. Warshaw (eds.), *Principles and Practice of Pediatrics*. Philadelphia: Lippincott, 1990, pp. 1513–1525.

PLATT, O. Hematologic problems. In R. A. Dershewitz (ed.), *Ambulatory Pediatric Care*. Philadelphia: Lippincott, 1993, pp. 474–493.

U.S. DEPARTMENT OF HEALTH AND HUMAN SERVICES. *Clinician's Handbook of Preventive Services: Put Prevention into Practice*. Washington, D.C.: U.S. Government Printing Office, 1994.

U.S. DEPARTMENT OF HEALTH AND HUMAN SERVICES. *Healthy People 2000: National Health Promotion and Disease Prevention Objectives*. (DHHS Publication No. (PHS) 91-50212). Washington, D.C.: Author, 1990.

WHEBY, M. S. Sizing up the seriousness of anemia. *Emergency Medicine* 21(14):179–181, 184, 186, 1989.

WINGATE, A. Anatomy and physiology of the hematologic system. In D. Jackson and R. Saunders (eds.), *Child Health Nursing: A Comprehensive Approach to the Care of Children and Their Families*. Philadelphia: Lippincott, 1993, pp. 1069–1076.

WOFFORD, L. Nursing planning, intervention and evaluation for altered hematologic function. In D. Jackson and R. Saunders (eds.), *Child Health Nursing: A Comprehensive Approach to the Care of Children and Their Families*. Philadelphia: Lippincott, 1993, pp. 1093–1136.

WONG, D. L. *Nursing Care of Infants and Children*. St. Louis: Mosby, 1995.

$\mathcal{H}$ELPFUL INTERNET SITES

PEDINFO: An Index of the Pediatric Internet at http://www.pedinfo. org   This is an excellent site that covers nearly all topics within this review. It has a wealth of information and is worth a visit. It is written for health care professionals but others could also use the information. Congenital syndromes, congenital malformations, and inborn errors of metabolism are covered.

Massachusetts General Hospital Web Site at http://cancer.mgh. harvard.edu/medOnc/sickle.htm   Interesting site dedicated to issues and problems surrounding sickle cell disease.

Emory University's Sickle Cell Site at http://www.emory.edu/PEDS/ SICKLE/index.htm   This site provides sickle cell patient and professional education, news, research updates, and worldwide resources.

International Journal of Pediatric Hematology and Oncology at http:// www.biomednet.com   One can log-in as a "visitor" (password: biomednet) to view abstracts. Members can view the full text of this and other publications. To fully use this site you need to become a member, which requires paying a subscription fee.

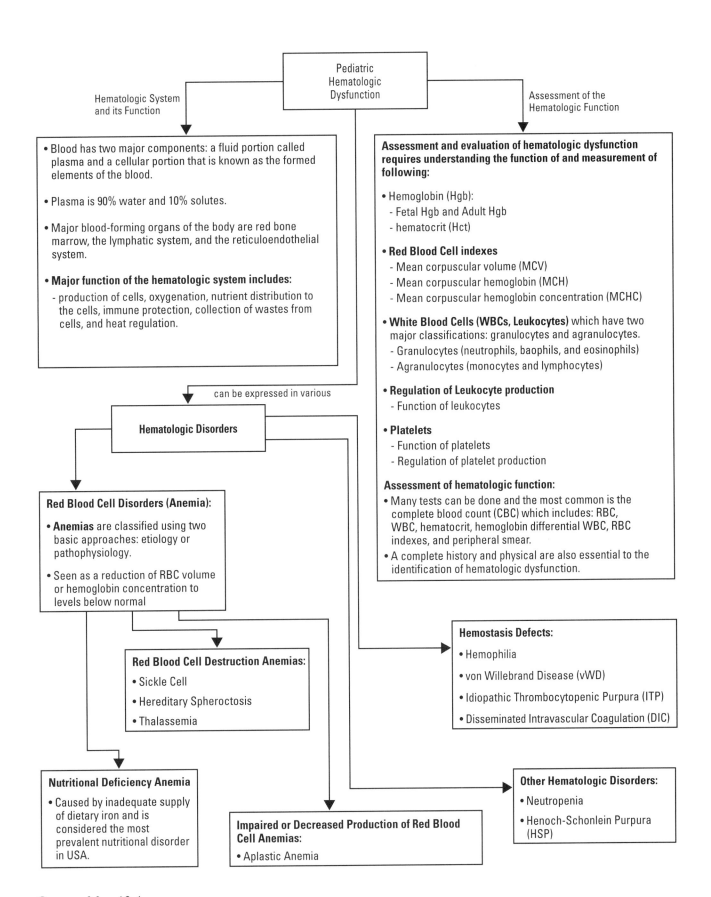

Pediatric Hematologic Dysfunction

Hematologic System and its Function

- Blood has two major components: a fluid portion called plasma and a cellular portion that is known as the formed elements of the blood.

- Plasma is 90% water and 10% solutes.

- Major blood-forming organs of the body are red bone marrow, the lymphatic system, and the reticuloendothelial system.

- **Major function of the hematologic system includes:**
  - production of cells, oxygenation, nutrient distribution to the cells, immune protection, collection of wastes from cells, and heat regulation.

Assessment of the Hematologic Function

Assessment and evaluation of hematologic dysfunction requires understanding the function of and measurement of following:

- Hemoglobin (Hgb):
  - Fetal Hgb and Adult Hgb
  - hematocrit (Hct)

- **Red Blood Cell indexes**
  - Mean corpuscular volume (MCV)
  - Mean corpuscular hemoglobin (MCH)
  - Mean corpuscular hemoglobin concentration (MCHC)

- **White Blood Cells (WBCs, Leukocytes)** which have two major classifications: granulocytes and agranulocytes.
  - Granulocytes (neutrophils, baophils, and eosinophils)
  - Agranulocytes (monocytes and lymphocytes)

- **Regulation of Leukocyte production**
  - Function of leukocytes

- **Platelets**
  - Function of platelets
  - Regulation of platelet production

Assessment of hematologic function:
- Many tests can be done and the most common is the complete blood count (CBC) which includes: RBC, WBC, hematocrit, hemoglobin differential WBC, RBC indexes, and peripheral smear.
- A complete history and physical are also essential to the identification of hematologic dysfunction.

can be expressed in various

Hematologic Disorders

Red Blood Cell Disorders (Anemia):

- **Anemias** are classified using two basic approaches: etiology or pathophysiology.

- Seen as a reduction of RBC volume or hemoglobin concentration to levels below normal

Red Blood Cell Destruction Anemias:
- Sickle Cell
- Hereditary Spheroctosis
- Thalassemia

Nutritional Deficiency Anemia
- Caused by inadequate supply of dietary iron and is considered the most prevalent nutritional disorder in USA.

Impaired or Decreased Production of Red Blood Cell Anemias:
- Aplastic Anemia

Hemostasis Defects:
- Hemophilia
- von Willebrand Disease (vWD)
- Idiopathic Thrombocytopenic Purpura (ITP)
- Disseminated Intravascular Coagulation (DIC)

Other Hematologic Disorders:
- Neutropenia
- Henoch-Schonlein Purpura (HSP)

Concept Map 12-1

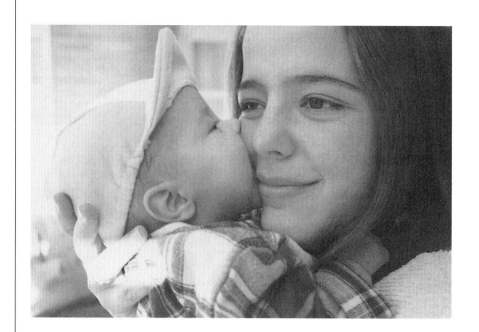

C H A P T E R   1 3

ℐNFECTIOUS DISEASES

ℐNTRODUCTION

The body continuously regenerates, repairs, and restores cells. The disease potential of a microorganism depends on its ability to invade and destroy cells, produce toxins, and produce damaging hypersensitivity reactions. Survival of a microorganism also depends on its ability to **proliferate**.

Bacterial survival and growth depend on the effectiveness of the body's **defense mechanisms** (the immune system), and its ability to recognize and destroy the invading microorganism. This "war" is carried out by the immune system. Natural immunity is present at birth; acquired immunity is gained after birth by active or passive immunity. Active acquired **immunity** is produced by the **host** after either natural exposure to an **antigen** or immunization. Passive acquired immunity does not involve the body's own immune response; rather, it is performed by, for example, maternal-infant antibodies transferred by breast milk.

The cells that defend the body are called phagocytes. **Phagocytosis** is the process of engulfment and destruction of microorganisms, dead cells, and foreign particles. Inflammation of the invasion site attracts phagocytes to attack the microorganism, antigen, or any other identified object deemed invasive. Leukocytes, which include granulocytes, neutrophils, eosinophils, and basophils, are called to the inflammatory process. Monocytes (immature blood cells) and macrophages (immature cells in tissue) all are capable of phagocytosis. Once these cells respond to an antigen invader (foreign substance), they "remember" and are able to recognize the invader if it appears again. T cells and B cells are killer, helper, and suppressor cells in

Proliferation. Ability to reproduce and invade a medium rapidly and repeatedly grow new parts, as by cell division.

Defense mechanism. Mechanism used to offer resistance or protection as means of self-defense.

Immunity. Defense or protection from a disease, especially an infectious disease. Usually induced by having been exposed to the antigenic maker on an organism that invades the body.

Antigen. A protein marker on the surface of cells that identifies the cell as "self" or non-"self."

Phagocytosis. A process of engulfment and destruction of microorganisms.

Virus. A minute organism that is entirely dependent on nutrients inside cells for its metabolic and reproductive needs.

Viral infections. Infection caused by a virus.

Infection. The spread of a disease.

Contagious. A communicable transmittable infection.

Transmission. Condition in which the organism that transmits the causative agent of a disease plays an essential role in the life of a parasite.

Incubation period. Interval between exposure to infection and the appearance of the first symptom of the disease.

Communicable. A transferable infection from a person to a person or from a person to an animal or vice versa.

antigen/antibody immune responses. This is particularly important in subsequent encounters with the same organism. This immunity provides a lasting protection against specific antigens. These cell-mediated immune responses are thymus-dependent and rely on the lymph glands and bone marrow for cell development.

Fever is caused by the release of endogenous pyrogen from macrophages or circulating white blood cells. Fever is also caused by the release of biochemicals during the inflammatory phase.

Viruses are intracellular parasites that take over host cells and use them for survival and replication. **Viral infections,** which include the common cold, are the most common afflictions of humans. The hard protein coat resists phagocytosis but does evoke a strong immune response.

Children are exposed to many different organisms: bacterial, viral, fungal, protozoal, and helminthic. Some of the more common **infections** will be discussed in this chapter. (See Concept Map 13-1.)

$\mathcal{E}$RYTHEMA INFECTIOSUM

Erythema infectiosum (fifth disease) is a mild, minimally febrile, **contagious** virus illness caused by Parvovirus B 19 (Figure 13-1; Color Insert 10). Erythema infectiosum is also known as fifth disease because of its clinical presentation of the 5 classical common infections of childhood. It occurs everywhere in the world, especially in schoolchildren between ages 5 and 15. Family and/or institutional outbreaks of fifth disease tend to occur in the late winter and early spring. **Transmission** is usually through contact of respiratory secretions from an infected person. The **incubation period** for the infection varies, ranging from 4 to 20 days to the development of the rash. **Communicability** is believed to be the greatest before the onset of the rash and probably not after the onset of the rash.

Human Parvovirus B 19, which causes erythema infectiosum, has been implicated in arthritic syndromes, particularly in adults, and is the cause of aplastic crises in patients with chronic **hemolytic** disorders. Intrauterine Parvovirus infection may produce hydrops and fetal death. Infection in immunocompromised patients may lead to chronic infection and anemia.

The initial symptom is the **rash,** which appears in three stages. Stage 1: The rash first appears on the face with a "slapped cheek" appearance in nature. The child also exhibits circumoral pallor that lasts 1 to 4 days. Stage 2: A lacy maculopapular eruption appears on the face, arm, thighs, and buttocks. Stage 3: After the rash disappears, there may be periodic recurrence precipitated by heat or cold. The rash lasts 3 to 7 days and may recur over 1 to 3 weeks. Children are no longer infectious by the time the rash appears, but the incubation period before the rash appears is approximately 4 to 14 days, during which time the child is contagious. Other symptoms that may be present, include headache, **pruritus,** and arthralgia.

Treatment is not indicated in uncomplicated cases; however, a child who has a hemolytic disease may require a blood transfusion. In the case

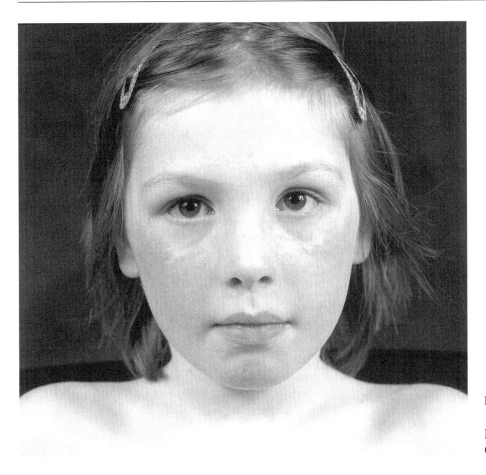

FIGURE 13-1

◩

Erythema infectiosum. (See also Color Insert 10.)

of **disease-immune response, immunoglobulin** may be effective. Supportive treatment for discomfort such as arthralgia, fever, or pruritus can be done at home without hospitalization.

ℋUMAN IMMUNODEFICIENCY VIRUS

The human **immunodeficiency** virus (HIV) is a retrovirus that functions by carrying genetic information through the ribonucleic acid (RNA) rather than the typical carrier deoxyribonucleic acid (DNA). This changes the genetic molecule and allows takeover of the target cell. With the enzyme reverse transcriptase, the HIV RNA is transformed to DNA.

A seroconversion illness or "window period" usually occurs within 1 month of being infected with the HIV virus, which is transmitted through infected blood and body fluids, excluding saliva and tears. The most prevalent modes of transmission are in utero from mother to fetus or via breast milk. On average, it takes 7 to 9 years for symptoms to develop in the adult; however, clinical symptoms are usually present by time an infected child is 2 years old.

Hemolytic. The breakdown of red blood cells.

Rash. A reaction manifested in the skin to an allergen.

Pruritus. Severe itching; may be a symptom of a disease process, such as an allergic reaction.

Disease-immune response. Resistance to immunization.

Immunoglobulin. A preparation used intravenously in patients with immunodeficiency syndromes and in immuno-suppressed recipients of bone marrow transplants.

Immunodeficiency. Decreased or compromised ability to respond to antigenic immunity reaction.

Opportunistic infections. An infection that is developed due to favorable conditions for the microorganism.

HIV surpasses the immune system's ability to contend with the invasion of the virus, weakening the immune system beyond its functional level. In addition to the effects on the immune system, HIV has the potential to infect other organs and cause serious problems within the host. The clinical descriptors of children with AIDS include flulike symptoms: fever, diarrhea, significant weight loss, and poor appetite; followed by adenopathy, developmental delay, or encephalopathy; and, inevitably, **opportunistic infections.** It is hypothesized that early exposure to the HIV infection, via the mother, is cause for increased mortality before age 2 or 3. When one or more opportunistic infections develop in conjunction with a drop in the CD4 count to 200 cells/mm or less (normal is a reading in excess of 800 cells/mm), the patient's diagnosis changes from carrier of HIV to AIDS. The range for CD4 counts is 350 to 1334.

Features found more commonly in children are recurrent bacterial infections, such as otitis media, sinusitis, and bacteremia. Additionally, parotitis, microcephaly, sepsis, and pneumonitis are common findings. With drug therapy leading to prolonged life, malignancies that previously were seen only in adults are now observed in children. Adults and children may present with hepatosplenomegaly, hepatitis, progressive renal disease, chronic eczemoid rashes, thrombocytopenia, and neurologic abnormalities.

Opportunistic infections include *Candida* or thrush, which is a common fungal infection of the mouth, manifesting itself as a white curdlike coating on the tongue, gums, palate, and esophagus, and is sometimes found in combination with oral hairy leukoplakia, an infection caused by the Epstein-Barr virus. *Candida* often causes discomfort and difficulty swallowing and can be one of the earliest signs of an HIV infection, occurring most often when CD4 levels decrease to a level of 200 to 500 cells/mm.

Diagnosis is usually made via clinical findings, and then confirmed by laboratory testing. An HIV-exposed infant is considered uninfected when two or more antibody tests are negative and the child is free of symptoms; however, it is recommended that a final test be performed when the child is 24 months old. Testing is repeated at that age because maternal antibodies may still be present in the child until about 18 to 24 months.

Inhibitors. Chemical substances that stop enzyme activity.

Drugs that have proven to be the most beneficial in the fight against the HIV virus are the antiretroviral drugs. Suggested treatment for adults now includes triple drug therapy, which is a combination of 2 nucleoside reverse transcriptase inhibitors plus 1 protease inhibitor. The action of antiretroviral drugs is to **inhibit** the activity of reverse transcriptase, the primary enzyme required for HIV replication, thereby rejecting transmutation to the virally tainted DNA. The only drugs currently approved for use in the treatment of pediatric patients include the use of antiretroviral agents, such as zidovudine (ZDV), formerly known as azidothymidine (AZT), and ddI (2'3' dideoxyinosine). ZDV is preferred for initial treatment of children. Those receiving ZDV therapy should be monitored for neutropenia and anemia. Children who are exposed to varicella should receive the varicella-zoster immune globulin (VZIG) within 72 hours of exposure, unless intravenous gamma globulin (IVIG) was given within the past 3 weeks.

Parents and patients need to be given appropriate, age-specific information on the transmission of the disease. Adolescents need to be educated about sexual practices that put them at risk for infection and/or spreading the disease. The combination of drugs and alcohol use in adolescents has reportedly led to an increased number of cases of promiscuous sexual activity, which in turn has led to a documented rise in the number of teenagers with HIV.

Education is the key to preventing this illness. The parents of HIV/AIDS-infected children and adolescents should be instructed on instilling good hygienic habits for the child to follow, such as hand washing, oral care, and routine bathing. Household pet immunizations also need to be kept up-to-date, and children should be taught to avoid contact with excretions. Family members need to be taught that HIV is not transmitted through casual contact, such as shaking hands, touching, hugging, or holding an infected baby, interacting with peers (playing), sharing utensils, using public toilet seats, bites from insects, or from kissing without rough penetration of the oral cavity.

The Influenza Virus

The influenza virus, commonly called the "flu," has three types: A, B, and C. Types A and B are responsible for epidemics of respiratory illness that occur almost every winter and are often associated with hospitalizations and deaths. Type C usually has mild respiratory illness or no symptoms. Influenza viruses mutate, so previously developed antibodies may be only slightly effective against the mutated virus. Influenza Type A undergoes two kinds of changes. One is a series of gradual mutations called an antigenic "drift." The other is an abrupt change in the protein of the virus, called a "shift." Type B undergoes only the gradual drift.

Transmission of the influenza virus occurs from direct contact with infected perspiration droplets, nasopharyngeal secretions, and/or airborne transmission. The incubation period is short, only 1 to 5 days. Symptoms can last 3 to 4 days, but the cough may persist longer. Most children recover within 2 weeks.

Typical clinical features include a fever in children that can be as high as 103°F or higher, respiratory symptoms, nonproductive cough, clear nasal discharge, myalgia, malaise, sore throat, and headache. Children are also likely to experience gastrointestinal symptoms including nausea, vomiting, and diarrhea.

Treatment for fever and myalgia is usually supportive. Cough suppressants with codeine are also suggested. Amantadine HCl (Symmetrel) is given for Type B influenza for children younger than 9 years of age or who weigh less than 45 kilograms. Parents should be advised that the best treatment for influenza in their child is rest, and an increase of fluid intake is necessary to prevent dehydration. For children with chronic disorders of the pulmonary or cardiovascular system, including asthma, the influenza vaccine is recommended.

$\mathcal{H}$ERPES SIMPLEX

Lesions. A circumscribed area of pathologically altered tissue.

There are two types of herpes simplex viruses: type 1 (HSV-1) and type 2 (HSV-2). These viruses typically produce a subclinical or clinical primary infection, followed by latent persistence in the sensory ganglia. In herpes simplex virus type-1, reactivation can be caused by emotional factors including stress, fever, and menses. Contact with infected saliva or **lesions** transmits the herpes viruses. Lesions are usually around the mouth and face but can be seen on the hands of young children who are thumb suckers. Seventy-five percent of cases of HSV-1 occur above the waist. HSV-1, in its recurrent form, is often seen in children as acute herpetic gingivostomatitis. Seventy-five percent of herpes simplex virus type 2 occurs principally on the genitals and lower parts of the body. HSV-2 is one of the most common sexually transmitted diseases (STD) in children and adults. Recurrence is frequent, but subsequent outbreaks decrease after the first year.

In HSV-1, the incubation period is 2 to 12 days, at which time small transparent vesicles form on an erythematous base, and they become cloudy and purulent. The vesicles dry, become crusted over, and then may crack and bleed. The common name is the "fever blister" or "cold sore." These are often found on lips or nose, but may occur anywhere on the body. For HSV-1, there is no scientific documentation that any treatment decreases healing time. However, symptoms may be alleviated by topical ointments to prevent cracking and/or bacterial superinfections. (See Figure 13-2; Color Insert 11.)

FIGURE 13-2

🔯

Herpes simplex virus infection: neonatal. (See also Color Insert 11.)

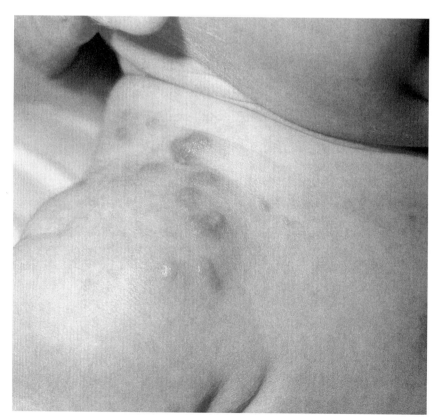

HSV-2 differs in appearance from HSV-1, in that there can be small groupings with gray-white ulcerations, which appear within 1 to 3 days. The infected child will complain of extreme tenderness in the area of the lesion before it appears, and occurrences can be in areas other than the primary site. The primary infection lasts 15 to 42 days and recurrent infections last approximately 6 days. For HSV-2, there is no **prophylaxis** or cure. Treatment is aimed solely at pain control. Anesthetics such as benzocaine or lidocaine can be used. Zovirax (acyclovir) ointment or capsules are the treatment of choice for primary, recurrent, and chronic suppressive therapy. Education is important in both types of herpes simplex viruses. For type 1, family members should be made aware of methods of transmission and the length of communicability.

Prophylaxis. Measures necessary to prevent disease.

Infectious Mononucleosis

Infectious mononucleosis is a viral disease that infects the B-lymphocytes, which then manifest symptoms of an immune response within multiple body systems, including the immune system. Infectious mononucleosis is caused by the Epstein-Barr virus (EBV), a DNA virus, which is one of the known herpesviruses. It invades and replicates in the salivary glands in the B-lymphocytes, resulting in proliferation of the lymphocyte cells. In persons with normal immune response mechanisms, responses by the T cells and the killer cells usually inhibit this proliferation, and the person does not exhibit symptoms of the infection. In persons with altered immunity, however, the proliferation may result in disseminated infection or in B-cell lymphomas. Infectious mononucleosis is commonly known as "mono," or "the kissing disease." Transmission of the virus occurs when a person comes in contact with the saliva of an infected individual.

In adolescents and young adults, the illness usually develops slowly. Early symptoms are vague; they include fatigue; exudative pharyngitis; tonsillar enlargement; lymphadenopathy, especially of the posterior cervical chain nodes; pain behind the eyes; hepatosplenomegaly; and fever of 101° to 105°F for approximately 5 days and intermittently for 1 to 3 weeks. Other accompanying symptoms seen less frequently include a rash (typically a petechial rash seen on the palate), aseptic meningitis, Guillain-Barré syndrome, headache, splenic rupture, edema of eyelids, thrombocytopenia, hemolytic anemia, and myocarditis. Systemic involvement can include thrombocytopenia, agranulocytosis and hemolytic anemia, aseptic meningitis, and encephalitis.

Antibiotics are ineffective against viruses and should not be given for mononucleosis itself. Should streptococcal (bacterial) throat infection develop, however, antibiotics would be the course of treatment. Ninety percent of mononucleosis is benign and uncomplicated. Education on the mode of transmission of the disease, which includes kissing and sharing drinking glasses, should be given to all members of the family. Epstein-Barr virus does not cause chronic fatigue syndrome and does not usually recur.

Rubeola

Rubeola (measles) (see Figure 13-3; Color Insert 12) is an acute, highly communicable disease transmitted by direct contact with infectious droplets. The age range for the highest incidence of the disease is between 2 and 14 years. The incubation period is 8 to 14 days, with the majority of cases occurring 10 days after exposure. This virus crosses the placenta of a pregnant woman to infect the fetus, with sometimes catastrophic results, from birth defects to stillborn fetuses.

Fever is usually the first sign of measles, with temperatures that range from 101° to 104°F. The temperature tends to be higher before the rash appears. Sore throat, nasal discharge (coryza), and dry barking cough are common prodromal signs. Nonpurulent conjunctivitis appears toward the end of the prodrome and is accompanied by photophobia. Koplik's spots (fine white spots on a faint erythematous base) appear on the buccal mucosa opposite the first and second upper molars 2 to 4 days after the onset of fever. The blotchy, irregular macular erythema and red patches vary in size and shape. They appear on the face first, then behind the ears, spreading to the chest, abdomen, and extremities. The rash usually appears on the third to fifth day after the onset of symptoms. Petechiae (bleeding spots) and ecchymoses (bruises) can occur with very severe rashes.

Complications occur when rubeola is compounded by bacterial infections. Otitis media, tracheobronchitis, bronchopneumonia, thrombocytopenia, and encephalitis are some of the complications of this infection. Children with rubeola are more vulnerable to strep infections, and rubeola can reactivate and worsen tuberculosis.

Treat children symptomatically with Tylenol or Motrin for pain, decrease exposure to light for patients with photosensitivity, and always ensure adequate fluid intake. Usually, isolation is recommended through

FIGURE 13-3

Measles, maculopapular erythematous rash. (See also Color Insert 12.)

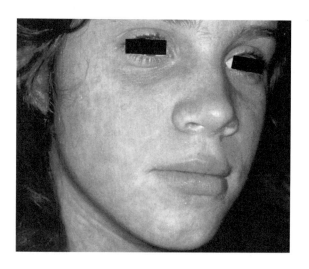

the seventh day after the onset of the rash. Secondary bacterial infections are usually treated with antibiotics. Vaccinations are recommended for children. Live measles virus vaccine should be given at 12 to 15 months of age. A second vaccine is usually given before the child enters school, at about 5 years of age. The vaccine can also be given within 72 hours of exposure, which may be effective as a postexposure prophylaxis. However, the measles vaccine is contraindicated in immunocompromised children and for children allergic to eggs or the drug neomycin. Parents should be educated on the importance of keeping immunizations of other children up to date and/or immunizing sexually active teenage girls. Pregnant women should avoid exposure to measles because of the complications it could cause to their unborn fetus.

*L*YME DISEASE

Lyme disease is a multisystem infection caused by a spirochete, which is transmitted to humans by the bite of an infected tick. Incidence/prevalence of the disease in the United States is May to September, occurring in all ages, but most commonly in children younger than age 15, and in adults 25 to 44 years old, with no apparent difference with regard to gender. The first sign of localized Lyme disease is a ring-shaped rash (called erythema migrans) (see Figure 13-4; Color Insert 13), which appears at the site of the bite. Within a week or two, the rash can spread to a diameter of 6 inches. Children may have accompanying fever, arthralgia, headaches, red eyes, swollen glands, or a generally sick feeling. If left untreated, Lyme disease can cause meningitis and facial palsy and can infect the pericardium. The most common late manifestation problem is large joint, self-limited oligoarthritis, often affecting the knees.

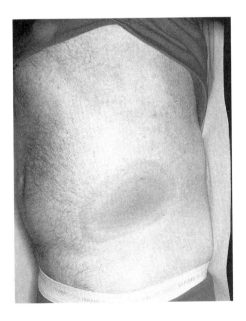

FIGURE 13-4

◙

Erythema migrans (Lyme disease). (See also Color Insert 13.)

Oral antibiotic therapy (tetracycline) is effective for early localized infection and should also avoid discoloration and mottling of permanent teeth if they have erupted. Intravenous therapy is recommended for the more serious systemic infections such as nervous system involvement. Education for parents should include the admonition for children to wear tick repellent when entering the woods. Dress children in long-sleeved shirts and tuck pants legs into socks. Light-colored clothing will contrast with the dark color of the tick and make identification easier.

ℛOCKY MOUNTAIN SPOTTED FEVER

Systemic infections. Diseases that are present in body systems.

Rocky Mountain spotted fever is caused by bacteria called *Rickettsia*, a gram-negative coccobacillus that replicates within the endothelial cells. This **systemic**, febrile illness is generally caused by a tick bite. The tick must attach and feed on blood for approximately 4 to 6 hours to cause infection in humans. People living in the eastern and southern plains regions of the United States are most at risk, especially during the spring and summer months. The incubation period ranges from 3 to 14 days.

Rocky Mountain spotted fever causes generalized fever, headache, and a rash that begins as blanchable macular rash observed first on the forearms, wrists, and ankles, and progresses to a papular rash. (See Figure 13-5; Color Insert 14.) This rash may also appear on the palms of the hands and soles of the feet, and spread to the arms, thighs, and trunk, but usually not the face. Lesions may coalesce and form ecchymoses or petechiae, and as the condition worsens nausea, vomiting, abdominal pain, hepatosplen-

FIGURE 13-5

▧

Rocky Mountain spotted fever rash: erythematous macules on wrists, hands, forearms, and legs. (See also Color Insert 14.)

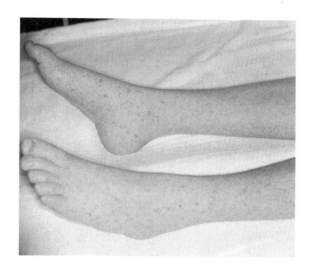

omegaly, lymphadenopathy, arthralgia, stupor, confusion, and coma can follow.

The organism seems to proliferate in the cells of capillaries, causing vascular necrosis, microinfarcts, and thrombosis of these vessels. The vasculitis may spread to small arteries and veins, and may progress to produce disseminated intravascular coagulopathy (DIC) and hypotension, which may be fatal.

It is important to treat infected persons with antibiotics, and it should be noted that mortality increases if treatment is delayed after the sixth day. Children older than 2 weeks are usually given chloramphenicol until they are afebrile for at least 2 to 3 days.

Recommended treatment for children older than 8 years is to give oral Vibramycin until the child is afebrile; the course is usually 6 to 10 days. Client education should include preventive measures such as clearing tall grass from play areas, making certain the child is wearing light-colored clothing so ticks can be easily seen, and tucking pants legs into socks. If any ticks are seen on the child, remove them with tweezers. Pull straight back with a slow, steady force. Disinfect skin before and after the tick is removed. Do not use nail polish, alcohol, or matches to remove ticks.

ROSEOLA

Roseola (Table 13-1) is an acute viral infection caused by the human herpesvirus 6 (HHV-6). Also known as exanthema subitum or sixth disease, roseola is an acute disease of young children between the ages of 6 months and 3 years, with 90% of the cases involving 2-year-olds. The mode of transmission is not known, but it is believed to be spread via respiratory secretions and it can be isolated from peripheral blood.

If children are infected early in life, symptoms often go unrecognized. Children with roseola are at risk for febrile convulsions, and are often anorexic, listless, and irritable, but do not appear seriously ill. The fever usually appears between 5 and 15 days after exposure to an infected individual. The fever can be as high as 105°F, without apparent cause, and remain elevated approximately 3 to 5 days. The fever is followed by a maculopapular, nonpruritic rash that blanches. Often the rash fades within hours. Rhinitis, cough, and conjunctivitis occur during prodrome, and Koplik's spots appear on the second to fourth day of the prodromal period.

The plan of care for children with roseola is to alleviate uncomfortable symptoms caused by the fever and soothe the itching with antipyretics and tepid baths, allowing the child's skin to air dry, which will facilitate heat loss. Educating parents on the importance of adequate hydration is vital. In addition, isolating other family members who have not been exposed before should be cautioned. Roseola is usually not recurring; therefore, permanent immunity occurs from the self-limiting exposure.

TABLE 13-1
COMMON SKIN LESIONS

Lesion	Description	Lesion	Description

A Macule

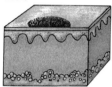

Lesion is small (less than 1 cm or 0.4 in), appearance is flat, is different from adherent skin. Example: freckle.

F Vesicle

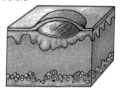

Lesion is small (less than 1 cm or 0.4 in), raised, fluid-filled mass. Example: herpes simplex, varicella.

B Papule

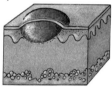

Lesion is small (less than 1 cm or 0.4 in), solid, raised mass. Example: small nevus.

G Bulla

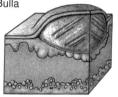

Lesion is raised fluid-filled mass; larger than a vesicle. Example: second-degree burn.

C Nodule

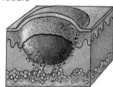

Lesion is solid, raised mass; slightly larger (1-2 cm or 0.4-0.8 in) and deeper than a papule.

H Pustule

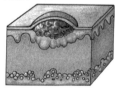

Lesion is vesicle containing purulent exudate. Example: acne, impetigo, staphylococcal infections.

D Tumor

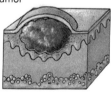

Lesion is solid, raised mass; larger than a nodule; may be hard or soft.

Secondary Lesions (arise from changes in primary lesions)

I Scale

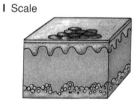

Thin flakes of exfoliated epidermis. Example: psoriasis, dandruff.

E Wheal

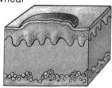

Lesion is irregularly shaped, transient area of skin edema. Example: allergic reaction.

J Crust

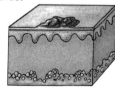

Dried residue of serum, blood, or purulent exudate. Example: eczema.

SCARLET FEVER

Scarlet fever infection is caused by *Streptococcus pyogenes*, one of the group A β-hemolytic streptococci (GAS). This streptococcal bacterium affects the skin and gastrointestinal tract from an erythrogenic toxin. Scarlet fever is a disease seen most often in children between the ages of 6 and 12 years, and can occur more than once in a single patient. A complication of this disease can be rheumatic fever.

Scarlet fever manifests symptoms of a sore throat, headache, vomiting, abdominal pain, and fever, followed by "beefy red" tonsils, white or red "strawberry tongue" (rough, erythematous, swollen tongue) (see Figure 13-6; Color Insert 15), and petechiae on the palate. The manifestations include a skin rash with an eruption of puncta, orange-red lesions with a texture like sandpaper, beginning on the chest and arms and spreading down to the abdomen, groin, and buttocks. (See Figure 13-7; Color Insert 16.) Desquamation follows about 1 week later. The face has circumoval cyanosis contrasting with the flushed coloring of the cheeks. Red streaks across the folds of the abdomen, axillae, and antecubital spaces are called Pastia lines (increased erythema in skin folds of the face).

Treatment is usually penicillin V or benzathine penicillin intramuscularly, single dose, and acetaminophen (Tylenol) for fever. Schoolchildren should stay out of school until they have been on antibiotics for at least 24 hours. Educate family members to avoid contact with infected persons.

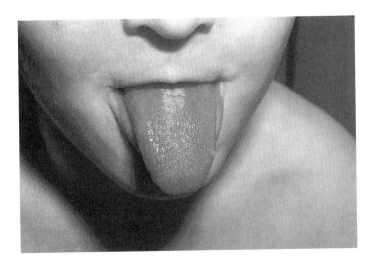

FIGURE 13-6

🔘

Strawberry tongue in scarlet fever. (See also Color Insert 15.)

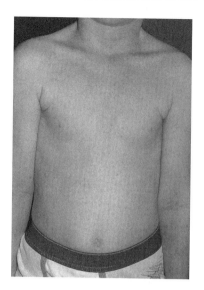

FIGURE 13-7

▨

Generalized exanthem in scarlet fever. (See also Color Insert 16.)

SEXUALLY TRANSMITTED DISEASES

Gonorrhea

Sexually transmitted disease (STD) is a catchphrase for a number of viral, parasitic, and bacterial diseases. The most common bacterial STD is gonorrhea, caused by *Neisseria gonorrhoeae*. This aerobic, non-spore-forming, gram-negative coccal (round) microorganism is usually found in pairs. It attaches to the epithelial surface during sexual intercourse (oral or anal sex). Transmission of the gonococcal (GC) infection can be by body fluids of an infected person, especially via vaginal fluids, semen, saliva, and secretions from the rectum. Newborns can acquire gonococcal infections if delivered vaginally from an infected mother, and the infection in newborns occurs in the infants' eyes.

The highest rate of gonococcal infections is in young men, followed by teenage males and females age 15 to 19. The incubation period is approximately 2 to 5 days in men and 5 to 10 days in women. Treatment for all STDs should include the treatment of all sexual partners of the infected person.

Gonorrhea often has no clinical symptoms, except for painful urination in men and boys, and a cloudy discharge from the penis in men or from the vagina in women. This discharge my be thick and may have a greenish-yellow color. In either sex, gonorrhea affects the rectum, causing pain, especially during bowel movements. In males, untreated gonorrhea can cause scars that form inside the urethra. The inner surface of the cervix is the most common site where the infection occurs in females. Damage occurs to the mucosa by an inflammatory process, and an exudate appears at the site of infection. Further complications occur with colonization of the bacterium in the Skene and Bartholin glands in the fallopian tubes, and in the ovaries, causing acute pelvic inflammatory disease (PID), which can potentially result in infertility.

Syphilis

Syphilis is caused by an anaerobic bacterium, *Treponema pallidum*. Under a microscope, these bacteria look like corkscrews with a tight, rotary motion. The average incubation period after exposure is 21 days. The most prevalent group affected is 15- to 34-year-olds. This microorganism is transmitted through microabrasions occurring during intercourse and can be transmitted from an infected mother to her fetus during the first trimester.

Syphilis has local and systemic effects and if untreated continues to develop in stages. During primary syphilis, 2 to 6 weeks after sexual contact with an infected person, a painless "chancre" appears, usually on the genitalia, mouth, or rectum. Because of the immune system's response, the lymph gland nearest to the chancre becomes enlarged. Without treatment, the chancre heals within 4 to 6 weeks.

Then, secondary syphilis begins, which is characterized by a rash, fever, headache, loss of appetite with resulting weight loss, sore throat, muscle aches, joint pain, and general "ill" feeling. Grey or white wartlike patches of skin called condylomata lata can appear on the moist areas around the anus and vagina.

It is during the third stage that the liver, kidneys, and eyes are affected. Meningitis may occur. Late or "latent" stage syphilis is asymptomatic in some infected persons, while others continue to develop more severe debilitating symptoms, including amnesia, loss of balance, difficulty walking, urinary incontinence, impotence, visual disturbances, and cardiac abnormalities.

In a person with syphilis for less than 1 year, the treatment is 1 dose of penicillin. Additional therapy is usually required if the patient has had the disease for longer than a year.

Chlamydia

Chlamydia is considered the most common STD reported to the Centers for Disease Control (CDC) in the United States. Chlamydia occurs most often in young adults (25 years old and younger) who have had multiple sexual partners, have a gonococcal infection, and are of low socioeconomic status. *Chlamydia trachomatis* is a gram-negative, intracellular bacterium that lacks the ability to reproduce independently. Like a virus, it needs a host cell. Chlamydia organisms are always pathogens and are not part of the normal flora found in the urogenital tract. *C. trachomatis* disrupts epithelial tissue but does not destroy deeper tissue or organs. This organism can also be passed to an infant from an infected mother.

Chlamydia can affect the eyes, respiratory tract, and urogenital area, depending on the age of the person and the mode of transmission. Asymptomatic chlamydia is common, but can affect the urethra, cervix, and Bartholin glands. Women may have vaginal redness and a discharge; men may experience a discharge from the urethra and dysuria. When chlamydia is passed from an infected mother, the baby can develop chlamydia conjunctivitis, which has a thick yellowish discharge from the eyes, which are red and swollen. Infected persons with *C. pneumoniae* have tachypnea and may have a cough and vomiting, and appear to have blue or grayish skin, but no fever.

Chlamydia and gonococcal infections are also treated with a 1-dose antibiotic, especially for adolescents, as compared to commonly used 7-day oral medications, to reduce noncompliance, and depending on the organism involved and any allergies the infected person may have. All exposed individuals should also be treated whenever possible. Washing the genitals, urinating, or douching after sex does not prevent STDs. Educate clients on the methods of prevention of sexually transmitted diseases, including the most basic one of using barrier contraception (condoms).

Toxoplasmosis

Toxoplasmosis is caused by the protozoan *Toxoplasma gondii*. The host for this disease is the domestic cat, bird, and other animals that can be regarded as opportunistic. The toxoplasmosis protozoan also can be found in soil contaminated by cat feces and in undercooked meat, particularly pork. Maternal-fetal transmission occurs during pregnancy by an infected mother. Symptoms of a congenitally infected infant include microcephaly, hydrocephalus, seizures, mental retardation, hepatosplenomegaly, jaundice, thrombocytopenia, pneumonitis, rash, fever, chorioretinitis, and cerebral calcifications. Chorioretinitis is a sequela of congenital infection with symptoms noted in the second or third decade of life.

Most of the human population infected are asymptomatic. Once exposed, antibodies form and toxoplasmosis does not cause the disease; however, if the immune system is compromised, the disease can invade the respiratory tract, retina of the eye, heart, pancreas, liver, colon, and testes. The most serious site is inflammation of the brain. Toxoplasmic encephalitis can cause hemiplegia, fever, seizures, confusion, personality changes, nausea, vomiting, and syncope.

Treatment is indicated for immunocompromised patients and pregnant patients, because of teratogenic effects on the fetus. Educate the family in the proper techniques of food preparation, including washing fruits and vegetables and cooking meat thoroughly. Pregnant women should take protective measures when cleaning litter boxes and gardening.

Varicella

Varicella is a herpesvirus called varicella-zoster. (See Figure 13-8; Color Insert 17.) The varicella is responsible for the chickenpox part of the

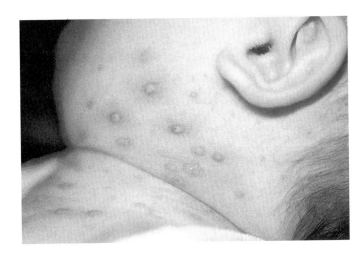

FIGURE 13-8

⊠

Varicella (chickenpox). (Courtesy of Lawrence B. Stack, MD.) (See also Color Insert 17.)

infection and the zoster component causes shingles. The shingles virus remains latent, but can be reactivated later in life. Ninety percent of varicella patients are younger than 10 years old and by 15 years old have already contracted varicella. The virus is transmitted by an infected person by direct contact from fresh drainage from open sores, droplets, and airborne transmission. The incubation period is 10 to 21 days. The period of communicability is 1 to 2 days prior to the eruption of the rash, and until the lesions have scabbed over and dried.

Varicella (chickenpox) is characterized by fever up to 102°F, malaise, and pruritic maculopapular skin eruptions that last for a few hours, then become vesicular. The vesicles break easily, creating open sores that eventually crust over. The lesions start on the scalp and travel to the trunk, which is the area of greatest concentration, then to the extremities. An existing irritation of diaper rash, poison ivy, eczema, or sunburn can yield pruritus. These lesions can also present on the buccal mucosa, palate, trachea, conjunctiva, vagina, and anus. Symptoms tend to appear 14 to 16 days after the initial exposure but can occur any time from 10 to 21 days after contact. Lesions progress in different stages in 1 area over a 6- to 8-hour period and then scab over in 2 to 4 days. There can be as many as 200 to 400 lesions during the outbreak.

The recommended treatment is to be supportive and alleviate discomfort as much as possible. Oral and/or topical medication administered for pruritis can be an advantage to prevent scratching, which will serve to decrease the exposure to other infections. Modifications to the course of the infection can be altered by the administration of varicella-zoster immune globulin (VZIG), if given within 96 hours of exposure. Education as to the mode of transmission should be communicated to all family members. It should further be stressed that indirect transmission from articles of clothing is also a problem.

The virus can resurface late in life as shingles (zoster). The chickenpox vaccine is recommended for children around 1 year of age; however, children who are immunocompromised should not be given the vaccine.

Summary

During childhood and adolescence a multitude of infections occur. Infants and children generally experience a whole gamut of these diseases. Many of them are normal immune responses to viruses, bacteria, parasites, and fungi, while others, although rare, can become devastating illnesses caused by primary infections. Children who are in general good health go on to recovery, but the ones who are not in good health have problems with their immunologic response and therefore succumb to more complicated illness. Except in the very young infant, a careful history and physical examination can reveal infections. In this chapter common infectious diseases in children were discussed. Understanding the pathophysiology of the conditions, including the differences among them, assists the nurse in identifying the appropriate nursing interventions for the child and his/her family.

Critical Points in the Care of the Child with an Infection

Infectious conditions are prevalent in children; there is not one child that escapes some kind of infection. Viruses are the number one cause of the infections, and in early childhood and in infancy the most prevalent are upper respiratory and gastrointestinal. Most of these infections are transient and are resolved quickly without having to hospitalize the child. The role of the nurse in the management of these conditions is to teach the parents how to take care of the conditions at home, and then to serve as a support system for the parents and the child. The nurse also plays an important part in the diagnosis and prevention of further complications. His/her skill is best used in performing a thorough assessment of the child and the family, and then preparing a plan of care based on the family's resources, stressing necessary parenting skills.

Along with the treatment of the disease, parents are confronted with the reality that with this kind of condition, the child will also have a high fever. Fever can be a devastating experience for first-time parents or young parents. A nurse's clear understanding of fever management as it relates to the child's illness will help alleviate parental anxiety and secure a prompt recovery for the child.

Although the management of the disease is most important, it is also critical that the nurse use prophylactic measures. Prophylaxis is aimed at enhancing the host's defense mechanisms, minimizing the damage that infections can cause and reducing the colonization by the organism, and suppressing potentially pathogenic organisms currently colonizing the patient. The most important preventive factor in organism colonization is good hand washing by everybody involved in the care of the ill child.

QUESTIONS

Diagnosis: Varicella (Chickenpox)

History: Annie is a 3-year-old with no significant past medical history. She developed a fever and blisters on her back, which have spread to her trunk and face. Annie attends day care. Her mom takes Annie to the clinic for an evaluation.

Plan: Evaluation to rule out chickenpox. Interventions.

Nursing problems: Compliance; prevention of complications; pruritis; explanation of disease process; communicability.

1. Annie is diagnosed with chickenpox. Her mother asks how she might have gotten the disease. What is the most appropriate reply?
   A. "Chickenpox is an expected childhood illness that everyone gets."
   B. "It is transmitted from direct contact, droplet spread, and contaminated objects."
   C. "It is inherited and transmitted through the genes."
   D. "It is possibly a side effect of recent immunizations."

2. The progression of the lesions is best described as:
   A. macule, papule, vesicle, crust
   B. crust, macule, papule, vesicle
   C. vesicle, papule, crust, macule
   D. papule, vesicle, macule, crust

3. Annie's mom is concerned when she learns that chickenpox is contagious. The nurse informs her that the child could pass on the disease 1–6 days before the eruption of lesions to 6 days after the first crop of vesicles when crusts have formed. When is Annie not contagious?
   A. When the vesicles are still visible.
   B. When all the vesicles have crusted.
   C. When the trunk vesicles have crusted but not those on the face.
   D. When there are still waterlike blisters on all Annie's extremities.

4. For the fever and itching, the nurse advises the mother to administer which of the following?
   A. Dimetapp
   B. Aveeno baths with sponging
   C. Aspirin and sponge baths
   D. Acetaminophen, Benadryl, and oatmeal baths

5. Exposure to chickenpox would pose the greatest danger in which of the following disease states?

   A. Pneumonia
   B. Asthma
   C. HIV
   D. Emphysema

Diagnosis: Scarlet Fever

History: Melanie is a 5-year-old who is taken to the clinic for her immunizations and physical examination. Her mom also decided to take her at this time because Melanie has been experiencing high fever and sore throat for 3 days now. She has no medications and no significant history. She is not vomiting but has decreased appetite.

Plan: Assessment; confirm diagnosis; intervention.

Nursing problems: Complications; compliance; supportive measures; communicability.

1. During the physical examination, which of the following findings is expected in a patient with scarlet fever?

   A. Red strawberry tongue, enlarged tonsils with white patches
   B. Maculopapular rash that begins on the head and spreads downward
   C. Vesicular rash that appears in crops
   D. Petechial rash that begins on the wrists and ankles

2. A throat culture is obtained. To confirm the diagnosis of scarlet fever, which organism is found in the culture?

   A. Varicella-zoster
   B. Group A β-hemolytic streptococci
   C. *H. influenzae*
   D. RSV

3. Penicillin (Bicillin G, IM or po) is the usual treatment of choice, but Melanie is allergic to penicillin. Which of the following drugs may be used?

   A. Amoxicillin
   B. Rocephin
   C. Ceftin
   D. Erythromycin

4. Which of the following instructions to the mother, made by the nurse, is the most appropriate to relieve Melanie's sore throat?

   A. Do nothing; it will go away by itself.
   B. Give lozenges and chloraseptic sprays.
   C. Give Robitussin and Listerine.
   D. Give ice cream and cold drinks.

5. Melanie has brothers and sisters at home. Her mom asks how to protect them from scarlet fever. The nurse's response is based on the understanding that scarlet fever is:

A. Not contagious
B. Transmitted by the fecal-oral route
C. Transmitted by direct contact or droplet spread
D. Transmitted through the genes

ANSWERS

Varicella (Chickenpox)

1. *B.* Chickenpox is transmitted from direct contact, droplet spread, and contaminated objects.

2. *A.* The lesions progress from macule to papule to vesicle and then to crust.

3. *B.* The child is not contagious when *all* vesicles have erupted and crusted.

4. *D.* Dimetapp is for coughing; Aveeno baths with sponging would irritate the vesicles and spread them; aspirin is controversial.

5. *C.* HIV patients are immunocompromised.

Scarlet Fever

1. *A.* The presenting signs of scarlett fever are red strawberry tongue and enlarged tonsils with white patches.

2. *B.* Scarlet fever is caused by group A β-hemolytic streptococci.

3. *D.* Erythromycin; all the others are penicillin-based.

4. *B.* To relieve throat discomfort, lozenges are the most appropriate.

5. *C.* Scarlet fever is transmitted through direct contact with an infected person, or droplet spread, and is contagious.

GLOSSARY

antigen   a protein marker on the surface of cells that identifies the cell as "self" or non-"self."

communicable   a transferable infection from a person to a person or from a person to an animal or vice versa.

contagious   a communicable transmittable infection.

defense mechanism   mechanism used to offer resistance or protection as means of self-defense.

disease-immune response   resistance to immunization.

hemolytic   the breakdown of red blood cells.

immunity   defense or protection from a disease, especially an infectious disease. Usually induced by having been exposed to the antigenic maker on an organism that invades the body.

immunodeficiency   decreased or compromised ability to respond to antigenic immunity reaction.

immunoglobulin   a preparation used intravenously in patients with immunodeficiency syndromes and in immunosuppressed recipients of bone marrow transplants.

incubation period   interval between exposure to infection and the appearance of the first symptom of the disease.

infection   the spread of a disease.

inhibitors   chemical substances that stop enzyme activity.

lesions   a circumscribed area of pathologically altered tissue.

opportunistic infections   an infection that is developed due to favorable conditions for the microorganism.

phagocytosis   a process of engulfment and destruction of microorganisms.

proliferation   ability to reproduce and invade a medium rapidly and repeatedly grow new parts, as by cell division.

prophylaxis   observance of rules necessary to prevent disease.

pruritus   severe itching; may be a symptom of a disease process, such as an allergic reaction.

rash   a reaction manifested in the skin to an allergen.

systemic infections   diseases that are present in body systems.

transmission   condition in which the organism that transmits the causative agent of a disease plays an essential role in the life of a parasite.

viral infections   infection caused by a virus.

virus   a minute organism that is entirely dependent on nutrients inside cells for its metabolic and reproductive needs.

𝓑IBLIOGRAPHY

AMERICAN ACADEMY OF PEDIATRICS, COMMITTEE ON PEDIATRIC AIDS. Evaluation and medical treatment of the HIV-exposed infant. *Pediatrics* 99(6):909–917, 1997.

AMERICAN HEALTH CONSULTANTS. PHS draft guidelines recommend triple drugs as initial therapy. *AIDS Alert* 12(5):49–60, 1997.

BARTLETT, J. G. *Pocket Book of Infectious Disease Therapy.* 7th ed. Philadelphia: Williams & Wilkins, 1996.

BOYTON, R. W., DUNN, E. S., AND STEPHENS, G. R. *Manual of Ambulatory Pediatrics.* 3rd ed. Philadelphia: Lippincott, 1994.

BURNS, C. E., BARBER, N., BRADY, M. A., AND DUNN, A. M. *Pediatric Primary Care: A Handbook for Nurse Practitioners.* Philadelphia: Saunders, 1996.

BUTEL, J., JAWETZ, E., MELNICK, J., ADELBERG, E., BROOKS, G., AND ORNSTON, L. *Medical Microbiology.* 18th ed. Norwalk, CT: Appleton & Lang, 1989.

CENTERS FOR DISEASE CONTROL AND PREVENTION. Technical guidance on HIV counseling. *Morbidity and Mortality Weekly Report* 42(RR–2): January 15, 1–10, 1993.

CENTERS FOR DISEASE CONTROL AND PREVENTION. Division of STD Prevention. Chlamydia Facts [on-line]: http://www.CDC.gov/hchstp/dstd/fact_sheets_ home.htm.

CENTERS FOR DISEASE CONTROL AND PREVENTION. Division of STD Prevention. Syphilis Facts [on-line]: http://www.CDC.gov/nchstp/dstd/syphilis_facts.htm.

CHAMBERS, H. F., AND SCHECTER, G. F. Mycobacterium tuberculosis infection. *The AIDS Knowledge Base* [on-line]: http://hivinsite.ucsf.edu/akb/1997/06tb. 1997.

EL-SADR, W., OLESKE, J. M., AND AGINS, B. D. *Managing Early HIV Infection: Quick Reference Guide for Clinicians.* Rockville, MD: U.S. Department of Health & Human Services, 1994.

HANSON, C., AND SHEARER, W. Pediatric HIV infection and AIDS. In R. D. Feigin and J. D. Cherry (eds.), *Textbook of Pediatric Infectious Disease.* 3rd ed. Philadelphia: Saunders, 1992, pp. 990–1008.

HARTY-GOLDER, C. *HIV/AIDS Primer: Science, Law, and Policy.* Sarasota, FL: Bert Rodgers School of Continuing Education, 1997.

JACOBSON, M. Mycobacterium avium complex. *The AIDS Knowledge Base* [on-line]: http://hivinsite.ucsf.edu/akb/1997/06mac/index.html. 1997.

KLAUS, B. D., AND GRODESKY, M. J. HIV and HAART in 1997. *The Nurse Practitioner* August: 139–143, 1997.

LEE, B., AND TAUBER, M. Cryptococcosis. *The AIDS Knowledge Base* [on-line]: http://hivinsite.ucsf.edu/akb/1994/6-8/index.html. 1994.

MARLOW, D. R., AND REDDING, B. A. *Textbook of Pediatric Nursing.* 6th ed. Philadelphia: Saunders, 1988.

MAWSON, A. R., WARRIER, R. P., KUVIBIDILA, S., AND SUSKIND, R. Pediatric AIDS and nutrition. In R. M. Suskind and L. Lewinter-Suskind (eds.), *Textbook of Pediatric Nutrition.* New York: Raven, 1993, pp. 447–453.

MCCANE, K. L., AND HUETHER, S. E. *Pathophysiology: The Biologic Basis for Disease in Adults and Children.* 2nd ed. St. Louis: Mosby-Year Book, 1994.

MEDICINENET INC. Diseases and Treatments: Influenza [on-line]: http://www.medicinenet.com/art.asp?li=mni&ag=y&artilekey=365. 1995–1997.

MEDICINENET INC. Diseases and Treatments: Chicken Pox [on-line]: http://www.medicinenet.com/art.asp?li=mni&ag=y&artilekey=319. 1995–1997.

MEDICINENET INC. Diseases and Treatments: Measles (Rubeola) [on-line]: http://www.medicinenet.com/art.asp?li=mni&ag=y&artilekey=6242. 1995–1997.

MOYLE, G. *A Guide to the Medical Treatment of HIV-Related Diseases.* London: Avert, 1997.

NATIONAL INSTITUTE OF ALLERGY AND INFECTIOUS DISEASES. Pneumocystis carinii pneumonia. *Fact Sheet* [on-line]: http://www.niaid.nih.gov/factsheets/pcp.htm. 1994.

NATIONAL INSTITUTE OF ALLERGY AND INFECTIOUS DISEASES. Infectious Mononucleosis. *Fact Sheet* [on-line]: http://www.niaid.nih.gov/factsheets/info/infmono.htm. 1997.

NATIONAL INSTITUTE OF ALLERGY AND INFECTIOUS DISEASES. Microbiology and Infectious Diseases: Sexually Transmitted Diseases. *Fact Sheet* [online]: http://www.niaid.nih.gov/facts/mwhhp2.htm. 1997.

NATIONAL INSTITUTE OF ALLERGY AND INFECTIOUS DISEASES. Toxoplasmosis. *Fact Sheet* [on-line]: http://www.niaid.nih.gov/factsheets/tox.htm. 1994.

NORMAN, J. *HIV/AIDS: The Florida Requirement.* Sacramento, CA: CME Resource, 1997.

PIZZO, P. A., AND WILFERT, C. M. Markers and determinants of disease progression in children with HIV infection. *Journal of Acquired Immune Deficiency and Human Retrovirology* 8(1):30–40, 1995.

Publication Manual of the American Psychological Association. 4th ed. Washington, DC: American Psychological Association, 1995.

SHANK, S. *HIV/AIDS in the '90s.* Roseville, CA: National Center of Continuing Education, 1997.

UPHOLD, C. R., AND GRAHAM, M. V. *Clinical Guidelines in Family Practice.* Gainesville, FL: Barmarrae Books, 1994.

WOOD, G. E. Antiretroviral therapy in infants and children with HIV. *Pediatric Nursing* 21(3):291–296, 1995.

$\mathcal{H}$ELPFUL INTERNET SITES

PEDINFO: An Index of the Pediatric Internet at http://www.pedinfo.org   This is an excellent site that covers nearly all topics within this review. It has a wealth of information and is worth a visit. It is written for health care professionals but others could also use the information.

National Center for Infectious Disease at http://www.cdc.gov/ncidod/ncid.htm   An excellent site that has a host of materials and links that are highly useful for those interested in infectious disease issues and research.

Centers for Disease Control (CDC) site at http://www.cdc.gov   A great resource site that has a vast amount of information concerning issues and research on disease control and prevention.

HIVdent Pediatric Health Care at http://www.hivdent.org/pediatrics/pediatric.htm   This site has some excellent links to information concerning pediatric HIV as well as other pediatric health care issues and includes an excellent link to current news updates about pediatric health care concerns. Updates are from multiple sources and include updated treatments. This site is aimed at health care professionals rather than the lay public.

Centers for Disease Control (CDC) site concerning Immunization at http://www.cdc.gov/nip   A good starting point to find information on this national program.

Guidelines for Treatment of Sexually Transmitted Disease at http://www. cdc.gov/nchstp/dstd/STD98TG.HTM   This site has guidelines for treatment of sexually transmitted diseases, which includes teenagers.

Virtual Naval Hospital Information for Providers at http://www.vnh. org/Providers.html   This site is part of the University of Iowa's health care site and is linked to a large set of databases that can be used by health care providers. The site covers a larger number of links to other sources on health care issues and problems. This is an excellent starting place to discover information on various common diseases and their treatments.

CRITICAL POINTS IN THE HUMAN IMMUNE SYSTEM

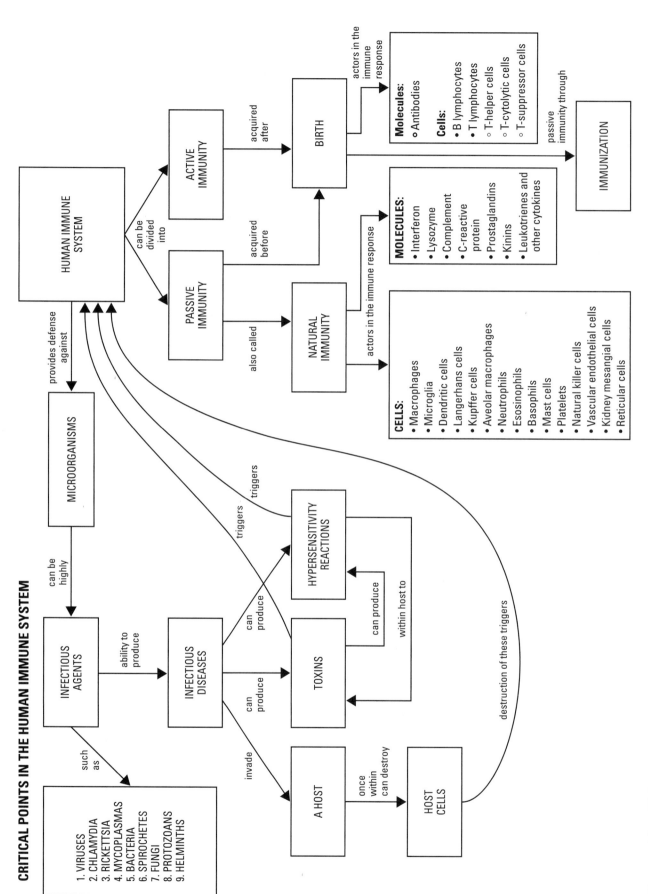

Concept Map 13-1

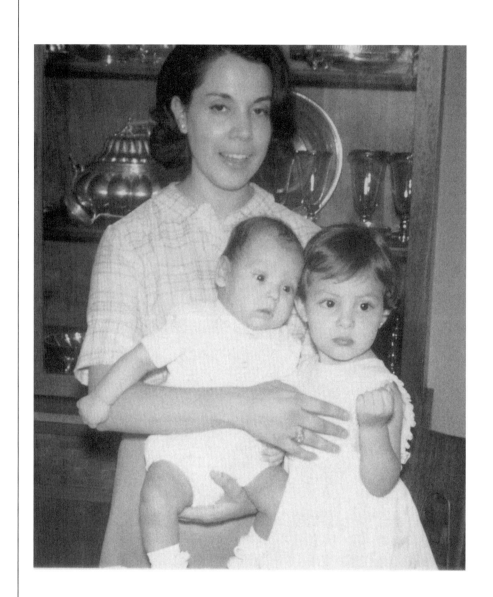

C H A P T E R   1 4

☙

𝒟ERMATOLOGICAL DISORDERS

𝒥NTRODUCTION

The skin is the largest and most important organ in the body. It has multiple functions. The condition of the skin affects us physically as well as emotionally and psychologically. Skin provides a protective layer against injury and physical harm to the inner organs of the body, and homeostasis is conserved through the skin, as is thermoregulation. Skin development is constant throughout the entire life of an individual, beginning in the embryonic period and continuing until death.

The skin is composed of 3 major layers: the epidermis, the dermis, and the subcutaneous tissue layer. The **epidermis** or outer layer, which is responsible for much of the protection and strength of the skin, has 5 layers itself. Melanin, produced in the basal layer of the 5 layers, contributes to skin color. The second major layer of skin, called the dermis, contributes strength, support, and elasticity to the skin. The dermis is primarily composed of fibrous connective tissue, with some elastic fibers and a mucopolysaccharide gel. Also in this layer are inflammatory cells, blood and lymph vessels, and cutaneous nerves. Underneath the dermis is the third layer, the subcutaneous tissue, composed of adipose tissue or fat, which insulates or serves as a cushion for trauma and is a source of energy and hormone metabolism.

Skin appendages, which include the hair, sweat glands, **sebaceous glands,** and nails, are also present in the skin. The hair follicles are found all over the body except for the palms of the hands and feet, knuckles, distal and interdigital spaces, lips, prepuce of the penis, and areola of the nipples.

Epidermis. Outermost portion of the skin, consisting of 2 layers: stratum corneum and cellular stratum.

Sebaceous glands. Small sacculated organs in the dermis that secrete sebum.

Disruptions of the skin are demonstrated by a variety of disorders that are usually caused by infections (bacteria, fungal, and viral), allergic reactions, infestations, vascular reactions, congenital disorders, and hair and nail disorders. When the skin is being attacked, it is the outermost layer, the epidermis, that provides the first line of defense against any kind of injury. Although the epidermis and dermis provide protection against injury to the inside of the body, they also prevent microorganisms from invading the body. The subcutaneous tissue provides insulation and cushioning.

CONTACT DERMATITIS

Contact dermatitis is acute or chronic inflammation of the skin due to contact with an irritant or allergen. There are 2 types of contact dermatitis: irritant contact dermatitis and allergic contact dermatitis. Irritant contact dermatitis is an eczematous response, where there is damage to the epidermis caused by irritants such as chemicals, dry cold weather, or friction. A rash develops within a few hours of exposure and reaches its peak of severity in 24 hours.

Allergic Contact Dermatitis

Allergic contact dermatitis is also called delayed-type dermatitis. The T lymphocyte-mediated hypersensitivity occurs in 2 phases: (1) the sensitization phase, and (2) the elicitation phase. The sensitization phase occurs when the allergen penetrates the epidermis and produces a proliferation of the T lymphocytes. The elicitation phase occurs when the antigen-specific T lymphocytes within the skin combine with the subsequent exposure to the allergen to produce inflammation. This has a delayed onset of 18 hours, peaks at 48 hours, and can last 2 to 3 weeks, even if exposure to the offending allergen is discontinued.

Erythema. Redness or inflammation of the skin or mucous membrane.

Fissures. Linear cracks or breaks from the epidermis to the dermis.

Blister. A vesicle or bulla.

The symptoms inherent in irritant contact dermatitis vary with the intensity of inflammation, which in turn depends on the concentration of the irritant and the exposure time to it. If the irritant is mild, the child presents with **erythema**, dryness, and **fissuring** of the skin. If there is a chronic exposure, the child presents with **blisters** and oozing, weeping lesions. Blisters often are linear in the acute onset with their distribution often providing clues for diagnosis. This type of allergic contact dermatitis is seen in children who have come in contact with poison ivy, poison sumac, and poison oak.

The nurse must obtain a family history of allergies, confirm if any treatment has been tried prior to coming to the office, and what effect, if any, it had on the dermatitis. It is important to inquire about exposure to chemicals, poison plants, or new soaps, perfumes, or detergents. A determination of the first location of the eruption, the time and rate of the onset, and any associated symptoms should be made after questioning both the parents and the child. With the above information gathered, the nurse must determine the primary lesion during the physical examination. Diagnostic tests used include the skin allergy patch test and potassium hydroxide (KOH) preparation to rule out fungus.

Treatment is determined according to the cause of the dermatitis and is based on the time of the exposure to the allergen. Parents should be instructed to wash the exposed area as soon as possible with cold water and soap (preferably 15 minutes after exposure). The nurse should instruct the parent to bathe the child with allergic contact dermatitis from exposure to poison ivy, poison oak, or poison sumac in an oatmeal bath in order to reduce inflammation. (Make sure that the child is not allergic to oats.) After the bath, apply a drying lotion such as calamine lotion. The child should be given medications for pruritus (hydroxyzine 0.5 mg/kg/dose tid as needed). After the blistering stage, apply 2.5% hydrocortisone cream tid for 1 to 3 weeks. For severe cases, prednisone 1 to 2 mg/kg/day orally for 14 to 21 days can be used.

Parents and children should be educated as to how to recognize the plant that has caused the dermatitis. Children with this condition do not need follow-up, unless the case is severe.

Atopic Dermatitis

Atopic dermatitis, also called infantile eczema (see Figure 14-1; Color Insert 18), is a hereditary disorder characterized by intensive **pruritic**, often **excoriated, maculopapular** inflammation. Seventy to 80% of children with atopic dermatitis have a personal or family history of asthma or allergic rhinitis; of these children 80% have an increased serum IgE level and positive immediate skin tests.

Pruritic. Itching.

Excoriated. Linear or hollowed-out crusted epidermis, leaving dermis exposed.

Maculopapular. Combination of macular and papular lesions.

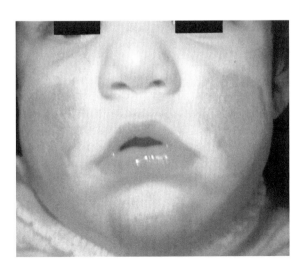

FIGURE 14-1

❧

Atopic dermatitis in infancy. (See also Color Insert 18.)

Papular. Solid, elevated area less than 1 cm in diameter; top may be pointed, rounded, or flat.

Lichenification. Rough, thickened epidermis causing accentuated skin markings.

Eighty-five percent of cases occur within the first 5 years of life, but most parents bring the child to the clinic or doctor's office between 3 and 6 months of age. The child presents with lesions that vary from erythematous and **papular** to scaling; in chronic cases the child presents with vesicular and oozing **lichenification** lesions. The child who has severe pruritus has a chronic course and frequent exacerbations. The rash appears primarily on the face, scalp, trunk, and extensor surfaces of arms and legs. Epidermal cracks allow water out of the skin, and irritation leads to further drying and cracking and increases the urge to rub and scratch. Eczema has an itch-rash-itch cycle. The itching is what provokes the rash.

The diagnosis is based on the personal and family history of allergic rhinitis, asthma, and atopic dermatitis. It is also important to determine the age of the onset of itching and the appearance of the lesions at that time. The nurse should also inquire about bathing practices and the brand of skin care products the family uses. During the physical exam the nurse must examine the skin thoroughly over the entire body, always looking for erythema, scaling, and lichenification. There are no specific laboratory tests that help with the diagnosis of this condition. IgE antibodies are not clinically relevant.

The treatment for this condition is basically to teach the family about care and prevention. Parents are advised to control exacerbating factors that promote dryness or increase the child's need to scratch. The child's environment should be cool; he/she should not use high-fat-content soaps such as Dove; and he/she should not wear wool or synthetic clothing. The best fabric for the child's clothing is 100% cotton. Foods known to exacerbate the eczema should be avoided. The child should be bathed at least once a day with nonirritating soap and should be rinsed thoroughly. Excessively dry areas should be coated with cream such as Euricin or emollients such as Aquaphor. Parents should also be told to lubricate the skin more during the winter months and to maintain humidity in the home environment.

If the child presents with inflammation, topical corticosteroids—hydrocortisone cream 2.5% (1% on face)—can be applied thinly, bid, until controlled (up to 14 days). The parents should be instructed to apply lubricant to the inflamed area tid along with topical corticosteroid. Once the inflammation has subsided, they need only continue with the lubricant.

The main emphasis for the medical team is to teach parents to use medication cautiously for pruritus, and to return to the office with the child for follow-up in 1 week.

Seborrheic Dermatitis

Seborrheic dermatitis is a common chronic, recurrent inflammation of the skin with characteristic patterns for each different age group. The cause is unknown. Inflammation occurs in areas with large numbers of sebaceous glands; however, there is no proof it occurs secondary to increased sebum production. The child usually has scalp lesions ("cradle cap") that are scaling, adherent, thick, yellow, and crusted over an erythematous base that can spread over the ears and down near the neck. This condition commonly involves the scalp, eyebrows, eyelids, ear canals, nasolabial folds, axillae, chest, and back. It occurs predominantly in the newborn and at puberty, ages at which there is an increase stimulation of sebum production. In adolescents, it can escalate hair loss.

The diagnosis is based on the history of the onset, duration, and location of the lesions. The nurse usually asks the parents what kind of treatment was tried before coming to the office. The management of the disorder is tailored according to the age of the child. For cradle cap the parents are instructed to rub petroleum jelly or mineral oil on the scalp for 20 to 30 minutes prior to using shampoo; this softens the crusts. The baby ought to have his/her head shampooed with baby shampoo daily, with a soft brush, to remove the sebum. For toddlers and adolescents, parents must use an antiseborrheic shampoo such as Selsun Blue or Sebulex every other day. The child should be brought to the clinic or doctor's office after 1 week for a follow-up visit. If the child has inflammatory or extensive lesions, the parents should be given a corticosteroid lotion (Valisone lotion) to be used daily. For lesions on areas other than the scalp, 1% hydrocortisone cream should be used 2 to 3 times a day, continuing the treatment for several days after the lesions disappear. Parents should be instructed to return the child to the clinic if the condition does not improve in 1 week.

Diaper Dermatitis

Diaper dermatitis, the most common contact dermatitis seen in pediatrics (see Figure 14-2; Color Insert 19), is an inflammatory disorder of the skin due to breakdown of the skin. The factors that contribute to this condition include a chemical irritation caused by urine, feces, diapers, and/or rubber pants. The introduction of a new lotion can cause diaper dermatitis, or the inflammation may be caused by a medication the baby is taking, such as antibiotics. But the most common cause of this condition is poor hygiene, and it usually starts after the first month of life.

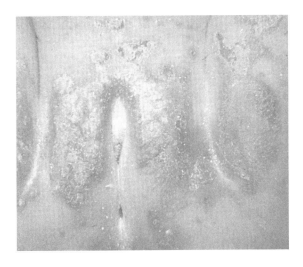

FIGURE 14-2

◙

Diaper dermatitis. (See also Color Insert 19.)

Management of diaper dermatitis includes frequently changing soiled diapers and practicing appropriate hygiene. If the condition is acute, the nurse should teach the parents to give the child warm sitz baths at least 3 times a day; use Burrow's solution soaks or compresses 4 times a day if the skin is weepy; expose the irritated area to air; apply hydrocortisone 0.5% or 1% 3 times a day for no more than 3 days, especially if the skin is dry; and force fluids to the child so that the urine will not be concentrated. The child should be seen for a follow-up so that secondary bacterial infections do not occur.

Sunburn

Sunburn is an injury to the skin caused by overexposure to the ultraviolet rays of the sun. It is connected with the development of skin cancer. Overexposure of the skin to the sun causes a change in the blood flow of the skin. Primary damage to the skin results in erythema, pigmentary and texture changes, and potential carcinogenesis (Coody, 1987).

Light-skinned children are more sensitive than dark-skinned children to sunburn because of the latter's increased amount of melanin. Children should not be allowed to stay outdoors without a hat, especially between 11 A.M. and 3 P.M.

Parents should be instructed that the incidence of skin cancer is increasing in children and adolescents, and 90% of it is attributed to excessive sun exposure in childhood.

Warts

Warts are a common skin condition during childhood. They are more a cosmetic problem than a health problem. Warts occur in about 10% of children. Warts are produced by a virus that creates one or more skin-colored, raised or flat, irregular nodules. Most warts resolve spontaneously between 12 and 24 months. Warts are transmitted by skin contact. Parents should be instructed that warts disappear over time. The decision to treat should be based on the location and discomfort; there is no treatment that brings resolution. The treatments available include liquid nitrogen, which is applied to an area 1 to 3 mm beyond the wart for 20 to 30 seconds. Salicylic acid paints with concentration higher than 20% applied once or twice a day for 2 to 4 weeks are also used. Also, warts can be removed surgically by snipping with scissors (not a scalpel).

$\mathcal{P}$ITYRIASIS ALBA

Stratum corneum. The horny, outermost layer of the skin, composed of dead cells converted to keratin. Continually flakes away.

Pityriasis alba, also called common idiopathic dermatosis, is the thickening in the **stratum corneum** leading to edema. The thickening stratum corneum reduces the penetration of ultraviolet light; therefore, the pigment transfer from **melanocytes** to **keratinocytes** is interrupted by the edema. The lesions are exaggerated by suntanning. This condition occurs primarily in children and adolescents.

The skin exhibits round or oval, scaly, macular areas of hypopigmentation with distinct borders, usually seen on the cheeks. Other areas that may be affected are the extensor surfaces of the upper arms and the upper portions of the trunk. If left untreated, the lesions can become pruritic.

The size of the lesions varies from 5 to 20 mm in diameter and commonly the child exhibits 10 to 20 lesions. The diagnosis is done by KOH exam to exclude tinea versicolor. The treatment is the use of a topical steroid cream—triamcinolone acetonide, 0.025% (Aristocort)—twice a day for 14 days. After the treatment a moisturizer (Moisturel) should be used at bedtime to control the scaling. The child should be seen after the treatment in order to evaluate its efficiency.

Melanocyte. A body cell capable of producing melanin.

Keratinocytes. Epidermal cells that synthesize keratin and other proteins and sterols.

CAFÉ-AU-LAIT SPOTS

Café-au-lait spots (see Figure 14-3; Color Insert 20) are a light brown (dark brown on dark skin), oval macule of patches that can be found anywhere on the body. The condition is caused by an increased amount of melanin in the melanocytes of the base cell layer; it occurs for unknown reasons. This condition is normally benign but if several café-au-lait spots more than 1.5 cm in their longest diameter develop simultaneously, it may be an indication of neurofibromatosis, an autosomal dominant disease. This condition is found in approximately 10% of white and 22% of black children, and may be present at birth. The lesions persist throughout life and may increase in number and size with age.

The diagnosis is based on family history of neurofibromatosis, including onset and duration, as well as any change in number and/or size of the lesions. There is no specific test for this condition. The most important

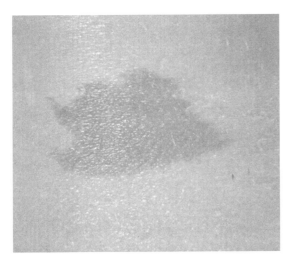

FIGURE 14-3

▣

Café-au-lait spot. (See also Color Insert 20.)

nursing intervention is to instruct the parent to bring the child to the clinic if there is a change in the number or size of the lesions. Also, the parents should be told the importance of keeping appointments for yearly health maintenance examinations, so that the lesions can be evaluated. While doing the physical examination the nurse must carefully count, measure, and evaluate the lesions and diagram their location on a chart. If there are any larger than 5 mm, neurofibromatosis should be considered as a possibility.

$\mathcal{V}$ITILIGO

Macules. Circumference less than 1 cm in diameter; lesions with color change in flat skin.

Vitiligo is a result of a lack of pigmentation in the skin, causing white areas. Vitiligo commonly occurs with autoimmune disease. This condition can be present at birth or it can occur in conjunction with a disease or following trauma. The exact cause is unknown. Usually milk-white **macules** and papules with scalloped borders are observed on the face and trunk. There is no specific test nor treatment for this condition. Broad-spectrum sunscreens are used in order to decrease the tanning effect on normal skin. Mild to moderate steroids are successful on one-half of patients.

$\mathcal{S}$CABIES

Ectoparasitic. Organisms that live outside the body of the host.

Scabies (see Figure 14-4; Color Insert 21) is a highly contagious dermatosis caused by *Sarcoptes scabiei*, an **ectoparasitic** mite. A fertilized female mite excavates a burrow into the stratum corneum in which to deposit eggs and fecal pellets. The larvae hatch and reach maturity in about 14

FIGURE 14-4

▨

Scabies, with its linear lesions and tiny black dots representing the mite, eggs, and/or fecal material in the small vesicle. (See also Color Insert 21.)

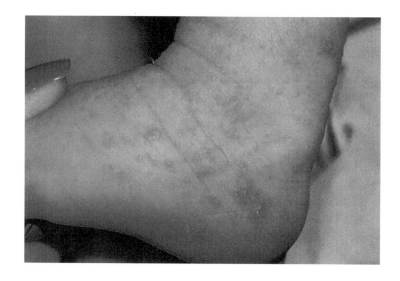

days, mate, and repeat the cycle. A hypersensitivity reaction to the ova and feces of the mite occurs about 1 month after initial infestation, which is the reason a child develops a rash and intense pruritus. The primary infestations are noted approximately 4 to 6 weeks after infestation, while reinfestation symptoms are noted within 24 hours. The child exhibits a symmetric distribution of lesions, dozens to hundreds of pruritic **vesicles, pustules,** and linear burrows that may end in a vesicle or papule. The entire skin is susceptible, but the most predominant areas are the fingers, flexor surfaces of wrists, and antecubital fossae. The biggest problem for the parents and for the children is that pruritis is more intense at night. In small children this may mean waking up or irritability at night.

In doing the assessment or the physical exam, the nurse should inquire about the onset, duration, and distribution of lesions, when the pruritis is most intense, and if any other member of the family is having the same symptoms. It is also important to find out what kind of treatment has been used, if any. While doing the exam, the nurse should have good lighting.

The diagnosis is confirmed by microscopic examination of the mite, eggs, and feces from skin scrapings done using a sterile surgical blade. Scrapings from interdigital areas are usually the most effective. Impetigo can be present as a secondary infection and often obscures the lesions of the scabies.

While instituting the treatment for the child, the family needs to treat the whole household simultaneously, because this condition is highly contagious. The child and the whole family should bathe and dry their skin before the scabicides are applied. The cream used in the treatment of scabies is a 5% permethrin called Elimite. It should be applied lightly and evenly over the entire body. Care should be taken to avoid getting the cream in the child's eyes. It should remain on the skin for 8 to 14 hours, and then be removed with a warm bath. Elimite is not recommended for the treatment of children under 2 years of age, and should not be used by a pregnant mother: substitute 10% Crotamiton. Crotamiton should be applied over the entire body of the child from the neck down, for 2 nights, and should be washed off thoroughly 24 hours after the second application. If the child complains of excessive pruritis, topical corticosteroids may be used after the treatment for a short period of time.

The most important nursing intervention for this condition is to educate the caregiver on the importance of laundering clothing and bedding in hot water and using the dryer's hottest setting. Clothing or items that cannot be laundered should be placed in a plastic bag and stored for at least 1 week. These parasites are unable to live off the skin for longer than 3 to 4 days. Children can return to school after the treatment has been completed. Follow-up should be done in 7 to 10 days if the child is symptom free. However, if the child complains of the same symptoms or develops a secondary infection, he/she should be brought back to the clinic immediately. In treating scabies-infected children, the nurse should remember that the parents and child may feel embarrassed about having this condition; so the nurse should let them know that this condition affects all socioeconomic groups and all ages. There should be a prophylactic treatment for all family members, and all should be treated at the same time in order to avoid reinfection.

Vesicle. Lesion less than 1 cm in diameter; elevated, circumscribed, superficial, and filled with serous fluid.

Pustules. Elevated, superficial, and purulent filled lesions.

𝒫EDICULOSIS

Pediculosis (lice) is infestation with one of the three species of lice that infest humans: *Pediculus humanus* var. *capitis* (head lice), *P. humanus* var. *corporis* (body lice), and *P. pubis* (pubic or crab lice). The female lice deposit 3 to 10 eggs daily on their human host. They can lay approximately 150 to 300 eggs in a month. The ova are attached to hair or fibers of clothing until they hatch. Once hatched it takes lice another 2 weeks to mature. Larvae will die unless they feed within 24 hours of hatching and then again in a few days. The lice feed on human blood and deposit their fecal matter on the skin, which causes intense pruritis. Transmission of head lice is the result of sharing combs or using an object that has come in contact with the infested person. Using the same clothing commonly transmits body lice, while pubic lice are transmitted by sexual contact. If a child has pubic lice, it is an indicator of sexual abuse, and appropriate documentation should be made.

Head lice (see Figure 14-5; Color Insert 22) are most commonly seen in children; African Americans are less likely to become infested. Nits (eggs) are most commonly seen in the hair at the back of the neck and around the ears. Excoriation from scratching and cervical adenopathy are often present. Body lice (see Figure 14-6; Color Insert 23) are not commonly seen in children. Pubic lice (see Figure 14-7; Color Insert 24) are seen on the pubic hair, and can also be seen on the chest, abdomen, and thighs. The pubic area may be excoriated and small bluish macules may be present. The diagnosis is based on observation of the nits. The nurse should identify when and where the child became infested, because it is not uncommon to have an outbreak at school. The physical exam can be aided with the use of Wood's lamp, which makes it easier to identify the nit on the hair shaft.

FIGURE 14-5

◪

Pediculus capitis. (See also Color Insert 22.)

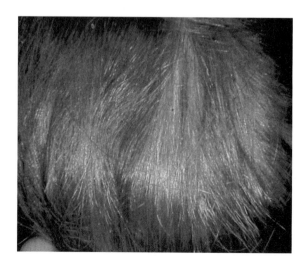

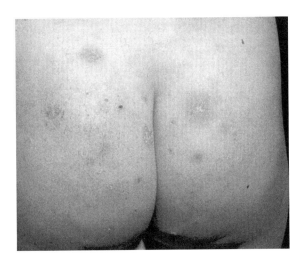

FIGURE 14-6

◙

Pediculus corporis. (See also
Color Insert 23.)

The most accepted treatment is Permethrin. Hair should be shampooed
prior to the treatment and Permethrin should be left on the hair for 10
minutes, then rinsed thoroughly. Hair should not be washed again for 24
hours after the treatment. For pubic lice, the same treatment should be
used. The second step of the treatment is ensuring the removal of the nits
by using a fine-toothed comb called an Alice comb. Parents should be
instructed do this for 20 minutes or more, in order to remove all the nits.
The last step is the treatment of the family, which should be done at the
same time in order to avoid reinfestation. Children can go back to school
once the treatment has been done and the doctor clears them. One of the
most important nursing interventions for this condition is to educate
the caregiver on the importance of laundering clothing and bedding in hot
water and also washing hairbrushes with hot water.

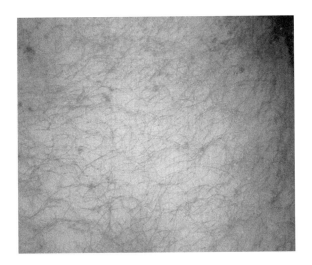

FIGURE 14-7

◙

Pediculus pubis. (See also Color
Insert 24.)

Acne Vulgaris

Keratinization. Process in which epithelial cells exposed to the external environment lose their moisture and are replaced by horny tissue.

Proliferation. Multiplication of similar forms.

Comedones. Two kinds: open (blackheads) and closed (whiteheads). Blackheads are caused by accumulation of keratin and sebum within the opening of a hair follicle.

Cysts. Encapsulated, elevated, palpable, and circumscribed fluid-filled semisolid material.

Acne vulgaris is a common form of acne seen predominantly in adolescents and young adults. Acne is an effect of androgenic hormones and *Propionibacterium acnes* in the hair follicle. There is usually an abnormal **keratinization** of the follicular epithelium; also there is excessive sebum production and a **proliferation** of *P. acnes*. **Comedones** formation is secondary to accumulation of keratin and sebum.

Acne vulgaris affects 85% of the population between the ages of 12 and 25 and the incidence is identical for both sexes. However, severe cases of the disease affect males more frequently. Some children may be more genetically susceptible to acne. Follicles are located primarily on the face and upper parts of the chest and back. The acne lesions are divided into two categories: (1) noninflammatory (closed and open comedones) (see Figure 14-8; Color Insert 25) and (2) inflammatory (pustules, papules, cystic nodules) (see Figure 14-9; Color Insert 26). There is also a possible severe scar formation secondary to rupture of the **cysts**.

The diagnosis is based on the history as disclosed by the adolescent. It is important to determine the onset, type, and distribution of the lesions. Often, the child will disclose that his/her parents had acne as adolescents. Females should be assessed if there is a relationship with exacerbation of acne and menstrual cycle, and also if the adolescent is taking oral contraceptives. The history should include what kinds of treatments were tried and the results of those treatments.

When doing the physical exam, the nurse should determine what kind of lesions the teen has, and if they are mild, moderate, or severe. No diagnostic tests are needed, but before initiating treatment, the nurse should explain the mechanism of acne to the parent and to the adolescent. After they understand the mechanics of the disease, the teen should be made aware that there will not be much improvement for 4 to 8 weeks, and that

FIGURE 14-8

ⓈⓈ

Noninflammatory acne in the newborn characterized by closed comedones. (See also Color Insert 25.)

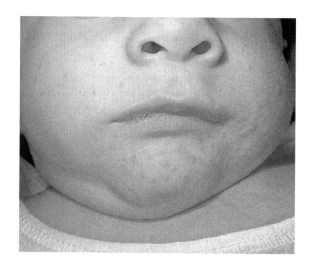

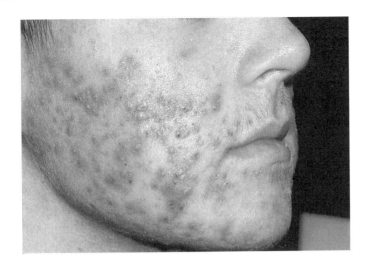

FIGURE 14-9

⌗

Inflammatory acne vulgaris with papules, pustules, and cystic nodules. (See also Color Insert 26.)

it is crucial not to manipulate the lesions to avoid scarring. The teen should be instructed not to use any oil-based cosmetics, face creams, and/or hair sprays. Before applying any topical agent to the face, the teen should gently wash his/her face with mild soap and dry it thoroughly. However, this should be done no more than 3 times per day. The literature states that there is no relationship between dietary restrictions and development of acne. Drug therapy is related to the condition for mild acne (mainly comedonal with occasional papules and pustules). The topical agents that are used are benzoyl peroxide gels (Desquam-X; 2.5%, 5%, and 10%) 2 times daily. Add retinoic acid cream (Retin-A; 0.025% and 0.05%) once every second and third night for more persistent cases and advance to nightly application as tolerated. For clients more than 14 years old, tetracycline 500 mg p.o. bid for 3 to 6 weeks is recommended. The tetracycline must be taken on an empty stomach and the patient should be warned about photosensitivity and teratogenic effects. The tetracycline ought to be tapered off to 250 mg bid for an additional 6 weeks, and then gradually to once a day or every other day for the next month or as the condition improves. If the condition does not improve with the tetracycline, the patient should be switched to topical antibiotic therapy, which is composed of erythromycin 2% solution or gel bid or clindamycin 1% solution, gel, or lotion bid. Severe cases of acne should be referred to a dermatologist.

𝒴EAST INFECTIONS

Tinea Versicolor

Tinea versicolor (see Figure 14-10; Color Insert 27) is a common superficial infection caused by a yeastlike fungus, *Pityrosporum orbiculare*, which is a normal bacterial skin flora, but when it overgrows it causes an

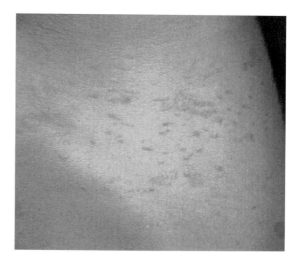

FIGURE 14-10

⬚

Tinea versicolor with small scaly hyperpigmented macules and patches. (See also Color Insert 27.)

Scales. Heaped-up keratinized epidermal cells.

infection. The reason for the overgrowth is unknown. The child usually presents lesions found primarily on the trunk. Characteristically, they are polycyclic connected hypopigmented macules with very fine **scales**; they usually are tan or reddish brown but can vary from white to brown. Usually they do not cause any pruritis.

The diagnosis is made on the basis of microscopic examination of the scales in KOH fungal preparation. If it is tinea versicolor, short, curved hyphae and clusters of round budding yeast are revealed. The aim of treatment is to eradicate the infection. Selium sulfide 2.5% lotion (Selsun) is applied to the skin from the neck down for 7 days. The lotion should be left on the skin for 10 to 20 minutes or overnight and should be rinsed off thoroughly. The treatment should be repeated monthly until the skin looks normal. The nurse should explain clearly to the patient that the treatment does not repigment the skin, and that it takes anywhere from 1 to 6 months for the repigmentation to occur, once the infection has cleared.

Candidiasis

Plaque. An elevated, flat, circumscribed area greater than 1 cm.

Candidiasis is an infection of the skin and/or the mucous membranes caused by the yeastlike fungus *Candida albicans*, which is a normal bacterial flora of the skin and mucous membranes. Overgrowth of *Candida* occurs when there is a breakdown or an overgrowth in intact epithelial barriers and invasion into the epidermis occurs, secondary to moisture and warmth and breaks in the barrier. The child usually develops adherent, curdlike **plaques** in inflamed oral mucosa (tongue, buccal mucosa, gingiva, and throat). The plaques are not easily removed, and bleeding may occur when one tries to wipe them away. The child may present cracks or fissures in the corners of his/her mouth. Candidiasis can also be found in conjunction with diaper rash. The diaper rash often occurs secondary to

Candida, and the diaper area becomes beefy red and shiny with sharply defined borders. Satellite lesions are mainly erythematous papules and/or pustules. Candidiasis may also be found in intertriginous areas (neck, axillae, umbilicus, and inguinal body folds appear red, moist, and glistening with plaque). Diagnosis is made based on location of the lesions, if the child has been in antibiotic therapy recently, if the child has immunosuppression, and whether or not the mother has had vaginal candidiasis. In doing the exam, the nurse should palpate for adjacent lymph nodes. Confirmation of the diagnosis is based on KOH fungal preparation being positive for yeast cell and pseudohyphae.

Treatment is based on the location of the candidiasis. For oral candidiasis, nystatin oral suspension (100,000 μ/ml) 1 ml on each side of the mouth is given qid for 7 to 10 days. Another alternative is gentian violet 1% aqueous solution painted in the oral cavity 1 to 2 times a day. The mouth should be rinsed prior to the application of the medication. If possible the large plaques should be removed with a warm moist cotton swab. All the nipples and pacifiers ought to be sterilized, all the toys should be washed in order to prevent further infection, and anyone handling the baby should wash his/her hands thoroughly prior to touching the child. If the baby is being breast fed, the mother's nipples ought to be checked for infection, and cleansed thoroughly before and after feeding. The most important nursing intervention is to educate the caregiver.

For diaper dermatitis, nystatin cream should be applied liberally to the area, but if Monistat cream is used only a small amount should be applied twice a day. The most important nursing intervention is to educate the caregiver on the cause of the infection and its prevention: Change diapers frequently; keep the baby clean and dry; avoid plastic pants; avoid the use of cornstarch—it may be metabolized by the microorganisms; maintain careful handwashing techniques; and continue medication for at least 2 days after the rash has disappeared.

$\mathcal{D}$ERMATOPHYTE INFECTIONS

Fungi that cause superficial infection thrive on keratin. Fungal disorders are known as mycoses. When they are caused by dermatophytes, they are termed tinea. Tinea capitis (infection of the scalp) and tinea corporis (infection of the body) are more common in children than in adults. The stratum corneum is invaded by the dermatophyte and an inflammatory response occurs, secondary to the release of toxins by the dermatophyte. The causative organisms are *Microsporum canis* or *Trichophyton tonsurans*, which cause tinea capitis, and *M. canis* or *T. mentagrophytes*, which cause tinea corporis. *M. canis* (carried by dogs) transmission does not occur from human to human, but such transmission occurs with *T. tonsurans*.

Tinea Capitis or Ringworm of the Scalp

Ringworm (see Figure 14-11 and Color Insert 28), the common name for tinea capitis, is mainly seen in children age 2 to 10 years old. The scalp lesions are circular, slightly erythematous, and scaling, with raised borders. Children who have this condition have partial alopecia from 1 to 5 cm in diameter.

Tinea Corporis or Ringworm of the Body or Face

Ringworm of the body or face (see Figure 14-12; Color Insert 29) is found on children age 2 to 10 years old. The lesions are found on nonhairy parts of the body, and are most commonly found on the face, neck, and arms. The lesions are flat, erythematous, round or oval, scaling patches that spread peripherally and have a clearing center, creating the ring appearance. Children that have this infection complain of pruritis. This infection is seen more in warm climates than in cold ones.

The diagnosis is based on history, including the onset, duration, and distribution of the lesions, as well exposure to others (including exposure to cats and dogs) with similar lesions or symptoms. Also, it is very important to find out if the child has been treated previously and what the treatment was.

In doing the physical exam, the nurse should examine the entire skin to determine the type and distribution of lesions. Wood's light may be used as an aid in the exam. It is important not to depend on it solely since some species do not fluoresce; for example, *T. tonsurans* is not visible with Wood's light. Some species of the infecting organism cause tinea to fluoresce pale or brilliant green. However, hair products containing petrolatum also fluoresce a bluish or purplish color. The diagnostic test used to

FIGURE 14-11

◙

Tinea capitis with patches of alopecia, crusting, and scaling. (See also Color Insert 28.)

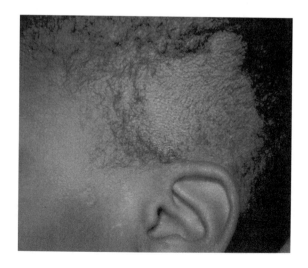

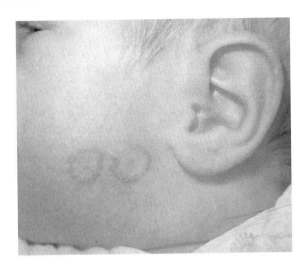

FIGURE 14-12

Tinea corporis (facial) with ring shape at periphery of the lesion. (See also Color Insert 29.)

detect this infection is KOH fungal preparation, which is used to examine scrapings from lesion borders, and also a fungal culture.

The treatment varies in accordance with where the lesion is located. If it is found on the scalp (tinea capitis), the treatment is with griseofulvin ultramicronized 15 mg/kg every day p.o. for 1 to 2 months or longer. The side effects of griseofulvin are insomnia and headaches. Also caution should be exercised because it is not safe for children younger than 2 years of age. The nurse should instruct the parents that this medication needs to be taken with milk or fatty foods to augment absorption. Another alternative treatment is ketoconazole 6 mg/kg/day every 12 hours. The side effects of ketoconazole are headache, nausea, vomiting, and abdominal discomfort. Along with this medication, children need to use selenium sulfide shampoo twice a week for 2 weeks to decrease chances of infectivity. It is important to teach parents that topical antifungal medications are not effective on the scalp, that the child can go back to school in 1 week, and that no one should share the combs or the brushes of the infected child. The child needs to be reassured that the hair will grow again but that it is a lengthy process. The child needs to be seen for a follow-up visit 2 weeks after the start of treatment, and then again 1 month after the treatment is stopped. The follow-up visits are needed to evaluate the effectiveness of the treatment.

If the lesion is tinea corporis, topical clotrimazole 1% cream or econazole nitrate 1% cream should be applied twice a day for 14 to 28 days, and for 1 week after the lesions have disappeared, the skin must be kept dry as much as possible. The nurse should teach the parents that no one else in the household ought to wear the clothing of the infected child. Prior to the treatment, the clothing of the infected child should be washed with hot water and dried in the dryer on the hottest setting. If there is a doubt that any other member of the family has worn the infected child's clothes, that child should be watched closely for symptoms.

*I*MPETIGO

Bulla. Circumscribed, elevated lesion greater than 1 cm in diameter, filled with serous fluid.

Impetigo (see Figures 14-13 and 14-14; Color Inserts 30 and 31) is a purulent bacterial skin infection caused by the invasion of pathogenic *Staphylococcus aureus, Streptococcus pyogenes*, or both, to the epidermis. Small breaks in the epidermal barrier allow the penetration of the pathogens. The staphylococci produce a bacterial toxin called exfoliate toxin (ET), which causes a disruption in cellular adhesion. The ET stimulates the formation of vesicles, which enlarge to form the **bullae.** The invasion is superficial; but if impetigo is not treated, it can develop into acute glomerulonephritis, which is a condition secondary to strains of nephritogenic streptococci. The small break in the epidermis begins as a 1 to 2 mm superficial vesicle with a fragile roof that is quickly lost, once the vesicle ruptures. It leaves a moist honey-colored crusted erosion. Usually multiple lesions are located on the face and around the nose and mouth; the hands and other areas also can be involved. There are two patterns of infection: (1) bulbous, which has a staph origin; and (2) vesicular, which has a strep origin. Impetigo is more commonly seen in mid- to late summer with increased incidence in hot, humid climates. It is also enhanced by poor hygiene or crowded conditions. Although impetigo is seen by itself, often it is seen after the child has had chickenpox, scabies, insect bites, or trauma.

The diagnosis is based on the history taken by the nurse. It is important to identify any other person in the family who has been infected with impetigo, and what treatment they had. The history should also include the location of the lesions, their onset and duration, and whether the child has had pruritis. The whole body should be inspected for lesions that have eroded and are covered by moist, honey-colored crusts. The nurse should also check for lymphadenopathy. The diagnosis is not as important as culturing the lesions if they are extensive or severe. The crust must be removed by gently washing the area with warm water and an antiseptic soap or

FIGURE 14-13

◙

Impetigo contagiosa (vulgaris). Lesions evolve from small vesicles to pustules to thick yellow crusted formations. (See also Color Insert 30.)

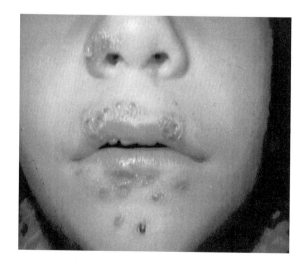

Plate 1 (see Figure 6-1). Bacterial conjunctivitis. Mucopurulent discharge, conjuctival injection, and lid swelling, in a 10-year-old with *Haemophilus influenzae* conjunctivitis. (Courtesy of Frank Birinyi, MD.)

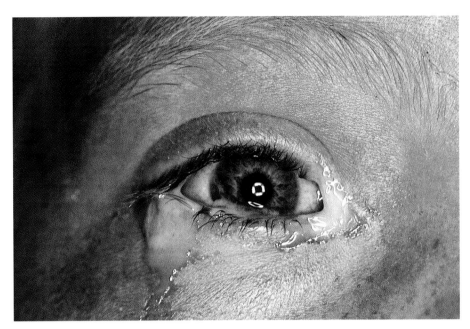

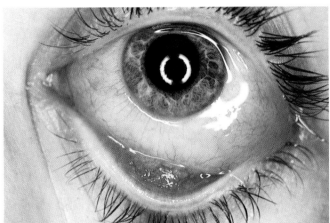

Plate 2 (see Figure 6-2). Allergic conjunctivitis. Conjunctival injection, chemosis, and a follicular response in the inferior palpebral conjunctiva in this patient with allergic conjunctivitis secondary to cat fur. (Courtesy of Timothy D. McGuirk, DO.)

Plate 3 (see Figure 6-3). Ophthalmia neonatorum from gonococcal infection. Copious and purulent drainage in a newborn with neonatal gonococcal conjunctivitis. (Reprinted with permission of American Academy of Ophthalmology. *Eye Trauma and Emergencies: A Slide-Script Program.* San Francisco, 1985.)

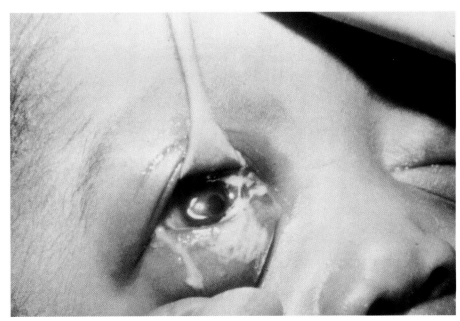

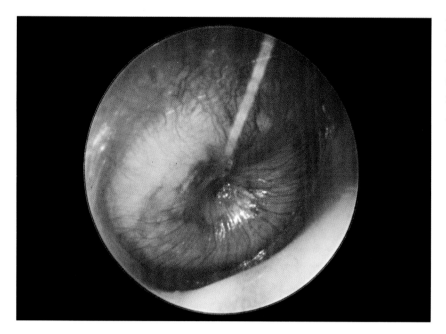

Plate 4 (see Figure 6-4).
Otitis media. The middle ear is filled with purulent material behind an erythematous, bulging tympanic membrane. (Courtesy of Richard A. Chole, MD, PhD.)

Plate 5 (see Figure 6-5).
Pharyngitis. Exudative pharyngitis showing erythema and tonsillar exudate in patient with viral mononucleosis. (Courtesy of George L. Murrell.)

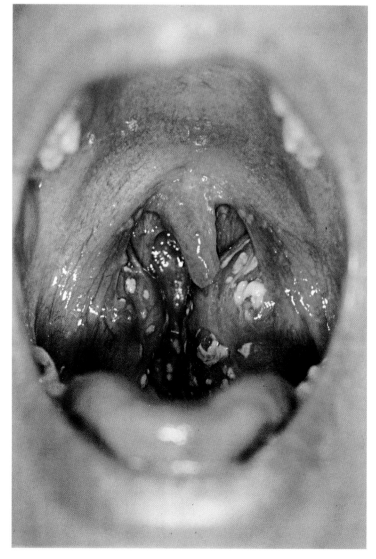

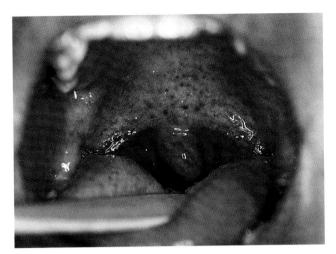

Plate 6 (see Figure 6-6).
Palatal petechiae. Palatal petechiae and erythema of the tonsillar pillars in a patient with streptococcal pharyngitis. (Courtesy of Kevin J. Knoop, MD, MS.)

Plate 7 (see Figure 6-7).
Oral candidiasis or thrush. Whitish plaques are seen on the buccal mucosa. These plaques are easily removed with a tongue blade, differentiating them from lichen planus or leukoplakia. (Courtesy of James F. Steiner, DDS.)

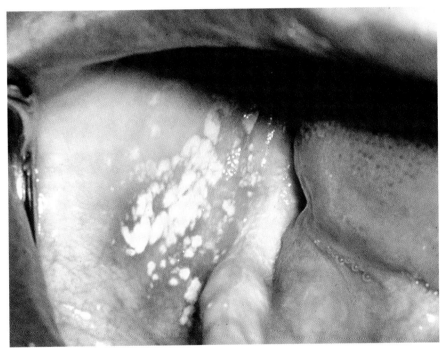

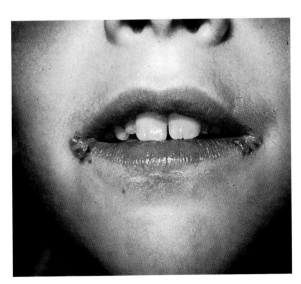

Plate 8 (see Figure 6-8).
Candidiasis. The angles of the mouth are also places where intertriginous conditions favor the overgrowth of ubiquitous *Candida albicans*, streptococci, staphylococci, and other ordinarily saprophytic but facultatively pathogenic microorganisms. The condition produced at the angles of the mouth is called *perlèche* or *angular stomatitis*. From such a beginning or even without it, the lips themselves may become involved.

Plate 9 (see Figure 10-4).
Gastric wave of hypertrophic pyloric stenosis. A gastric wave can be seen traversing the abdomen in this series of photographs of a patient with HPS. (Courtesy of Kevin J. Knoop, MD, MS.)

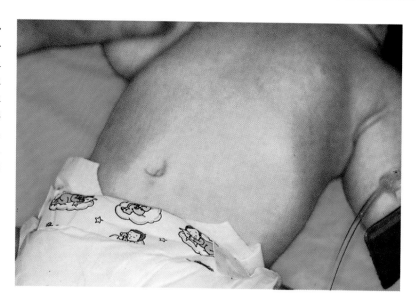

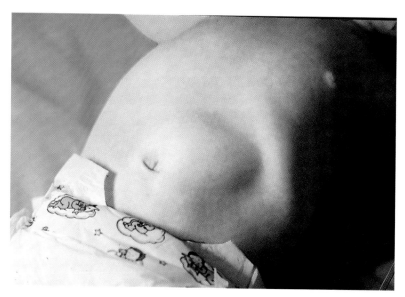

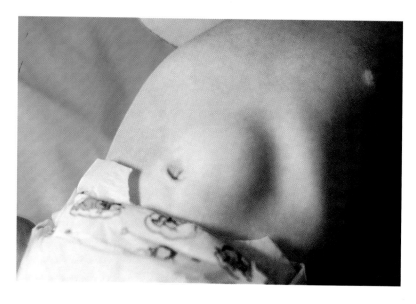

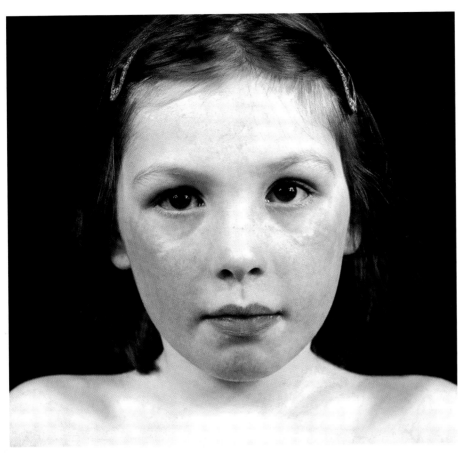

Plate 10 (see Figure 13-1).
Erythema infectiosum.

Plate 11 (see Figure 13-2).
Herpes simplex virus infection: neonatal.

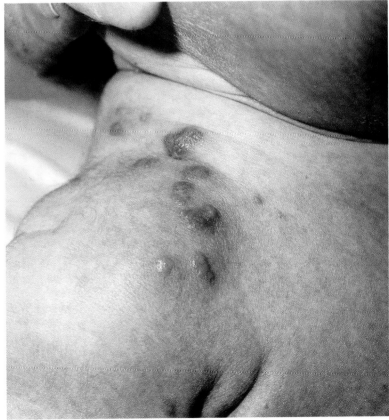

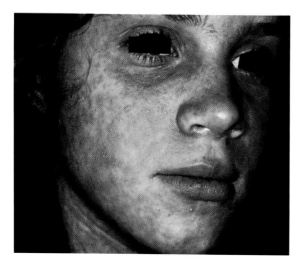

Plate 12 (see Figure 13-3).
Measles, maculopapular erythematous rash.

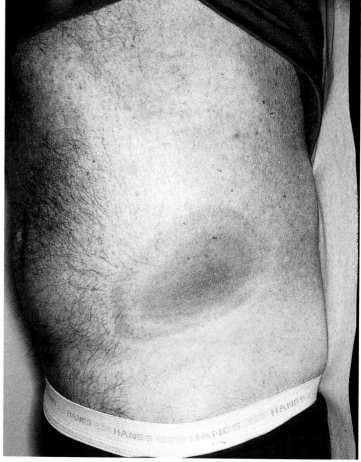

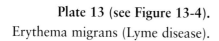

Plate 13 (see Figure 13-4).
Erythema migrans (Lyme disease).

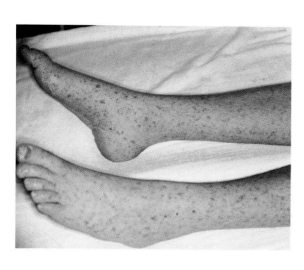

Plate 14 (see Figure 13-5).
Rocky Mountain spotted fever rash: erythematous macules on wrists, hands, forearms, and legs.

Plate 15 (see Figure 13-6).
Strawberry tongue in scarlet fever.

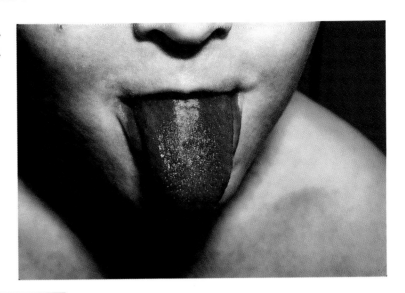

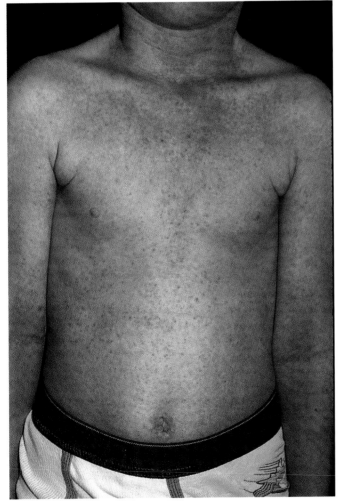

Plate 16 (see Figure 13-7).
Generalized exanthem in scarlet fever.

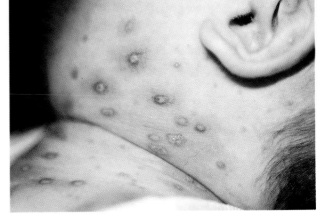

Plate 17 (see Figure 13-8).
Varicella (chickenpox).
(Courtesy of Lawrence B. Stack, MD.)

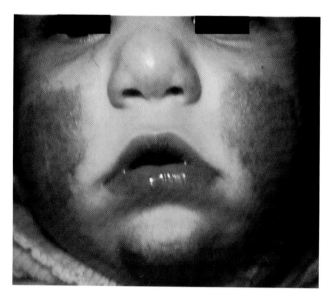

Plate 18 (see Figure 14-1).
Atopic dermatitis in infancy.

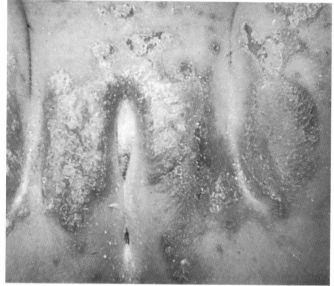

Plate 19 (see Figure 14-2).
Diaper dermatitis.

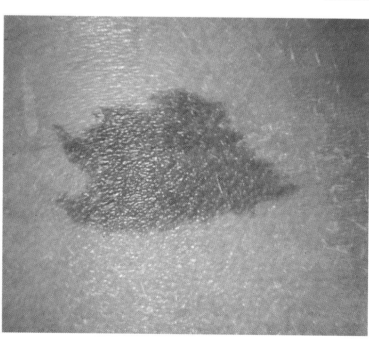

Plate 20 (see Figure 14-3).
Café-au-lait spot.

Plate 21 (see Figure 14-4).
Scabies, with its linear lesions and tiny black dots representing the mite, eggs, and/or fecal material in the small vesicle.

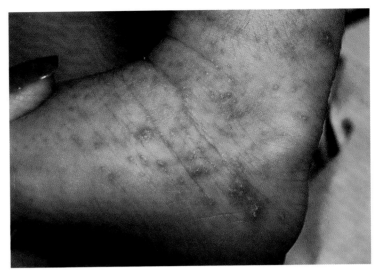

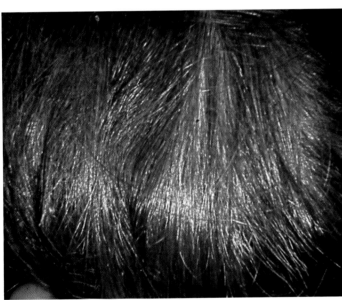

Plate 22 (see Figure 14-5).
Pediculus capitis.

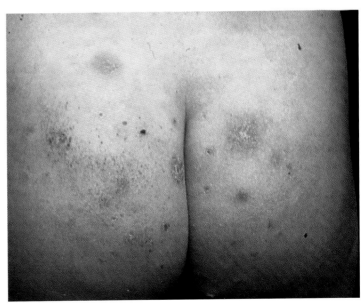

Plate 23 (see Figure 14-6).
Pediculus corporis.

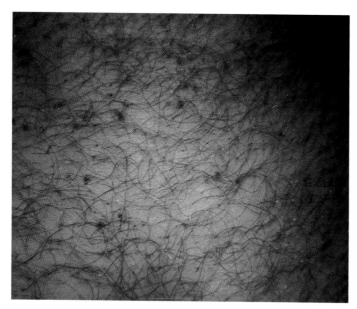

Plate 24 (see Figure 14-7).
Pediculus pubis.

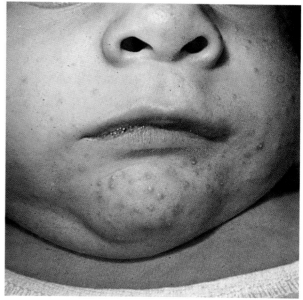

Plate 25 (see Figure 14-8).
Noninflammatory acne in the newborn
characterized by closed comedones.

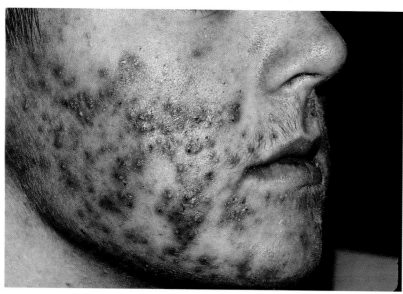

Plate 26 (see Figure 14-9).
Inflammatory acne vulgaris with
papules, pustules, and cystic nodules.

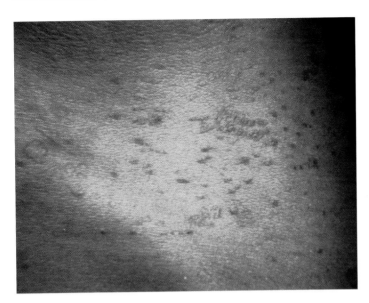

Plate 27 (see Figure 14-10).
Tinea versicolor with small scaly hyperpigmented macules and patches.

Plate 28 (see Figure 14-11).
Tinea capitis with patches of alopecia, crusting, and scaling.

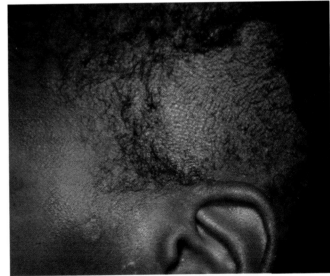

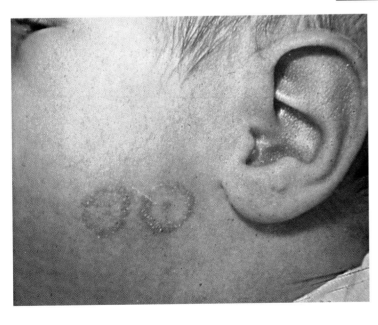

Plate 29 (see Figure 14-12).
Tinea corporis (facial) with ring shape at periphery of the lesion.

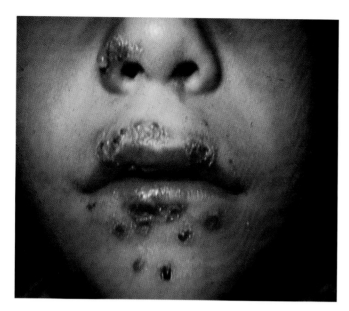

Plate 30 (see Figure 14-13).
Impetigo contagiosa (vulgaris). Lesions evolve from small vesicles to pustules to thick yellow crusted formations.

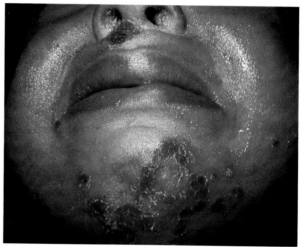

Plate 31 (see Figure 14-14).
Impetigo contagiosa (vulgaris). Shiny, bright red erosions where yellow thick crust is removed from lesion.

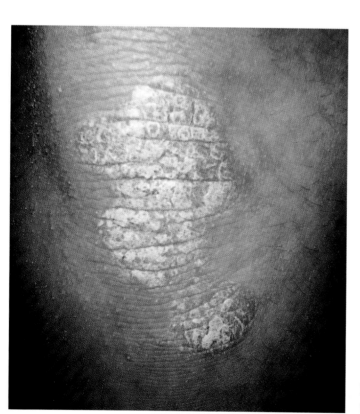

Plate 32 (see Figure 14-15).
Psoriasis with its silvery scale.

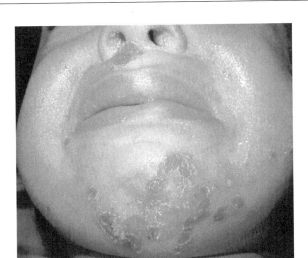

FIGURE 14-14

♲

Impetigo contagiosa (vulgaris). Shiny bright red erosions where yellow thick crust is removed from lesion. (See also Color Insert 31.)

cleanser such as Betadine or Hibiclens. Scrubbing the lesions has not been shown to be effective. The incubation time of the impetigo is 1 to 3 days, and it is not communicable after 48 hours of antibiotic therapy. The nurse should instruct the parents not to let anyone use the same towel as the infected child. The child's linen and clothes should be washed in hot water, and his/her fingernails should be cut as short as possible to prevent reinfection by scratching. Parents should be instructed to observe the child's urine for color: dark-colored urine may mean glomerulonephritis. Also, the child should be observed for decreased urinary output and edema.

Treatment varies according to the severity of the problem: If the child has 1 or 2 lesions, local treatment with a topical application of Neosporin ointment is indicated, usually 4 to 5 times a day for crusted lesions; or Bactroban ointment, which should be applied 3 times a day for bulbous lesions. If the child exhibits a large number of lesions, the treatment needs to be systemic. The systemic treatment encompasses giving the child Dicloxacillin 25 mg/kg/day in 4 divided doses for 10 days, or erythromycin 30 to 50 mg/kg/day in 4 divided doses for 10 days. The parents are instructed to make a follow-up visit in 10 days to 2 weeks after therapy is completed in order to determine the effectiveness of the treatment.

𝒫SORIASIS

Psoriasis (see Figure 14-15; Color Insert 32) is a chronic inflammatory skin disorder with spontaneous remissions and exacerbations. It is characterized by thick silvery scales, and the condition is usually linked to a family history. However, the mode of inheritance has not been established. The child's dermis and epidermis are thickened with cellular proliferation and inflammation, which results in plaque formation. The normal turnover time for shedding the epidermis is decreased from 26 to 30 days to 3 to 4

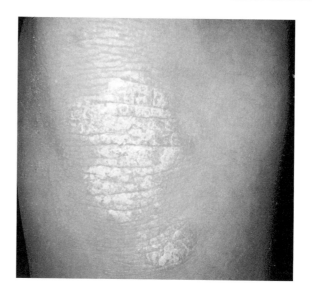

FIGURE 14-15

◙

Psoriasis with its silvery scale.
(See also Color Insert 32.)

days. There is increased vascularization to accommodate increased cell metabolism, which causes erythema. There is also a silvery lesion appearance, which is secondary to loosely cohesive keratin. This condition can appear at any age; it affects only 1 to 2% of the population, and is more common in white children. The typical lesion is a well-circumscribed thick, silvery, scaly, erythematous plaque surrounded by normal skin. The initial lesions are small erythematous papules that enlarge and coalesce into large inflammatory lesions. The lesions often involve the elbows, knees, scalp, and other areas of trauma, and sometimes the fingernails, where they are seen as pinpoint pits in the nail plate along with yellow discoloration. Guttate (droplike) psoriasis is a common form seen in children 2 to 3 weeks after an episode of streptococcal pharyngitis: 3 to 8 mm papules suddenly appear predominantly over the trunk and quickly become covered by white scales. Silvery scales may reveal bleeding points when removed. Five to 7% of individuals with psoriasis develop psoriatic arthritis.

The diagnosis is based on the family history, including information on onset, location, duration of appearance of lesions, bleeding if the scales were removed, nail pitting, or arthritis. The skin should be examined for lesions, and the nails and joints of the toes should also be examined for inflammatory changes.

There is no indicated diagnostic test. It is only when inflammation of the joints occurs that blood samples are drawn in order to examine the erythrocyte sedimentation rate and the uric levels. The main goal of therapy is to diminish epidermal turnover time. The parents are instructed that exposure to sunlight or artificial ultraviolet light may improve the condition. The therapy is guided to where the lesions are: If the lesions are in the scalp, the parent is instructed to use a tar shampoo (Penetrax, Polytar, Zetar), leaving it on for 5 minutes, rinsing, and then following with a commercial shampoo to remove the scales. The tar shampoo ought to be used twice weekly and the commercial shampoo daily if necessary to remove the scales. Triamcinolone lotion (0.1%) (Kenalog 0.1%) can be applied to stubborn areas of the scalp once a day at bedtime until controlled. The parents need to be instructed to avoid washing the face of these children when using these treatments. If the lesions are on the face and skin folds, the most common treatment is the application of hydrocortisone cream 1% twice a day for 4 weeks. If unresponsive, it should be increased to 2.5% and tapered back to 1% as soon as the condition improves. If the lesion is on the body, arms, or legs, the treatment of choice is triamcinolone acetonide, 0.025% cream twice a week up to 2 weeks. When using creams, the parents need to be instructed to avoid using the cream on normal skin. The child should be seen again in 2 months and the physician must be notified immediately if there is no improvement or if the child has any symptoms of psoriatic arthritis. Psoriasis is a chronic condition in which the child will experience remissions and exacerbations. Avoidance of cutaneous injury, streptococcal infections, sunburn stress, itching, bites, tight shoes and clothes, and oral steroids will help to prevent recurrence of the symptoms.

$\mathcal{S}$UMMARY

The skin is the largest organ of the body, and one of the most important because the skin reflects physical and emotional health, and plays a major role in defining an individual's identity as well as supporting his/her survival. A comprehensive assessment of the skin often reveals or provides important cues to underlying conditions.

Emotions are expressed when a person blushes or becomes nervous and sweats. The skin provides the sensory input as to the conditions of the external environment, such as heat, cold, pressure, and pain. Additionally, the skin provides a physiologic covering and is the first line of defense against injury from chemical, physical, and microorganic invaders. Thermoregulation and homeostasis are maintained through fluid regulation by the skin.

Disruptions in the skin account for 20 to 30% of all pediatric office visits. The nurse plays an important role in maintaining skin integrity by identifying and minimizing skin disruptions, maximizing healing, and teaching parents and children about the care of their skin.

The maintenance of skin hydration is essential for prevention and treatment of skin conditions. If overhydrated the bonds between cells at the stratum corneum are loosened and the barrier is broken. If too dry, the skin becomes cracked, and again the barrier is broken. Although less frequent bathing is often recommended, especially for dry skin or in dry climates, proper bathing may enhance addition and retention of water in the skin. The use of lukewarm rather than hot water is recommended. Bathing should not last long enough for the skin to become supersaturated, and in general mild soaps should be used. Bubble-bath solutions for children should be avoided since they can be especially irritating and drying to the skin. Drying should be done gently and even some sort of lubricating agent should be applied immediately after drying. Often if the child is going outdoors after bathing a sunblock/screen can be applied right after drying off.

Most sunblocks should not be rubbed into the skin but applied lightly without excessive rubbing, since hard rubbing reduces their effectiveness and lowers their ability to produce UV protection.

CRITICAL POINTS IN THE CARE OF DERMATOLOGICAL DISORDERS

The skin provides a protective covering for the body. It is composed of several functionally related layers, which allow several integral functions such as protection against microbial and foreign substance invasion and minor physical trauma. Skin textures among infants, children, adolescents, and adults vary. A proper examination of the skin requires that the entire surface of the body be palpated and inspected in good light. It is important to know and be able to recognize anatomic location, arrangement, type, and color of lesions along with the history of onset, duration, and changes, in order to diagnose and treat disorders of the skin.

Children with skin conditions have unique health and social needs. Many children with these conditions receive the majority of their treatment in clinics where they are seen one time, or where immediate care is given and there is no follow-up care. A child's self-concept and interpersonal skills greatly influence his/her adherence to treatment regimens. The most important contribution the nurse can give to families and children is a solid knowledge about skin and the ability for accurate assessment in order to arrive at a correct diagnosis. Going from one specialist to another usually misses the screening needed. In order to avoid sequelae, children need to be reminded that who they are comes from inside, not just from the way they look, especially if the skin problems are disfiguring, even if only temporarily.

Being misdiagnosed can be harmful to the child because of the treatment. In the case of inflammatory processes, for instance, the application of heat is only indicated in the presence of folliculitis and cellulitis. So the nurse needs to be alert in recognizing the different symptoms present in the different conditions. Being alert to the initial signs and symptoms of infection is an important skill for the nurse who can mentally amplify such signs and symptoms to arrive at an appropriate diagnosis.

All treatments for skin conditions are designed to provide relief from discomfort. The role of the nurse is in her support and teaching of the parents and children. Skin conditions always involve the parents. Since skin conditions are rarely treated in the hospital, the parents are the ones who institute the treatment; therefore, their understanding and knowledge of the process of the disease are most important. The nurse should give a clear and detailed explanation of how the treatment will work, concentrating on teaching unexplained reactions and what action to take if they do happen. The instructions should be written, so parents can review them whenever they need to, and the nurse should have the parents repeat the verbal instructions so any misunderstandings can be eliminated. Verbal instructions should always be backed up with written ones.

One sensitive issue is the fact that the skin is the most visible part of the body, and that parents and children are very uncomfortable with deviant physical appearance. The nurse should be prepared for these circumstances and provide the parents and the child with all the support and reassurance that they require. In order to ensure a good resolution of the skin condition, the nurse needs to do a continuous evaluation of her interventions, modifying them as the condition changes and always using her assessments as the basis for guidelines for expected outcomes.

$\mathcal{Q}$UESTIONS

Diagnosis: Oral Candidiasis

History: 8-month-old Teresa is brought to the clinic by her mother, who states that she has noticed white patches on Teresa's tongue and the sides of her mouth for the last 4 days. The nurse suspects that the baby may have candidiasis.

Nursing problems: Teach parents how to give medications. Teach parents sterilization of nipples and pacifier. Teach parents how to avoid recurrence.

1. What historical statement made by Teresa's mother supports the diagnosis?
   A. Teresa has been on oral antibiotics for a week.
   B. Teresa has bleeding of the tongue.
   C. Teresa also has a diaper rash.
   D. Teresa has had the patches for 4 days.

2. What characteristic presentation of symptoms would help to diagnose Teresa as having oral candidiasis (thrush)?
   A. Adherent, curdlike plaques on an inflamed oral mucosa
   B. Adherent, yellowish-white plaque on the tongue
   C. Nonadherent, curdlike plaque on the tongue
   D. Greenish spots on the gums

3. Teresa is diagnosed with oral thrush and a prescription for oral nystatin is written. How should her mother be advised to give the medication to Teresa?
   A. Place 2 cc of medication at the back of her throat and allow Teresa to swallow the medicine before feeding her.
   B. Mix 2 cc of nystatin with a small amount of her formula to ensure Teresa takes the medication.
   C. After Teresa has been fed, rinse her mouth out with water and place 1 cc of nystatin in each side of her mouth.
   D. Mix the medication with water to ensure Teresa takes the medication.

4. Her mother asks if she has to worry about Teresa becoming reinfected. Which of the following is the most appropriate response?

   A. No, the chances are very unlikely.
   B. Yes, there is a chance. Special precautions such as washing toys must be done to prevent reinfection.
   C. Most children develop this only once and then become immune.
   D. Teresa can only develop this condition again if she uses a pacifier.

5. The causative agent of oral thrush is:

   A. *Pityrosporum orbiculare*
   B. *C. albicans*
   C. *S. pyogenes*
   D. Tinea

Diagnosis: Diaper Dermatitis

History: Diaper dermatitis, which Teresa also had, commonly occurs concurrently with oral thrush. Her diaper area was beefy red, and shiny with a sharply defined border and small satellite papules along the margins.

Nursing problems: Teach parents good hygiene habits. Teach parents parenting. Ensure that parents understand treatment.

1. Which of the following is the treatment of choice for diaper dermatitis?

   A. Application of cornstarch with every diaper change.
   B. Application of zinc oxide to the diaper area with every diaper change.
   C. Application of nystatin cream twice a day.
   D. Do not apply anything; just change the diaper 6 times a day.

Diagnosis: Cradle Cap

History: 3-week-old Brian is brought to the clinic with a 1-week history of a scaly scalp. On examination, adherent, thick, yellow, crusted scalp lesions are noted on a slightly erythematous base to the front of the scalp. Diffuse hair loss is noted to the area. His mother states she has been applying baby oil to the scalp to relieve the scaliness.

Nursing problems: Teaching parents proper management of the condition. Education on control measures. Reinforcement of need for compliance with follow-up visits.

1. Which of the following questions would be important to ask?

   A. Has the infant been febrile?
   B. How long has the infant been losing hair?
   C. Is the infant taking any medications?
   D. Do any pets live in the home?

2. What characteristic symptoms would lead to the diagnosis of cradle cap (seborrheic dermatitis) rather than tinea capitis?

   A. Diffuse hair loss
   B. Scaling of the scalp
   C. Continuous pruritis
   D. No hair loss

3. In the absence of pruritus, what is the treatment of choice for seborrheic dermatitis?

   A. Selsun shampoo
   B. An antifungal shampoo
   C. Massaging petroleum antifungal medication on the scalp and using a soft brush to loosen scale before shampooing
   D. Brushing the scalp for 20 minutes before applying anything, before shampooing

Diagnosis: Tinea Capitis

History: 5-year-old Gary was diagnosed as having tinea capitis with the causative organism being *Microsporum canis*.

Nursing problems: Patient education and prevention. Monitoring of liver function tests and CBC. Education on medication management. Need to address compliance with office visits.

1. His mother ask if Gary possibly got the fungal infection from their pet. The nurse's best response is:

   A. Yes; Gary could have been infected from his grandparents' dog.
   B. No; more than likely he got the infection from a previous infection.
   C. This condition can only be obtained from another human.
   D. Animals like cats or dogs cannot infect humans.

2. Which laboratory test is used to confirm the diagnosis of tinea capitis?

   A. KOH scraping (positive)
   B. There is no lab test that confirm this condition.
   C. Skin biopsy
   D. Serum cortisol test

3. Which of the following, adjunct with 2.5% selenium sulfide shampoo, is the best treatment for tinea capitis?

   A. Clotrimazole 1% cream
   B. Griseofulvin 125 mg/5ml at 10–20 mg/kg/day once a day
   C. Ketoconazole 250 mg–30 mg/kg/day 4 times a day
   D. Corticosteroids p.o. for 10 days

Diagnosis: Acne

History: 15-year-old Pauline is having a physical in order to be on the school soccer team. Pauline states she is in healthy condition and her only complaint is ongoing acne. The physical examination is entirely normal except for her skin. Erythematous pustules are noted across her hairline along with a few cystic lesions on her cheeks and black-heads over her nose and cheeks.

Nursing problems: Teach the proper management of skin care. Control the inflammatory process. Teach the patient how to reduce obstruction of the sebaceous ducts.

1. Before the physical examination is done, it is important to:
   A. Have Pauline wash her face.
   B. Obtain a history from Pauline.
   C. Immediately write a prescription for the acne since this is Pauline's major concern.
   D. Call her parents so that they can be instructed about her care.

2. Pauline asks the nurse what foods she should avoid. The nurse answers:
   A. Avocados and nuts
   B. All soft drinks
   C. None; she can eat everything
   D. Chocolates and sweets

3. Where are lesions of acne vulgaris predominantly seen?
   A. Face and chest
   B. Neck and chest
   C. Chest and back
   D. Upper thigh

4. On physical examination, what determines the severity of acne?
   A. Primary sites of acne
   B. Inflammation and infection of lesions
   C. Distribution, type, and spread
   D. Presence or absence of scarring

5. Patient education is very important in the management of acne. How often should follow-up visits occur?
   A. Twice a month.
   B. Every week until the condition has improved.
   C. Only if the condition has not improved.
   D. Every 4 to 6 weeks until control is established.

6. What is the initial treatment for Pauline?
   A. Topical antibiotics
   B. Systemic antibiotics
   C. Topical and systemic antibiotics
   D. Antiandrogens and antibiotics

Diagnosis: Scabies

History: 7-year-old David is brought to the clinic by his mother, who states David has been intensely scratching his arms and hands for the past 2 days. His mother also states David's best friend was recently diagnosed with scabies.

Nursing problems: Pharmacological management. Teaching parents how to avoid recurrent infestations. Avoidance of complications. Reinforcement of the necessity of follow-up visits.

1. What is the diagnostic test used to confirm scabies?
   A. KOH test
   B. Microscopic examination
   C. Wood's light
   D. No test available

2. His mother asks if David can return to school once treatment is started. She should be informed that:
   A. Yes; David can return to school once treatment is initiated.
   B. No; David cannot return to school until the day after treatment is completed.
   C. No; David cannot return to school until 48 hours after treatment is initiated.
   D. David needs to stay at home at least for 1 week.

3. The most sensitive education that the nurse must give to David's mother is:
   A. Clothing and bedding need to be laundered in hot water and the hot drying cycle.
   B. Scabies affects all socioeconomic groups and all ages.
   C. Only household members who have the same symptoms need to be treated.
   D. Parasites causing scabies are unable to live off the skin for longer than 3 to 4 days.

*A*NSWERS

Oral Candidiasis

1. *A.* The patient usually gives a history of antibiotic use in the previous weeks, and has a rash. *Candida* is part of a normal flora of the skin. Disseminated infection is almost always preceded by prolonged broad-spectrum antibiotic therapy.

2. *B.* White plaques adhere to mucous membranes tightly.

3. *C.* Nystatin is the drug of choice. Infants are given oral nystatin suspension (100,000 units 4–6 times a day until resolution usually suffices). Apply it directly to the mucosa, and do not give the child anything to drink for at least 15 minutes.

4. *B.* Reinfection can occur if the child comes in contact with articles that have been infected previously, such as toys, nipples, cups, etc. All toys that the child can place on his/her mouth should be washed with soap and water.

5. *B. C. albicans* is the causative agent of oral thrush. It is ubiquitous and often present in small numbers on the skin and mucous membranes, or in the intestinal tract.

Diaper Dermatitis

1. *C.* Nystatin cream is the treatment of choice. Cutaneous infection usually responds to a cream or lotion containing nystatin, amphotericin B, or an imidazole. Cornstarch should be avoided because it can be metabolized by the microorganisms.

Cradle Cap

1. *B.* The presence of hair loss indicates a severe inflammatory process. Psoriatic lesions on the scalp can mimic seborrhea. A skin biopsy may be required for definite diagnosis.

2. *A.* Diffuse hair loss is noted with cradle cap, whereas hair loss with tinea capitis is more commonly circumscribed.

3. *C.* This is the treatment of choice for infants. Antiseborrheic shampoos are recommended for toddlers and adolescents.

Tinea Capitis

1. *A. Microsporum canis* is contracted from a pet that has ringworm.

2. *A.* KOH scraping is one of the tests used to diagnose tinea capitis. The others are fungal tests and Wood's light (which is positive with *M. canis*).

3. *B.* Griseofulvin is the best medication for this condition. It should be taken with fatty foods such as ice cream for 6–8 weeks.

Acne

1. *B.* Before performing a physical examination, obtaining a history is always important, since the condition could be linked to genetic factors.

2. *C.* Specific foods such as chocolate, soda, or french fries have not been shown to cause or worsen acne.

3. *A.* The most common places affected by acne are the face and chest.

4. *C.* The severity of the acne is determined by the quantity, type, and spread of the lesions.

5. *D.* Follow-up visits should occur at least every 4–6 weeks until control is established. Control is indicated by clearing lesions or only a few new lesions every 2 weeks.

6. *C.* Pauline has moderate acne. Oral antibiotics are used in addition to topical antibiotics. They must be taken for 1–3 months and it often requires 3–4 weeks to see improvement.

Scabies

1. *B.* Microscopic examination identifies mites, eggs, or feces from skin scrapings.

2. *B.* It is recommended that students do not return to school until the day after treatment is stopped to make sure treatment was successful.

3. *B.* Parents of children who have scabies usually feel ashamed and tend to think that the infestation is associated with poor hygiene or low socioeconomic status. The nurse must always be sensitive to parents' and children's feelings.

$\mathcal{G}$LOSSARY

blister   a vesicle or bulla.

bulla   circumscribed, elevated lesion greater than 1 cm in diameter, filled with serous fluid.

comedones   two kinds: open (blackheads) and closed (whiteheads). Blackheads are caused by accumulation of keratin and sebum within the opening of a hair follicle.

cysts   encapsulated, elevated, palpable, and circumscribed fluid-filled semisolid material.

ectoparasitic   organisms that live outside the body of the host.

epidermis   outermost portion of the skin, consisting of 2 layers: stratum corneum and cellular stratum.

erythema   redness or inflammation of the skin or mucous membrane.

excoriated   linear or hollowed-out crusted epidermis, leaving dermis exposed.

fissures   linear cracks or breaks from the epidermis to the dermis.

keratinization   process in which epithelial cells exposed to the external environment lose their moisture and are replaced by horny tissue.

keratinocytes   epidermal cells that synthesize keratin and other proteins and sterols.

lichenification   rough, thickened epidermis causing accentuated skin markings.

macules   circumference less than 1 cm in diameter; lesions with color change in flat skin.

maculopapular   combination of macular and papular lesions.

melanocyte   a body cell capable of producing melanin.

papular   solid, elevated area less than 1 cm in diameter; top may be pointed, rounded, or flat.

plaque   an elevated, flat, circumscribed area greater than 1 cm.

proliferation   multiplication of similar forms.

pruritic   itching.

pustules   elevated, superficial, and purulent filled lesions.

scales   heaped-up keratinized epidermal cells.

sebaceous glands   small sacculated organs in the dermis that secrete sebum.

stratum corneum   the horny, outermost layer of the skin, composed of dead cells converted to keratin. Continually flakes away.

vesicle   lesion less than 1 cm in diameter; elevated, circumscribed, superficial, and filled with serous fluid.

ℬIBLIOGRAPHY

BOYNTON, R., DUNN, E., AND STEPHENS, G. *Manual of Ambulatory Pediatrics.* 3rd ed. Philadelphia: Lippincott, 1994.

COODY, D. There is no such thing as a good tan. *Journal of Pediatric Health Care* 1(3):125–132, 1987.

HAY, W., JR., GROOTHUIS, J., HAYWARD, A., AND LEVIN, M. *Current Pediatric Diagnosis and Treatment.* 12th ed. Norwalk, CT: Appleton & Lange, 1995.

MCCANCE, K., AND HUETHER, S. *Pathophysiology: The Biological Basis for Disease in Adults and Children.* 2nd ed. St. Louis: Mosby, 1994.

NELSON, J. *1996–1997 Pocket Book of Pediatric Antimicrobial Therapy.* 12th ed. Baltimore: Williams & Wilkins, 1996.

SEIDEL, H., BALL, J., DAINS, J., AND BENEDICT, G. *Mosby's Guide to Physical Examination.* 3rd ed. St. Louis: Mosby, 1995.

UPHOLD, C., AND GRAHAM, M. *Clinical Guidelines in Family Practice.* 2nd ed. Gainesville: Barmarrae Books, 1994.

*H*ELPFUL INTERNET SITES

An Introduction to Basic Dermatology at http://www.vh.org/Providers/ Lectures/PietteDermatology/BasicDermatology.html   This site is part of the University of Iowa's health care site, "Virtual Hospital." It provides a good overview of basic dermatology and treatments.

Virtual Naval Hospital Information for Providers at http://www.vnh. org/Providers.html   This site is part of the University of Iowa's health care site and is linked to a large set of databases that can be used by health care providers. The site covers a larger number of links to other sources on health care issues and problems. This is an excellent starting place to discover information on various common diseases and their treatments.

Dermatological Image Bank at http://medstat.med.utah.edu/kw/derm   If you need a dermatological image, this is your site. The site includes anatomy and physiology, a large database of images, a comprehensive set of references, and a bibliography.

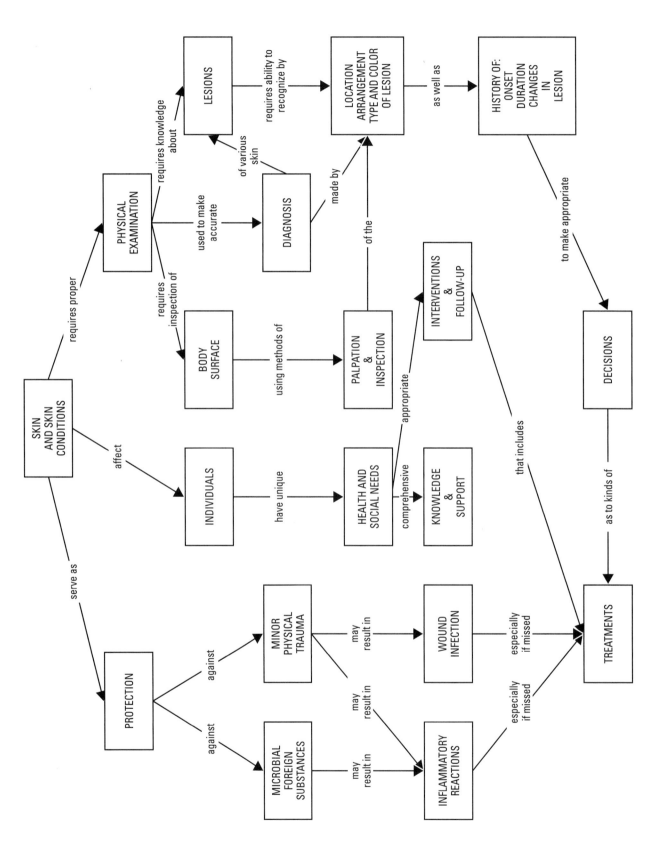

436

Concept Map 14-1

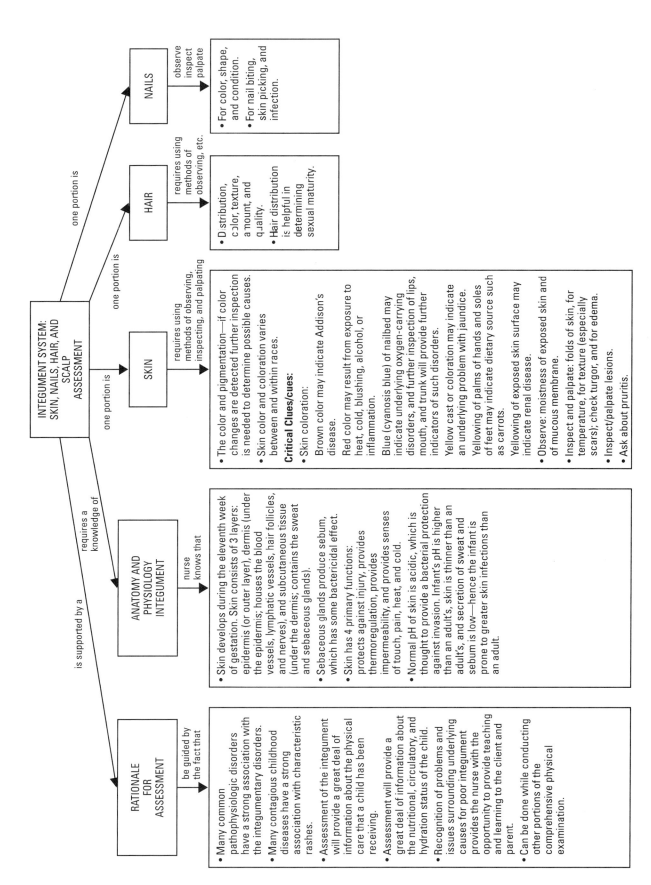

INTEGUMENT SYSTEM: SKIN, NAILS, HAIR, AND SCALP ASSESSMENT

one portion is → **NAILS** → observe inspect palpate
- For color, shape, and condition.
- For nail biting, skin picking, and infection.

one portion is → **HAIR** → requires using methods of observing, etc.
- Distribution, color, texture, amount, and quality.
- Hair distribution is helpful in determining sexual maturity.

one portion is → **SKIN** → requires using methods of observing, inspecting, and palpating

- The color and pigmentation—if color changes are detected further inspection is needed to determine possible causes.
- Skin color and coloration varies between and within races.

Critical Clues/cues:
- Skin coloration:

  Brown color may indicate Addison's disease.

  Red color may result from exposure to heat, cold, blushing, alcohol, or inflammation.

  Blue (cyanosis blue) of nailbed may indicate underlying oxygen-carrying disorders, and further inspection of lips, mouth, and trunk will provide further indicators of such disorders.

  Yellow cast or coloration may indicate an underlying problem with jaundice.

  Yellowing of palms of hands and soles of feet may indicate dietary source such as carrots.

  Yellowing of exposed skin surface may indicate renal disease.
- Observe: moistness of exposed skin and of mucous membrane.
- Inspect and palpate: folds of skin, for temperature, for texture (especially scars); check turgor, and for edema.
- Inspect/palpate lesions.
- Ask about pruritis.

is supported by a / requires a knowledge of → **ANATOMY AND PHYSIOLOGY INTEGUMENT** → nurse knows that

- Skin develops during the eleventh week of gestation. Skin consists of 3 layers: epidermis (or outer layer), dermis (under the epidermis; houses the blood vessels, lymphatic vessels, hair follicles, and nerves), and subcutaneous tissue (under the dermis; contains the sweat and sebaceous glands).
- Sebaceous glands produce sebum, which has some bactericidal effect.
- Skin has 4 primary functions: protects against injury, provides thermoregulation, provides impermeability, and provides senses of touch, pain, heat, and cold.
- Normal pH of skin is acidic, which is thought to provide a bacterial protection against invasion. Infant's pH is higher than an adult's, skin is thinner than an adult's, and secretion of sweat and sebum is low—hence the infant is prone to greater skin infections than an adult.

RATIONALE FOR ASSESSMENT → be guided by the fact that

- Many common pathophysiologic disorders have a strong association with the integumentary disorders.
- Many contagious childhood diseases have a strong association with characteristic rashes.
- Assessment of the integument will provide a great deal of information about the physical care that a child has been receiving.
- Assessment will provide a great deal of information about the nutritional, circulatory, and hydration status of the child.
- Recognition of problems and issues surrounding underlying causes for poor integument provides the nurse with the opportunity to provide teaching and learning to the client and parent.
- Can be done while conducting other portions of the comprehensive physical examination.

Concept Map 14-2

437

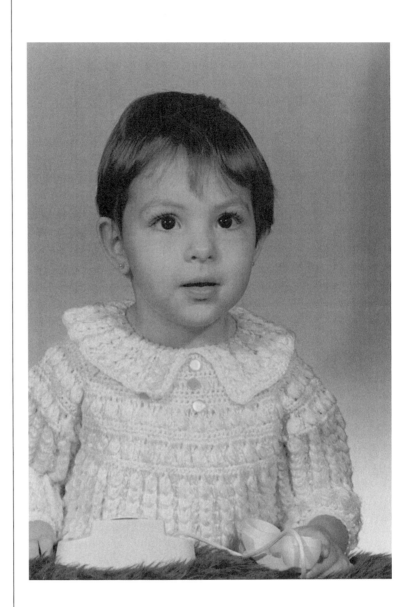

CHILDHOOD CANCERS

INTRODUCTION

The face of neoplastic disease has changed drastically in the last decade. It was once considered a fatal disease; today, the majority of children who contract cancer survive the disease and are able to grow and live a normal life. The big challenge for the nurse is the management of these children while they undergo treatment and adjust to the effects of the disease and the treatment.

Trauma is the leading killer of children. **Cancer**, though rare, is the second leading cause of death. Between birth and 15 years, there are an estimated 14 cases of cancer per 100,000 children per year, and 20 cases in 100,000 for adolescents between 15 and 19 years of age.

Leukemia is the most common malignancy in children and accounts for one-third of childhood cancers. Brain tumors are the next in frequency, and other malignancies, like neuroblastoma, Wilms' tumor (nephroblastoma), rhabdomyosarcoma, osteosarcoma, and Ewing sarcoma, may also occur. Embryonic tumors, which originate during intrauterine life, occur early in life and are usually diagnosed by age 5.

The warning signs of cancer in adults do not apply to children. Childhood cancers are extremely fast growing, with 80% metastasis at diagnosis. They are 10 to 25% more common in white children than black children. Carcinomas are rare in children because most are caused by long-term environmental exposure.

Causes are unknown, but host factors are helpful in identifying a child at risk. Congenital malformations with chromosome aberrations or single

Cancer. Uncontrolled growth of cells from the site of origin to distant sites; malignant growths.

Radiation. Process by which energy is propagated through space or matter.

gene defects and a positive family history are factors with tendencies for implicating cancer and leukemia in children. Prenatal exposure to some drugs, ionizing **radiation**, postnatal exposure to anabolic steroids, immuno-suppressive and cytoxic agents, and certain viruses are also implicated as environmental risk factors. Seventy percent of children with cancer are cured. Investigations into minimizing residual effects, finding less toxic treatments, and discovering genetic factors are continually being researched to help children with cancer. Cancer is viewed as a chronic disease, and the focus of treatment should be the quality of life.

$\mathcal{L}$YMPHOMAS

Lymphoma, the third most common type of cancer in children, is a malignancy of the lymphoid system. The most frequent origin is a lymph node in the neck, from which the cancer spreads to other organs of the body in weeks, months, or even years. In the United States, the annual incidence in children younger than 15 years is 4:1,000,000; 15% of all cases occur in children younger than 16 years of age; 60% occur between 10 and 16 years of age; and 3% in children younger than 5 years of age. It is more frequent in boys.

Hodgkin's Disease

The presence of multinucleated Reed-Sternberg cells confirms the diagnosis of Hodgkin's disease. It is divided into 4 pathologic-histologic types: (1) lymphocytic predominant, 10 to 20%; (2) mixed cellularity, 20 to 40%; (3) nodular sclerosing, 40 to 60%; and (4) lymphocytic depletion, 5 to 10%. Children with lymphocytic predominant and nodular sclerosing types have a better prognosis.

The most common symptom is painless cervical or supraclavicular adenopathy. It arises in the lymph nodes with variable growth rate; its size may grow over weeks or months. In pediatrics, lymphadenopathy is common, but an enlarged node greater than 2 cm in size, supraclavicular adenopathy, abnormal chest x-ray, and lymphadenopathy that increases in size after 2 weeks and is still unresolved in 4 to 8 weeks in the absence of infection in the region of the involved node warrants a biopsy. Unexplained fever of 38°C (100.4°F), night sweats, and 10% loss of normal body weight in 6 months are also significant symptoms in Hodgkin's disease.

Clinical staging and classification of the disease are based on physical assessment, clinical basis of history, and findings from diagnostic studies. Pathologic staging, laparotomy with multiple lymph node samplings, splenectomy, and liver biopsy may follow to confirm diagnosis. A blood count may show anemia, neutrophilia, eosinophilia, and thrombocytosis. An elevation in ESR (erythrocyte sedimentation rate) is also seen.

Therapy is multidisciplinary, involving the pediatric oncologist and radiation oncologist, diagnostic radiologist, pathologist, pediatric surgeon, pediatrician, and the nurse. **Combination chemotherapy,** like MOPP (mechlorethamine, Oncovin [vincristine], procarbazine, and prednisone) and ABVD (Adriamycin [doxorubicin], bleomycin, vinblastine, and dacarbazine), and **radiation therapy** are usually effective. With treatment, children in stages I and II have a 90% disease-free survival rate 5 years from diagnosis. Two-thirds of relapses occur within 2 years after diagnosis. With relapsed Hodgkin's disease, combination chemotherapy and radiation are used with autologous or allogenic **bone marrow transplantation** as an alternative.

A late effect of Hodgkin's disease secondary to therapy is a second malignant neoplasm. Acute myelogenous leukemia may occur in 4% of patients. Soft tissue and bone growth impairment from radiation, and hypothyroidism in more than two-thirds of children younger than 6 years may occur as consequences of mantle irradiation. Irradiation may also induce infertility and cardiopulmonary complications.

Nursing management includes educating and preparing the parents and the patient for therapeutic and diagnostic procedures and side effects of the treatment. The family should have a clear explanation of why each test is being performed, and of the seriousness of the diagnosis. Parents are always anxious when their child is undergoing any kind of procedure. It is most important that the nurse explain the procedure to the parents and the time that each procedure takes, to tell parents the truth about each procedure, and to be near in order to answer their questions. Side effects of radiotherapy or **chemotherapy** include stomatitis, alopecia, nausea and vomiting, diarrhea, constipation, and fatigue. Nurses are also responsible for emotional support and counseling, and discussing with adolescents their fears and beliefs about sexual functioning to help reduce the fear of sterility.

Combination chemotherapy. A combination of drugs used in the treatment of a disease; the application of chemical reagents that have a specific toxic effect upon the disease-causing microorganism.

Radiation therapy. A treatment that utilizes ionizing radiation.

Bone marrow transplantation. The replacement of a patient's destroyed marrow from a donor marrow. After graftment, donor marrow should produce functioning cells that are nonmalignant.

Chemotherapy. Treatment that involves substances taken orally or intravenously to combat cancer.

Non-Hodgkin's Lymphoma

Non-Hodgkin's lymphoma (NHL) is a group of solid tumors from any of the lymphatic tissues. The malignant cells are widespread, with diffused infiltration pattern, and poorly differentiated, with faster and frequent dissemination that may involve the mediastinum or the meninges. NHL constitutes 7 to 13% of malignancies in children younger than age 15 in North America, with 390 new cases seen yearly in the United States. Incidence increases with age; children 15 years old or younger account for only 3%, and it is uncommon in children younger than 5 years. There is a marked male predominance with a ratio of 3:1. The risk of developing non-Hodgkin's lymphoma is increased in children with severe combined immunodeficiency syndrome—HIV, Wiskott-Aldrich syndrome, X-linked lymphoproliferative syndrome, and immunosuppressive therapy, post bone marrow therapy, or solid organ transplants. Epstein-Barr virus has been implicated in the pathogenesis of Burkitt's lymphoma in Africa, but is vaguely linked in North America.

Non-Hodgkin's lymphoma is classified by the pattern of histologic presentation. The three major histologic classifications are lymphoblastic lymphoma, small noncleaved cell lymphoma (endemic or sporadic Burkitt's lymphoma), and large cell lymphoma. The origins of this cancer can be clarified and aid in histologic classification by cell membrane markers. Small noncleaved cell lymphomas have the B-cell phenotype; lymphoblastic lymphomas have T-cell surface markers; and large cell lymphomas may show either T or B cells. The clinical staging of NHL is given in Table 15-1.

Signs and symptoms may arise from any site of the lymphoid tissue, including Waldeyer's ring, Peyer's patches, thymus, liver, and spleen. They may also involve extralymphatic sites including bone, bone marrow, skin, testes, and the central nervous system (CNS). The symptoms are brief and depend on the anatomic site and extent of involvement. The lymphoid tumors may present airway obstruction, cranial nerve palsies, or spinal paralysis. Cough, dyspnea, orthopnea, or superior vena cava obstruction symptoms like facial edema, venous engorgement, plethora, and chemosis may present as symptoms with mediastinal disease. Metastasis to the bone marrow or central nervous system, on the other hand, may have the clinical manifestations typical of leukemia. Burkitt's lymphoma, which is typical in parts of Africa but rare in the United States, is a fast-growing neoplasm in the orbit, abdomen, or jaw. Noncleaved cell lymphomas present with abdominal pain, right lower quadrant mass, abdominal distention, and in children older than 5, intussusception. With abdominal disease, children may experience metabolic abnormalities, impaired renal function, urinary obstruction, and urate nephropathy.

In most children, NHL exists with widespread disease; biopsy with histopathologic examination, cytogenetic studies, and immunophenotyping are required to confirm the diagnosis. A complete blood count (CBC), liver and renal function tests, biochemistry panel (BCP) 7, and a thorough physical exam should also be done. Bone marrow aspiration,

✸

TABLE 15-1

STAGING SYSTEM FOR NON-HODGKIN'S LYMPHOMA

Stage	Identifiers
Stage I	Single tumor at a single site
Stage II	Single tumor with regional involvement on same side of abdomen
Stage III	Tumor on both sides of abdomen; also, all primary thoracic, intraabdominal, and paraspinal or epidural tumors
Stage IV	Any of the involvements in stages I and II, with central nervous system and/or bone marrow involvement

Source: Wong, D., and Whaley, D. *Whaley & Wong's Nursing Care of Infants and Children.* 5th ed. St. Louis: Mosby, 1991, p. 1693.

surgical biopsy, radiological studies, lumbar puncture, and computed tomography (CT) scans of the lungs and gastrointestinal organs also aid in diagnostic evaluation.

Therapeutic management includes aggressive irradiation and chemotherapy for 6 to 24 months. Children with lymphoblastic leukemia usually are given the LSA2-L2 protocol, which includes cyclophosphamide, intrathecal methotrexate, vincristine, prednisone, daunorubicin, 6-thioguanine, BCNU, cytosine arabinoside, and L-asparaginase. Nonlymphoblastic lymphoma is treated with cyclophosphamide and intermediate or high-dose methotrexate. Central nervous system **prophylaxis** with cranial radiation and combination intratracheal chemotherapy is also administered. Nursing management is focused on managing the side effects of the chemotherapy protocol.

Prophylaxis. Observance of rules necessary to prevent disease.

With localized disease, 90% of patients are long-term disease free. Patients with metastasis to the diaphragm, bone marrow, and CNS involvement with a primary site have a 70 to 80% failure-free survival rate.

Neuroblastoma

A neuroblastoma is a tumor arising from the neural crest tissue of the sympathetic ganglia or adrenal medulla, with the majority from the adrenal gland or retroperitoneal sympathetic chain. It occurs early in childhood, with 50% of the cases diagnosed in the first 2 years, and 90% before age 5, with a higher incidence in males. Neuroblastoma is the most common solid neoplasm outside the central nervous system and accounts for 7 to 10% of pediatric malignancies. Primary sites are usually seen in the abdomen, but the head, neck, chest, or pelvis may also be affected.

Signs and symptoms depend on the primary site and stage. Many children present with fever, weight loss, and irritability. Cervical and supraclavicular adenopathy may be an early presenting sign. Children older than 1 year may also report bone pain. A firm, fixed, irregular mass beyond the midline may also be palpated. Supraorbital ecchymosis, periorbital edema, may be seen in distant metastasis.

Locating the primary site and the extent of metastasis is the focus of diagnostic evaluation. Skull, neck, abdominal, chest, and bone CT scans with bone marrow tests may be utilized to locate the tumor. Intravenous pyelogram is effective in diagnosing adrenal neuroblastoma. Urinary catecholamines like vanillylmandelic acid (VMA), homovanillic acid (HVA), dopamine, and norepinephrine are elevated in 90% of patients at diagnosis. Lactate dehydrogenase (LDH) and ferritin may also be elevated at diagnosis. When the bone marrow is infiltrated, anemia and thrombocytosis maybe present.

The staging of neuroblastoma is given in Table 15-2.

Neuroblastoma is also termed the "silent tumor" because more than 70% of cases occur after metastasis. Non-primary-site involvement like the lymph nodes, bone marrow, skeletal system, liver, or skin are the origin of

⬙

TABLE 15-2

THE INTERNATIONAL NEUROBLASTOMA STAGING SYSTEM

Stage	Identifiers
Stage I	Localized tumor confined to the areas of origin, complete gross excision, with or without microscopic residual disease; identifiable lymph nodes negative microscopically.
Stage II	Unilateral tumor with incomplete gross excision; identifiable lymph nodes negative microscopically.
Stage III	Unilateral tumor with complete or incomplete gross excision; with positive ipsilateral regional lymph nodes; identifiable contralateral lymph nodes negative microscopically.
Stage IV	Dissemination of the tumor to distant lymph nodes, bone, bone marrow, liver, or other organs (except as defined in stage IVS).
Stage IVS	Localized primary tumor as defined for stages 1 or 2 with dissemination limited to liver, skin, or bone marrow.

Source: Wong, D., and Whaley, D. *Whaley & Wong's Nursing Care of Infants and Children.* 5th ed. St. Louis: Mosby, 1991, p. 1166.

the initial system. Prognosis is poor and depends on the age and the stage of the disease at diagnosis. Therapy involves surgery, chemotherapy, and radiotherapy. Cyclophosphamide, doxorubicin, etoposide, cisplatin, and vincristine are some of the active chemotherapeutic agents used and 80% of patients with this treatment achieve partial or complete remission. Surgical resection irradiation is used to remove large tumors in stages I and II.

Nursing care includes psychological and physical preparation for operative and diagnostic procedures, education and explanation of radiotherapy and chemotherapy, with side effects and prevention of postoperative thoracic, cranial, or abdominal surgery complications. This is a life-threatening disease with a high degree of metastasis at the time of diagnosis. Parents often suffer guilt, which is expressed as anger toward themselves or the professionals for not recognizing the symptoms earlier. The nurse should initiate support in coping with the disease, and also refer these families for counseling.

𝒲ILMS' TUMOR

Wilms' tumor (nephroblastoma) is the most common type of renal cancer. It occurs in 1 per 200,000 to 250,000 children; there are approximately 460 new cases annually in the United States, with peak incidence at age 3. It arises from the kidney and is composed of blastema, epithelium, and stroma. Aniridia, hemihypertrophy, hypospadias, cryptorchidism, and ambiguous genitalia are congenital anomalies that are implicated for the disease. Mental and growth retardation, microcephaly, pinna deformities, and pigmented and vascular nevi are also associated with Wilms' tumor.

Asymptomatic swelling or mass accounts for 83% of the most common presenting signs, with the mass confined to one side, firm, nontender, and deep within the flank. Fever, hematuria, anemia, anorexia, lethargy, hypertension from increased secretion of renin, genitourinary malformations, aniridia, and hemihypertrophy may also be reported. Metastasis to the lungs may manifest with symptoms of cough, shortness of breath, chest pain, and dyspnea.

Normal CBC, blood urea nitrogen (BUN), and serum creatinine are seen and urinalysis is positive for blood or leukocytes. A physical examination with emphasis on liver and spleen size, anemia indications, lymphadenopathy, and family history are the key to diagnosis. Specific tests like computed tomography (CT), intravenous pyelogram (IVP), hematologic and biochemical studies, and urinalysis are also done.

The histology of the tumor cells identifies them as belonging to one of two groups: favorable histology (FH) or unfavorable histology (UH). The latter accounts for only 12% of the disease, with a poorer prognosis and requiring a more aggressive treatment.

The staging of Wilms' tumor is noted in Table 15-3.

Surgical laparotomy of the abdomen is the initial treatment. There can also be radiation and chemotherapy with or without radiation, depending on the histological pattern and clinical stage of the disease. Vincristine and dactinomycin are used in all patients and doxorubicin is used in patients in stages III and IV. Chemotherapy is usually initiated within 5 days postsurgery and radiotherapy within 10 days.

❧

TABLE 15-3

STAGING CLASSIFICATIONS FOR WILMS' TUMOR

Stage	Identifiers
Stage I	Tumor limited to the kidney and completely excised.
Stage II	Tumor extends beyond the kidney but is completely excised. There is no residual tumor beyond the margins of excision.
Stage III	Residual nonhematogenous tumor confined to the abdomen. a. Lymph nodes are found to be involved. b. Diffuse peritoneal contamination by tumor. c. Peritoneal implants are found. d. Tumor beyond surgical margins (microscopic or gross). e. Unresectable tumor infiltrating into vital structures.
Stage IV	Hematogenous metastases; deposits are beyond stage III, namely, to lung, liver, bone, and brain.
Stage V	Bilateral renal involvement is present at diagnosis.

Source: Wong, D., and Whaley, D. *Whaley & Wong's Nursing Care of Infants and Children.* 5th ed. St. Louis: Mosby, 1991, p. 1167.

Nursing care is similar to that for other cancers with surgery: irradiation and chemotherapy. Preoperative and postoperative care emphasizes preventing trauma to the site and reinforcing familial support. Play therapy with puppets or dolls and drawing illustrations are helpful in dealing with the different procedures. Precautions should be taken to prevent injury to the kidney and contact sports should be avoided. Proper hygiene, adequate fluid intake to prevent urinary tract infections, and the importance of quick detection of genitourinary signs and symptoms are mandated.

$\mathcal{B}$ONE CANCERS

Bone cancers represent less than 1% of all malignant neoplasms, with osteosarcoma accounting for 60% of the cases. They are seen primarily in adolescents and young adults. Ewing's sarcoma is the second most frequent. Both are seen predominantly in males.

Bone cancers arise from any tissues involved in bone growth: the osteoid matrix, bone marrow elements, blood and lymph vessels, nerve sheaths, fat, and cartilage. The cardinal signs are localized severe or dull pains at the affected site after slight trauma. Mass formation and fracture through area cortical bone destruction are also implicated. Often, pain is relieved by a flexed position. Limping and the inability to bear weight and hold heavy objects are also signs that necessitate further evaluation.

Diagnosis is confirmed by radiologic studies, CT scan, radioisotope bone scans to evaluate metastasis, and bone biopsy to determine histologic pattern. Lung tomography is also mandated since pulmonary metastasis is the most common complication of bone tumors.

Osteosarcoma

Osteosarcoma arises, presumably, from the bone-forming mesenchyme that produces malignant osteoid tissue. The metaphysis of long bones in the lower extremities, the femur, humerus, tibia, pelvis, and phalanges are some of the growth sites. The traditional approach for treatment is surgical resection and amputation, depending on the affected area. Amputation of the affected area is at least 3 inches above the proximal tumor margin or joint proximal to the involved bone. Massive chemotherapy is then utilized. Antineoplastic drugs like methotrexate with citrovorum factor rescue, Adriamycin, actinomycin, bleomycin, cyclophosphamide, and cisplatin may be administered alone or in any combination pre- or postsurgery.

Nursing care depends on the type of surgery. Amputation has an overwhelming impact on the patient and the family, so straightforward honesty is essential. The nurse must think of the amputated limb as a loss for which the patient will grieve deeply; therefore, introduction of procedures and prostheses to the amputees and their parents should occur prior to surgery.

In addition, the nurse can aid in emotional support by being the sounding board for the fears and concerns of both the patient and the family.

The need for chemotherapy and the side effects of the drugs should also be explained. Since most patients are adolescents and young adults, radical body alterations can occur, such as hair loss, and encouraging the patient to shop for wigs prior to the surgery is helpful. The nurse also works with the physical therapist to help the patient with utilizing and maintaining prosthetic devices. Phantom limb pain is common after amputation and is manifested by tingling, itching, and pain in the amputated leg. Amitriptyline (Elavil) is used to help ease the pain. Early discharge planning is essential. The nurse should work with the physical therapists in evaluating the child's physical and emotional needs. The role of the nurse is to promote normalcy and to help the child regain realistic daily living activities with the use of wheelchairs and crutches. Accessibility with regard to environmental barriers should be discussed. Selecting clothing that best camouflages the prosthesis encourages the child to regain a feeling of self-identity.

Ewing Sarcoma

Ewing sarcoma arises in the marrow spaces of the bone. It originates in the shaft of long and trunk bones, including the humerus, ulna, fibula, tibia, vertebra, ribs, scapula, pelvic bones, and skull. It usually occurs between ages 4 and 25.

The treatment of choice is intensive irradiation combined with chemotherapy. The most widely used drugs are actinomycin D, vincristine, cyclophosphamide, and Adriamycin. Since this type of bone cancer does not require amputation, psychological adjustment is less traumatic to the patient and the family. Chemotherapy causes hair loss, peripheral neuropathy, nausea and vomiting, and possible cardiotoxicity. The aim of nursing care should be to help alleviate these symptoms and to maximize the resumption of normal lifestyle and activities.

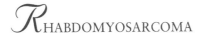

RHABDOMYOSARCOMA

Rhabdomyosarcoma (*rhabdo* meaning striated; *myo*, muscle) is the fourth most common solid tumor in children. It originates from the tendons, bursae, fascia, fibrous, connective, lymphatic, or vascular tissue or from undifferentiated mesenchymal cells in the body. Since the body is composed of multiple skeletal muscles, the tumor may arise at any site and may occur in all age groups. Incidence is higher in white children: 4.4 million per year younger than 15, and 1.3 million for black children in the same group. The four subtypes of rhabdomyosarcoma in order of the most common type are: (1) embryonal, found in the neck, abdomen, head, and genitourinary tract;

(2) alveolar, seen in the trunk and the deep tissues; (3) botryoid, which appears as clusters of grapelike polyps found in the ear, nasopharynx, vagina, and urinary bladder; and (4) pleomorphic, the rarest form, which usually occurs in the trunk and the soft parts of the extremities.

Diagnosis is difficult and sometimes requires immunocytochemistry, electron microscopy, and chromosomal analysis. A plain CT scan and MRI can be used to assess the extent of the primary tumor; and chest x-ray, lung mammograms, bone marrow aspiration, bone surveys, and lung tomograms are utilized to rule out metastasis. For head and neck tumors, a lumbar puncture is performed, and an excisional biopsy is done to confirm histologic type.

For planning, treatment, and prognosis, staging plays a major role. Staging is noted in Table 15-4.

Rhabdomyosarcoma is highly malignant and metastasis frequently occurs with diagnosis. A combined modality of chemotherapy and radiation is the treatment of choice. However, removal of the primary tumor is recommended when possible. In areas like those of the orbit, biopsy is only required when followed by chemotherapy and radiation. For chemotherapy, vincristine, actinomycin D, and cyclophosphamide with or without Adriamycin for 1 to 2 years are used, depending on the stage of the disease. Irradiations in high doses are recommended except for stage I tumors.

Nursing care and responsibilities are similar to those for other types of solid tumor cancers: careful assessment for signs of tumor, preparation for multiple diagnostic tests, pre-, intra-, and postsurgery, and supportive care through all stages of the disease and course of treatment.

There is a 93% 3-year disease-free survival rate with localized disease in a favorable site. Poor prognosis is noted in children classified in stage IV.

🐾

TABLE 15-4

THE INTERGROUP RHABDOMYOSARCOMA STUDY
CLINICAL GROUPING SYSTEM

Stage	Identifiers
Stage I	1. Localized, completely resected, confined to site of origin
	2. Localized, completely resected, infiltrated beyond site of origin
Stage II	1. Localized, grossly resected, microscopic residual
	2. Regional disease, involved lymph nodes, completely resected
Stage III	1. Local or regional grossly visible disease after biopsy only
	2. Grossly visible disease after ≥50% resection of primary tumor
Stage IV	Distant metastasis present at diagnosis

Source: Wong, D., and Whaley, D. *Whaley & Wong's Nursing Care of Infants and Children.* 5th ed. St. Louis: Mosby, 1991, p. 1171.

Summary

This chapter encompasses overall information concerning the survival rates of children from cancer. The most common malignancies in pediatrics and their treatments are discussed, including chemotherapeutic agents, signs and symptoms associated with pediatric malignancies, important nursing interventions during the diagnostic phase, nursing actions to support the child and the family during diagnostic treatment and recuperation, the treatment at the hospital and at home, and the use of nursing interventions to ameliorate or modify the problems that this disease brings. Each nursing intervention provides an opportunity for the nurse to synthesize and apply information on the nursing care of children with cancer, identify the procedures and tests associated with diagnostic procedures, and assist with interventions to modify the devastating outcomes of this diagnosis. It will also help the nurse to identify the major concerns for survivors of cancer; and, therefore, to apply the observed outcomes of care in evaluating the most useful nursing interventions.

Critical Points in Managing Cancer in Children

More than 8000 children are diagnosed with cancer each year in the United States. Of the 8000, more than 70% survive the disease if treated properly. Leukemia is the most common type of cancer in children. Second to this are brain tumors, which are more commonly seen in boys than in girls. The cause of childhood cancer is still unknown. The nurse working with these children needs to be aware of the complexity of the disease and its management, as well as the threat that this diagnosis brings to the life of the family and the child.

The role of the pediatric nurse in the management of the child with a diagnosis of cancer is to facilitate the transfer of the child to a pediatric cancer center. Since the initial history and physical exam are done on the pediatric floor of the hospital, the nurse must procure a complete history, including family history, developmental history, and psychosocial history. The physical exam ought to be head to toe, including all the laboratory findings that were done prior to transfer to the cancer center.

Nurses need to be aware that children with cancer have to deal not only with the disease, but also with the developmental delays caused by restrictive nutrition and restrictions in socialization. The number one problem faced by the families of children with cancer is the results from the decisions that the parents have to make while undergoing the most devastating experience in their lives. Many families decide to move their child to a medical center away from home. Later on these families are faced with a terrible economic burden and are without support. Others disengage from their spouses and end up in divorce after the child dies. The reality is that at the most critical point in their lives, these families only need to be told that any decision they make is the best and that the medical team is there to guide them and help them. Because cure is not certain, the nurse must focus on the care of the child and teaching the child and the family. In focusing on care of the child with cancer, the main goal of the nurse is to minimize the side effects of the treatment and of the disease, to maximize the child's strengths, such as psychological and cognitive, to his/her maximum potential. Children and families often harbor misconceptions regarding medical procedures, which can become a large obstacle in the management of the child's care. It is important that the nurse explain all procedures to the child with deference to his/her level of cognitive development, and to the family, according to their level of understanding.

The diagnosis of cancer brings with it fear, anxiety, hope, prayers, anger, guilt, and despair, but never acceptance or resolution. Therefore, attachment, self-concept, and religion play an important role in the adherence to treatment regimens. With regard to education, the primary goal of the nurse is to help prepare children in the development of self-care behaviors and also in the development of self-confidence in dealing with health care providers.

The most sensitive care that the nurse needs to prepare for is the reality that some of these children will die. Children do not deal well with separation, yet at this young age many are faced with the reality that they will be separated from their homes and parents forever. If seen from the child's perspective the process of preparing the child for the ultimate separation needs to be done according to his/her age and cognitive development. From the side of the parent, there is never a time that any parents are really ready to relinquish their child. The pain and devastation that the death of the child brings to families and to the medical staff are never resolved. The most that one can hope is that, as a professional, the nurse has the wisdom to facilitate this process with efficiency and with empathy.

QUESTIONS

Diagnosis: Hodgkin's Disease

History: Violeta, a 17-year-old with no significant past medical history, is diagnosed with stage II Hodgkin's disease. She has lymphadenopathy in the cervical and supraclavicular area with metastasis to the spleen.

Plan: Chemotherapy and radiation therapy.

Nursing problems: Side effects of chemotherapy. Immobility, fatigue related to radiation, and chemotherapy. Body image disturbance. Fear related to diagnosis and prognosis. Altered family process.

1. The most common finding in Hodgkin's disease is:

    A. Painful, enlarged, soft, tender, immovable node in the axillary area.
    B. Enlarged, firm, nontender, movable node in the supraclavicular area.
    C. Immovable, painful, firm node in the postcervical chain.
    D. Nontender, movable node in the occipital area.

2. Which of these histologic types, found in biopsy, confirms a positive diagnosis of Hodgkin's disease?

    A. Reed-Sternberg cell
    B. T cells
    C. B cells
    D. Stem cells

3. The most common side effects of chemotherapy include:

    A. Constipation, edema, bloating
    B. Nausea, vomiting, anorexia
    C. Diarrhea, fever, constipation
    D. Dry hair, seborrhea, conjunctivitis

4. The most common concern of adolescents about irradiation and chemotherapy is:

    A. Increased libido
    B. Dysmenorrhea
    C. Infertility
    D. Altered sexual function

Diagnosis: Wilms' Tumor

History: Nicholas was born with cryptorchidism. He is now 3 years old and losing weight. Upon physical assessment, a mass is found in his abdomen. He had radiographic studies and intravenous pyelogram and urinalysis. A diagnosis of Wilms' tumor was made.

Plan: Nicholas is admitted to the hospital to undergo surgery to remove one of his kidneys.

Nursing problems: Teaching about diagnostic tests, surgery. Support for the family. Anticipatory guidance postoperation.

1. The most common presenting sign of Wilms' tumor is:

    A. Fever, anemia
    B. Hematuria
    C. Firm, nontender mass confined to one side deep within the flank
    D. Movable, tender mass on the mid-axillary area

2. Nicholas is scheduled for surgery. The nurse explains to his parents that:

    A. The surgery is scheduled before school age.
    B. Surgery is scheduled within 24–48 hours.
    C. Nicholas will need emergency surgery.
    D. Not to worry, there will be no complications.

3. Postoperatively, Nicholas's tumor was stage II, but it was completely resected. After a few days, he is sent home. The best teaching for home care is:

A. Keep the child on bed rest.
B. Limit fluid intake.
C. Avoid contact sports that have high risk for injury.
D. Monitor for signs of urinary tract infection.

Diagnosis: Osteosarcoma

History: Roger, a 13-year-old, is in the clinic for his annual physical. He complains of pain in his upper leg, which was hit by a ball a few months ago. He is a varsity soccer player at school. He also has a positive family history of cancer. He is diagnosed with osteosarcoma.
Plan: Roger is to have his leg amputated, followed by chemotherapy.
Nursing problems: Grieving from loss of leg. Fear/anxiety, coping with new lifestyle. Body image alteration. Acceptance. Use of prosthetic devices.

1. After surgery, Roger is complaining of pain in the amputated leg. The nurse tells him and his parents that this common symptom is phantom limb pain. Phantom limb pain is:

A. Sensations of tingling, pain, and itching in the amputated leg.
B. Pain in the unaffected extremity.
C. Tingling sensation in the other extremity.
D. Psychosomatic pain.

2. Roger is to wear prosthetics. To assist him to maintain a positive body image, the nurse should:

A. Discourage him from going out.
B. Tell him to wear makeup so emphasis will be on his face.
C. Encourage long pants to camouflage the prosthesis.
D. Encourage the use of short pants.

3. A lung tomography is ordered after surgery, and Roger's parents are asking what the purpose of the test is. The nurse's best response is:

A. "The most common complication of bone tumor is lung metastasis."
B. "This is standard procedure."
C. "To test the lungs' capacity."
D. "Ask the doctor; he will tell you."

$\mathcal{A}$NSWERS

Hodgkin's Disease

1. *B.* The most common finding is an enlarged, nonpainful, firm, nontender, movable node in the supraclavicular area.

2. *A.* Reed-Sternberg cell is positive in the Hodgkin's histologic exam. The B and T cells are found in non-Hodgkin's disease.

3. *B.* Nausea and vomiting are the most common side effects of chemotherapy.

4. *C.* Irradiation and chemotherapy may cause infertility.

Wilms' tumor

1. *C.* Firm, nontender mass deep within the flank is the most common sign.

2. *B.* Surgery should be 24–48 hours after diagnosis of Wilms' tumor and should not be delayed.

3. *C.* The site should be protected from any trauma.

Osteosarcoma

1. *A.* Phantom pain is common. It is described as sensations of tingling, pain, and itching in the lost leg.

2. *C.* Encouraging Roger to camouflage his prosthesis would help his body image.

3. *A.* The most common complication in primary bone tumors is lung metastasis.

$\mathcal{G}$LOSSARY

bone marrow transplantation   the replacement of a patient's destroyed marrow from a donor marrow. After graftment, donor marrow should produce functioning cells that are nonmalignant.

cancer   uncontrolled growth of cells from the site of origin to distant sites; malignant growths.

chemotherapy   treatment that involves substances taken orally or intravenously to combat cancer.

combination chemotherapy   a combination of drugs used in the treatment of a disease; the application of chemical reagents that have a specific toxic effect upon the disease-causing microorganism.

prophylaxis   observance of rules necessary to prevent disease.

radiation   process by which energy is propagated through space or matter.

radiation therapy   a treatment that utilizes ionizing radiation.

$\mathscr{B}$IBLIOGRAPHY

Wong, D., and Whaley, D. *Whaley & Wong's Nursing Care of Infants and Children.* 5th ed. St. Louis: Mosby, 1991.

$\mathscr{H}$ELPFUL INTERNET SITES

The Association of Pediatric Oncology Nurses at http://www.apon.org The Association of Pediatric Oncology Nurses (APON) is the leading professional organization for registered nurses caring for children and adolescents with cancer and their families.

Pediatric Oncology Branch of the National Cancer Institute at http://www-dcs.nci.nih.gov/pedonc This Web site has a wealth of information and a large number of links for those interested in pediatric oncology issues and research.

International Journal of Pediatric Hematology and Oncology at http://www.biomednet.com One can log-in as a "visitor" (password: biomednet) to view abstracts. Members can view the full text of this and other publications. To fully use this site you need to become a member, which requires paying a subscription fee.

PEDINFO: An Index of the Pediatric Internet at http://www.pedinfo. org This is an excellent site that covers nearly all topics within this review. It has a wealth of information and is worth a visit. It is written for health care professionals but others could also use the information.

Project Decide at http://www2.allina.com/hnf/community.nsf/decide? OpenView This site concerns "Project Decide," which encompasses current issues of death and dying, from a seven-year Harvard study on the issues.

A Starting Point—University of Miami School of Medicine Web Site— Pediatric Neuro-Oncology at http://www.med.miami.edu/neurosurgery/ start_intro.htm A starting place for parents and health care professionals to find out about issues and research surrounding pediatric neuro-oncology.

Clinical Cancer Information from PDQ at http://cancernet.nci.nih.gov/ clinpdq/clinpdq.html This site is dedicated to providing clinical cancer information and is maintained by the National Institute of Health as part of "cancernet."

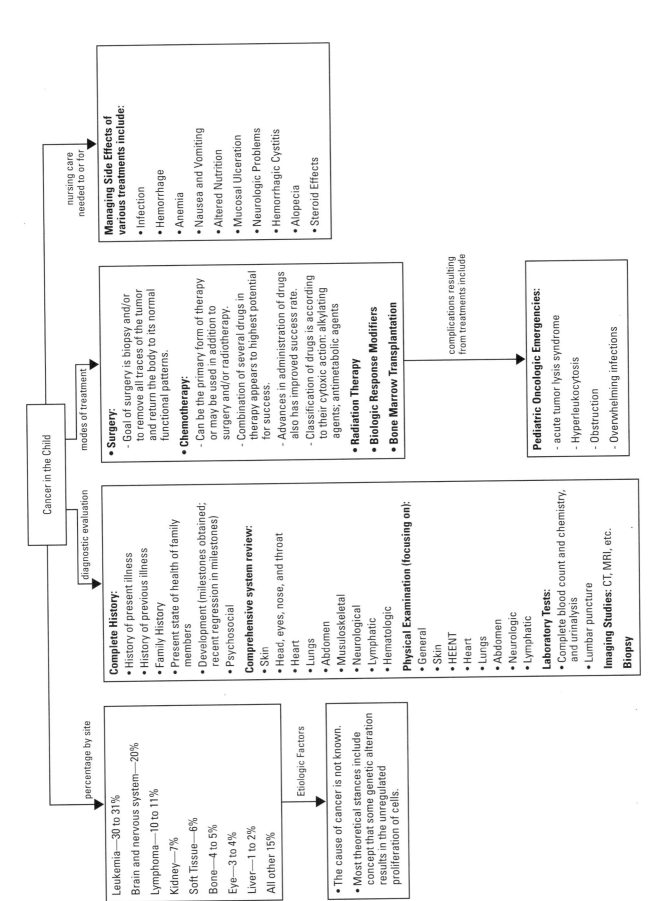

Cancer in the Child

percentage by site

Leukemia—30 to 31%
Brain and nervous system—20%
Lymphoma—10 to 11%
Kidney—7%
Soft Tissue—6%
Bone—4 to 5%
Eye—3 to 4%
Liver—1 to 2%
All other 15%

Etiologic Factors

• The cause of cancer is not known.
• Most theoretical stances include concept that some genetic alteration results in the unregulated proliferation of cells.

diagnostic evaluation

Complete History:
• History of present illness
• History of previous illness
• Family History
• Present state of health of family members
• Development (milestones obtained; recent regression in milestones)
• Psychosocial

Comprehensive system review:
• Skin
• Head, eyes, nose, and throat
• Heart
• Lungs
• Abdomen
• Musuloskeletal
• Neurological
• Lymphatic
• Hematologic

Physical Examination (focusing on):
• General
• Skin
• HEENT
• Heart
• Lungs
• Abdomen
• Neurologic
• Lymphatic

Laboratory Tests:
• Complete blood count and chemistry, and urinalysis
• Lumbar puncture

Imaging Studies: CT, MRI, etc.

Biopsy

modes of treatment

• **Surgery:**
  - Goal of surgery is biopsy and/or to remove all traces of the tumor and return the body to its normal functional patterns.
• **Chemotherapy:**
  - Can be the primary form of therapy or may be used in addition to surgery and/or radiotherapy.
  - Combination of several drugs in therapy appears to highest potential for success.
  - Advances in administration of drugs also has improved success rate.
  - Classification of drugs is according to their cytoxic action: alkylating agents; antimetabolic agents
• **Radiation Therapy**
• **Biologic Response Modifiers**
• **Bone Marrow Transplantation**

complications resulting from treatments include

Pediatric Oncologic Emergencies:
- acute tumor lysis syndrome
- Hyperleukocytosis
- Obstruction
- Overwhelming infections

nursing care needed to or for

Managing Side Effects of various treatments include:
• Infection
• Hemorrhage
• Anemia
• Nausea and Vomiting
• Altered Nutrition
• Mucosal Ulceration
• Neurologic Problems
• Hemorrhagic Cystitis
• Alopecia
• Steroid Effects

Concept Map 15-1

455

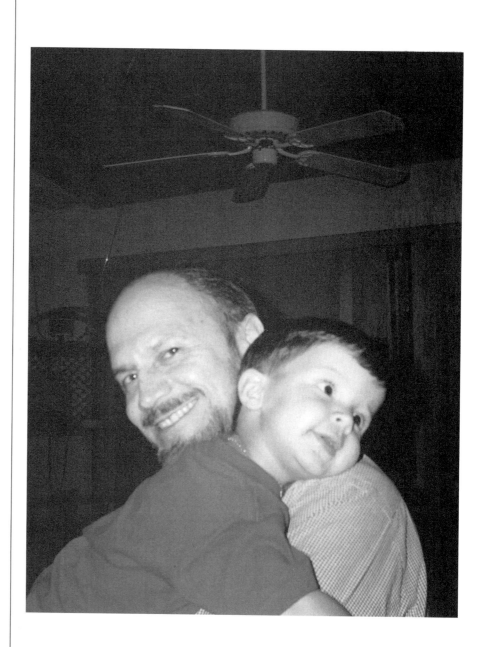

⚙

ℳETABOLIC DISORDERS

𝒥NTRODUCTION

The endocrine system controls or regulates metabolic processes, governing energy production, growth, fluid and electrolyte balance, response to stress, and sexual production. Hormones are released by endocrine glands into the bloodstream and carried to responsive or target tissue: another endocrine gland, an organ, or a tissue. The regulation of hormonal secretion is based on negative feedback. As a general rule, endocrine glands have a tendency to oversecrete their particular hormones. However, once the physiologic effect of the hormone has been achieved, this information is transmitted to the producing gland, inhibiting further secretion. If the gland undersecretes, the inhibition is relieved, and the gland increases production of the hormone. As a result, the hormone is secreted according to the amount needed.

The endocrine gland is primarily responsible for the stimulation and the inhibition of target glandular secretions in the anterior pituitary gland. Tropic hormones, secreted by the anterior pituitary, regulate the secretion of hormones from various target organs. As blood concentrations of the target hormones reach normal levels, a negative message is sent to the anterior pituitary to inhibit release of tropic hormones. The pituitary gland, in turn, is controlled by either hormonal or neuronal signals from the hypothalamus, alternately releasing and inhibiting hormones, which then stimulate the secretion of tropic hormones by the anterior pituitary. The central nervous system, by means of neural impulses, stimulates the hypothalamus to manufacture and secrete inhibitory hormones. These glands function interdependently; therefore, any malfunction affects the entire system.

Endocrine dysfunction may result because of an intrinsic defect in the target gland (primary) or because of diminished or elevated tropic hormones (secondary). Endocrine problems occur from hypofunctioning or hyperfunctioning of the glands.

$\mathcal{H}$YPOTHYROIDISM

Congenital hypothyroidism. A condition caused by deficiency of the thyroid secretion, resulting in a lowered basal metabolism. A lesser degree of cretinism.

Thyroid gland. A gland of internal secretion, which acts to control metabolic functions, located in the base of the neck on both sides of the lower part of the larynx and upper part of the trachea.

Hypothyroidism results from a deficient production of thyroid hormones, causing insufficient levels of the hormone available to maintain normal intracellular levels. Hypothyroidism is the most common thyroid illness. Hypothyroidism has a congenital variant and an acquired type. **Congenital hypothyroidism** (cretinism) is the irreversible failure of the **thyroid gland,** usually from the failure of the gland's migration during fetal development; it is also called permanent primary hypothyroidism. Transient primary hypothyroidism occurs when there is maternal iodine deficiency, fetal exposure to iodine, maternal antithyroid drugs, or maternal antibodies. Acquired hypothyroidism is the most common form and is likely to be autoimmune. The thyroid becomes shrunken and fibroid and does not function. Chronic lymphocytic thyroiditis (Hashimoto's hypothyroidism) is an inherited (genetic) condition in which the thyroid is usually enlarged (goiter), which diminishes the capacity to make thyroid hormones. This occurs in women 30 to 50 years old. Newborns, new mothers in the post-partum period, and individuals with autoimmune disease are also at risk for developing hypothyroidism.

The thyroid gland utilizes iodine to make thyroid hormones. The two most important thyroid hormones are thyroxine (T_4) and triiodothyronine (T_3). Thyroxine has 4 iodine molecules attached to its structure, while tri-iodothyronine has 3 iodine molecules attached. Iodine is found in seafood, bread, salt, and seaweed. Since the addition of iodine to table salt, iodine deficiency is rarely seen in the United States; however, it is estimated that 5 to 15% of the world's population has hypothyroidism.

In newborns with congenital hypothyroidism, symptoms may appear in the first 2 weeks of life, although some can be asymptomatic for the first month. Persistent jaundice, unstable temperatures, decreased activity, poor sucking ability, poor feeding, and delayed first stooling are some of the subtler symptoms. If the condition remains uncorrected for the first 3 to 6 months of life, symptoms likely to occur include thickened tongue, coarse facies, umbilical hernia, infrequent cry, hypothermia, combination of lethargy/irritability, delayed growth, linear growth retardation, short extremities, a short neck, sparse hair, periorbital puffiness, and persistent open posterior fontanels; irreversible mental changes may occur before these symptoms manifest. The severity of acquired hypo-thyroidism is relative to the length of time and the extent of the hormone deficiency. Symptoms range from apathy, dry skin, and hypothermia to constipation.

In acquired hypothyroidism patients have normal levels of the serum thyroid hormone but an elevation of thyroid stimulating hormone (TSH). Early symptoms have an insidious onset and consist of fatigue, dry skin, weight gain, cold intolerance, constipation, and heavy menses. Mental development is permanently retarded if left untreated.

Tests should be done to include levels of T_4 (low or borderline), T_3 resin uptake (low), and TSH (high if defect is in thyroid, low if defect is in pituitary or hypothalamus). The patient with hypothyroidism may be treated with oral sodium-L-thyroxine. In patients with congenital hypothyroidism, growth and motor development can be returned to normal with adequate replacement therapy.

The prognosis for mental development is guarded if treatment is delayed beyond 3 months of life. In patients with acquired hypothyroidism, restoration of physical and mental function to the predisease level is variable following replacement therapy. Overall treatment may produce accelerated skeletal maturation and craniosynostosis; osteoporosis is a concern in adults. Patients with hypothyroidism should be managed in conjunction with an endocrinologist. With medical treatment alone, prolonged remissions may be expected in about one-third of cases.

The slow progression of thyroid hypofunctioning followed by symptoms indicating thyroid failure is referred to as primary hypothyroidism. When the thyroid dysfunction is due to failure of the pituitary gland, the condition is known as secondary hypothyroidism; when the failure of the hypothalamus gland is the underlying cause, it is called tertiary hypothyroidism.

CRETINISM

Cretinism or congenital hypothyroidism is the insufficient production of the thyroid hormone thyroxine because of malformation or malfunction of the thyroid gland. Congenital hypothyroidism leads to severe, permanent neurological and developmental damage. Congenital hypothyroidism is usually from the failure of the thyroid gland to migrate during fetal development. In newborns with congenital hypothyroidism, symptoms and treatment are the same as for hypothyroidism.

In patients with congenital hypothyroidism, growth and motor development can be returned to normal with adequate replacement therapy. The prognosis for mental development is guarded if treatment is delayed beyond 3 months of life.

The initial screening is by radioimmunoassay (RIA), which measures the level of thyroxine (T_4). A nonisotopic, time-resolved fluoroimmunoassay (TR-FIA) that measures thyroid stimulating hormone (TSH) levels is low on initial (T_4) results. Affected infants have low T_4 and elevated

Cretinism. Congenital condition caused by lack of thyroid secretion.

TSH levels. Early treatment with supplemental synthetic thyroxin will result in normal development. An endocrinologist should continue to monitor hormone levels.

Hyperthyroidism

The thyroid gland is a butterfly-shaped organ located in the lower neck, anterior to the trachea. It consists of two lateral lobes connected by an isthmus. The thyroid hormone helps regulate growth and maintain basal metabolic rate (BMR). Hyperthyroidism is an autoimmune condition in which there is an excessive amount of thyroid hormones released in response to human thyroid stimulator immunoglobulin (TSI).

Normally, the rate of thyroid hormone production is controlled by the pituitary gland, located at the base of the brain. When there are insufficient thyroid hormones in the body for normal functioning, the cells in the pituitary gland release a thyroid stimulating hormone (TSH). In turn, TSH stimulates the thyroid gland to produce more thyroid hormones (feedback mechanism).

Hyperthyroidism in childhood is rare and accounts for less than 5% of cases of hyperthyroidism. **Congenital hyperthyroidism** or neonatal thyrotoxicosis occurs almost exclusively in infants of mothers with Graves' disease (a hyperthyroid disease characterized by protrusion of the eyeballs, increased heart action, enlargement of the thyroid gland, weight loss, and nervousness). Acquired hyperthyroidism is most often due to Graves' disease and is most likely to appear in childhood at 12 to 14 years of age.

Congenital hyperthyroidism may last several weeks to more than 6 months, and can be life threatening. Infants frequently have low birth weight and fail to gain weight. Clinical manifestations of hyperthyroidism also include hyperphagia, microcephaly, irritability, hyperactivity, tachycardia, tachypnea, protrusion of the eyes (ophthalmopathy), and thyroid enlargement. Other symptoms include vomiting, diarrhea, hepatosplenomegaly, jaundice, thrombocytopenia, and cardiac failure.

Immediate intervention and treatment of congenital hyperthyroidism is important to prevent the dangerous sequela of nervous system involvement. Treatment for children includes radioactive iodine, often in conjunction with antithyroid drugs. In certain cases, surgical intervention may be required. Nervousness associated with hyperthyroidism may require the use of sedatives or tranquilizers. Complications associated with the treatment of this disease sometimes include hypothyroidism; therefore follow-up and continued monitoring is necessary. Activity should be restricted in severe cases. Supportive measures include fluids, nutritional support, and electrolyte corrections. Medical treatment is usually effective within 2 to 3 years. With medical treatment alone, prolonged remissions may be expected in about one-third of cases. The risk of developing leukemia or carcinoma of the thyroid after treatment with radioactive iodide has not been determined.

Congenital hyperthyroidism.
A condition caused by excessive secretion of the thyroid gland, which increases the basal metabolic rate, causing increased demand for food to support the metabolic activity.

$\mathcal{D}$IABETES MELLITUS

Diabetes mellitus is a chronic disease for which there is no cure. It is estimated that in 1998 more than 180,000 people died from diabetes and its related complications.

Type I diabetes (previously referred to as juvenile diabetes and insulin-dependent diabetes mellitus) is a viral or immune-mediated disorder with a genetic predisposition. Peak incidence occurs during puberty, around 10 to 12 years old in girls and 12 to 14 years old in boys. **Diabetes mellitus type I** has a gradual onset and immunologic markers (islet cell antibodies [ICA], insulin autoantibodies [IAA], and other antibodies) may be present for years prior to the development of insulin dependency. The gradual destruction of the insulin-producing tissue (beta cells in the islets of Langerhans) of the pancreas limits the ability to metabolize carbohydrates, proteins, and dietary fats. The immune system has an antibody response against the beta cells because of a previous viral infection or other toxic agents.

Type I diabetes can mimic the flu in children. Abrupt onset of symptoms in children is common. Symptoms include extreme hunger, extreme thirst (polydipsia), extreme weight loss, failure to grow, weakness and tiredness, feeling edgy and having mood changes, "feeling sick," polyuria (osmotic diuretic effect from elevated serum glucose), and often bed-wetting.

If the condition goes unrecognized, diabetic ketoacidosis (DKA) (fat catabolism) may lead to anorexia, nausea/vomiting (presence of ketones), sweet-smelling breath, deep respirations (Kussmaul), air hunger (compensatory for metabolic acidosis), and, if left untreated, coma and death. One-third of children with diabetes develop joint contractures, particularly of the fifth finger. However, these are not disabling. Severe diabetic retinopathy and early nephropathy develop in one-third of pubertal adolescents and young adults who have had diabetes for 10 to 20 years. Microaneurysms are more common retinal changes. Large vessel involvement often puts diabetics at risk for cardiac problems, and tobacco use in adolescents increases their risk of developing thyroid disease.

Empowering the client and family is essential to the management of diabetes. The initial period usually takes approximately 3 days, depending on the client/family's rate of learning. Education includes the administration, storage, and disposal of insulin syringes. Injection sites including upper arms, anterior and lateral aspects of the thighs, the buttocks, and the abdomen (except 2 inches around the umbilicus) are preferred (rotating sites is no longer desirable). Finger-stick serum glucose monitoring, urine testing, meal preparation, and the treatments for hypoglycemia or DKA should also be taught to clients who have good cognitive and psychomotor functioning. A sugar-restricted diet for children gives them more freedom than the American Diabetes Association (ADA) exchange diet. If the diet is calculated by calorie, the rule is 1000 kcal/day and 100 kcal additional for each year of age up to 2500 kcal (an 11-year-old would require 2100 kcal/day). Insulin therapy for nonketoacidotic children begins with 0.25 units/kg/day; ketoacidotic children should start with

Diabetes mellitus (type I).
A disorder of carbohydrate metabolism, characterized by hyperglycemia and glycosuria, and resulting from inadequate production or utilization of insulin; sudden onset prior to age 25, usually difficult to regulate.

0.5 units/kg/day. Adolescents may need 1.25 to 1.5 units/kg/day during the pubertal growth spurt. Preschool children should remain within 90 to 140 mg/dL preprandially and 90 to 200 mg/dL postprandially. School-age children should remain within 80 to 120 mg/dL preprandially and 80 to 180 mg/dL postprandially. Strenuous activity tends to lower insulin requirements, and daily exercise in moderation without significant deviation is beneficial.

Type II diabetes is ketosis resistant and generally is not seen in children, except in obese adolescents.

Diabetes mellitus (type II). Same as type I, except gradual onset is after age 40, so it doesn't affect children.

𝒟WARFISM

Dwarfism. Condition of being abnormally small. May be hereditary or a result of endocrine dysfunction, deficiency disease, renal insufficiency, diseases of the skeleton, or other causes.

Pituitary gland. An endocrine gland secreting a number of hormones that regulate many bodily processes, including growth, reproduction, and various metabolic activities.

Dwarfism is a rare disorder that results from the body's inability to synthesize and utilize human growth hormone (hGH). This disorder is also called hypopituitarism or growth hormone deficiency. Human growth hormone is synthesized by the **pituitary gland** and promotes growth in the body and tissues. In addition, it has anabolic effects such as protein synthesis, lipolysis, and regulation of carbohydrate metabolism. The incidence of growth hormone deficiency is estimated at 1 in every 4000 school-age children. The congenital forms of multiple pituitary hormone deficiencies occur 3 or 4 times more often in boys than in girls. Idiopathic hypopituitarism is the most frequent.

It is believed that 70% of children with idiopathic hypopituitarism have histories of some form of perinatal insult, intrauterine growth retardation, Turner's syndrome, skeletal dysplasia, neural tube defects, chronic renal failure, and a variety of syndromes associated with short stature. Biosynthesis of hGH is used to treat causes of short stature, but certain metabolic disorders may also benefit from hGH therapy. Currently only classic hGH deficiency, due to undersecretion by the pituitary gland, is approved by the FDA for treatment with the synthetic hormone. If children are not screened for deficiencies of hGH, they could become pituitary dwarfs without treatment.

Infants with intrauterine hypopituitarism may present at birth with hypoglycemic seizures, prolonged jaundice, micropenis, and undescended testes. Because the majority of affected patients have idiopathic hypopituitarism, growth failure is often apparent by the end of the first year of life. Hypopituitary children are proportioned normally for their age; they tend to be overweight for their height and have prominent subcutaneous deposits of abdominal fat. The onset of puberty may be affected. Because adrenal secretion of mineralocorticoid is not dependent on pituitary ACTH, hypopituitary children rarely have electrolyte imbalances. Diabetes insipidus and hypothyroidism are rare in patients with idiopathic hypopituitarism. Delay in skeletal maturation is almost invariable and a considerable number of children have heights for their bone age that fall well below the fifth percentile.

Growth hormone replacement is usually given in a dosage of 0.06 or 0.10 mg/kg on alternate days, 3 times a week. Growth hormone can be given intramuscularly (IM) or subcutaneously (SQ). Growth hormone–deficient children typically increase their growth rate to 8 to 10 cm per year during the first year of therapy. In general, young children respond to growth hormone treatment better. Children who fail to respond should be evaluated for hypothyroidism or the formation of antibodies to growth hormone.

$\mathcal{P}$RECOCIOUS PUBERTY

Precocious puberty is defined as the onset of puberty before the age of 8 years in females and before the age of 9 years in males. (See Figures 16-1 and 16-2.) It is 5 times more common in girls than in boys, with 75% being idiopathic (no underlying abnormality can be found). Luteinizing hormone-releasing hormone (LHRH) is secreted in periodic bursts, which causes the pituitary gland to release hormones called gonadotropins. These gonadotropins in turn stimulate the gonads (ovaries and testes) to make sex hormones. The sex hormones cause sexual maturation, particularly estrogen in girls and testosterone in boys. Although boys are affected less often, the cause in their cases is usually organic.

There are three types of precocious puberty: (1) In isosexual precocious puberty, the hypothalamic pituitary ovarian axis is working normally but prematurely; (2) in heterosexual precocious puberty, the development of secondary sex characteristics of the opposite sex form; this is usually apparent at birth; and (3) in incomplete precocious puberty, there is a partial development of secondary sex characteristics, which can occur in girls from 6 months to 2 years of age. The process does not progress fully to puberty (ovulation and menstruation); premature adrenarche (growth of pubic hair) tends to occur between 5 and 8 years old.

Female children with central precocious puberty have complete sexual development including pubic hair, axillary hair, and breasts, and often menstruate. In male children, the testicles and penis enlarge, and pubic, underarm, and facial hair appears. Male children experience spontaneous erections. Both females and males have the potential to be fertile, high energy levels, and increased appetite, and can be emotionally labile because of the increase in hormone levels.

The goal in treating precocious puberty is to halt and even reverse sexual development, and to stop the rapid growth that results in short adult stature. Identifying the source and removing the excessive hormone is usually the treatment. These children are usually referred to an endocrinologist for treatment. Besides the premature development of secondary sex characteristics, the condition causes a cessation in long bone development. Therefore, the child might never reach his/her adult height potential.

Precocious puberty. Onset of puberty at an age much earlier than normal.

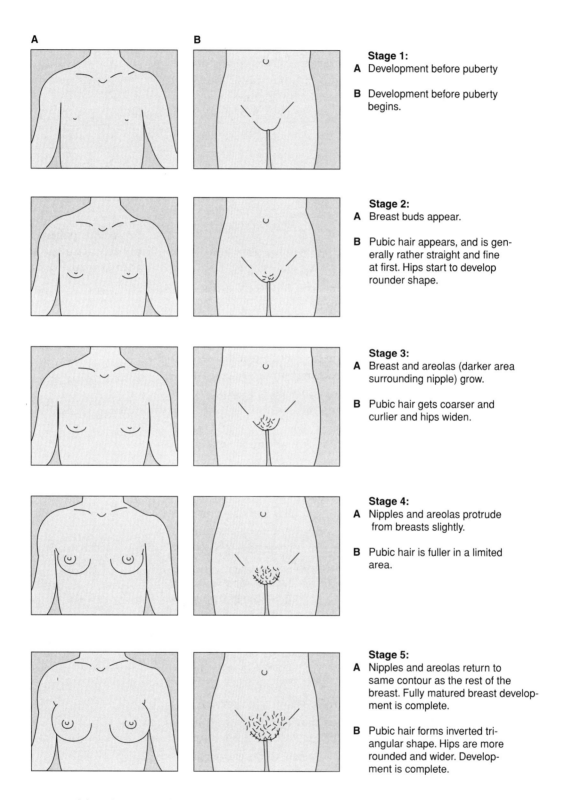

A   **B**

Stage 1:
A Development before puberty

B Development before puberty begins.

Stage 2:
A Breast buds appear.

B Pubic hair appears, and is generally rather straight and fine at first. Hips start to develop rounder shape.

Stage 3:
A Breast and areolas (darker area surrounding nipple) grow.

B Pubic hair gets coarser and curlier and hips widen.

Stage 4:
A Nipples and areolas protrude from breasts slightly.

B Pubic hair is fuller in a limited area.

Stage 5:
A Nipples and areolas return to same contour as the rest of the breast. Fully matured breast development is complete.

B Pubic hair forms inverted triangular shape. Hips are more rounded and wider. Development is complete.

FIGURE 16-1 Stages of female genital development.

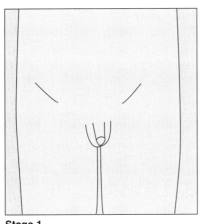

Stage 1

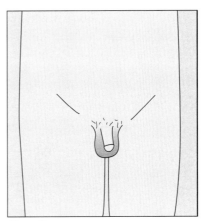

Stage 2

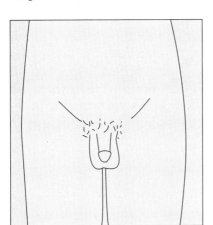

Stage 3

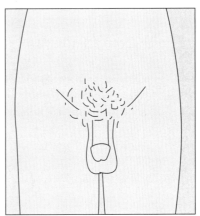

Stage 4

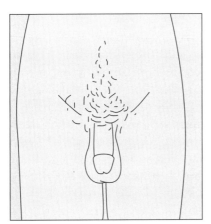

Stage 5

Stage 1: Development before puberty.

Stage 2: Pubic hair first appears at the base of the penis as testes increase in size. Scrotum becomes darker in darker skin people and redder in lighter skin people.

Stage 3: Pubic hair becomes coarser and curlier. Penis grows in length.

Stage 4: Pubic hair becomes fuller. Penis grows in width.

Stage 5: Matured stage of development.

FIGURE 16-2 Stages of external male development.

Education is extremely important in these sensitive cases. For a period of time the child will be more developed physically but not psychologically, so it is important to help the families of these children understand what is happening to the child and help them to deal with the issues that surround human sexuality within this context.

Summary

This chapter addresses concepts of the metabolic disorders, and discusses the congenital anomalies and the diagnostic tests as they apply to the metabolic disorders. The nursing care involved with problems associated with growth is included, which helps the nurse to identify signs of hypothyroidism in infants. In an effort to help the nurse to understand hormone regulation, this chapter describes the functions of the hormones secreted by the cortex and medulla of the adrenal gland as well as the pathophysiology and nursing care of the patient with diabetes.

The endocrine system is responsible for growth, maturation, reproduction, metabolic processes, and the reaction of the body to stress. Therefore, it is important that the nurse caring for children with metabolic disturbances develop a thorough understanding of the problems facing these children.

Critical Points in the Care of Children with Metabolic Disorders

The nurse taking care of the child with metabolic disorders has to realize that these conditions are sometimes complex, because the causes of these disorders are irreversible, and they range from mild to profound. When the nurse suspects the possibility of an inborn error of metabolism, he/she should encourage the parents to pursue medical diagnoses until they are certain that the disorder is present, or that it can be ruled out. A diagnosis made early may not change the condition, but definitely will have a great impact on the long-term outcome of the disease. An important fact for the nurse to remember is that these families need assistance with the management of symptoms. Although treatment directives are generally provided by a multidisciplinary team, the nurse plays the key role in the education of the child and his/her family, stressing anticipatory guidance.

Caregiver support is critical. The most important area for the nurse to be familiar with is assessment of the family support system and the availability of resources for them to utilize. In planning the care of the child, the nurse needs to plan realistic short-term and long-term goals in order to improve the family's functioning, and to help the family live as normal a life as possible. The nursing aim is to reduce anxiety and alleviate any guilt feelings on the part of the parents.

QUESTIONS

Diagnosis: Diabetes

History: Clarissa was diagnosed with diabetes mellitus type I at the age of 3; she is now 8½ years old and is in the second grade. Clarissa is having difficulty in reading and writing. She lives with her mom and step-dad and she has no other siblings.

Plan: Stabilize blood sugar levels. Prevent ketoacidosis. Prevent target organ damage.

Nursing problems: No compliance with diet. Potential for problems with growth and development. Teaching parents about disease process and progress. Teaching parents emergency treatments of diabetic coma and ketoacidosis. Dealing with fear and anxiety about chronic disease process.

1. Given Clarissa's age of 3 when diagnosed, what kinds of signs and symptoms would you expect to find?
   A. Increased hunger, thirst, and weight gain
   B. Bed-wetting, lethargy, poor appetite, and weight loss
   C. Weight loss, bed-wetting, lower leg cramping, lethargy
   D. Bed-wetting, increased thirst, hunger, and weight gain

2. You are the registered nurse working in the Endocrine Clinic. Clarissa and her mom have missed their last two appointments. Clarissa's mom is very apologetic about missing the previous appointments. In dealing with a chronic condition like this, what would be your best response to the apology?
   A. "It's okay, don't worry about it."
   B. "Don't let it happen again."
   C. "What happened that caused you to miss your appointments?"
   D. "I know it's difficult having a diabetic child, but you do want only the best for Clarissa, right?"

3. Clarissa's mom is very concerned about her newest problem, learning in school. She asks you if this problem is because of her diabetes. Your best response would be:
   A. "Diabetes does not have any effect on the brain, so don't be worried."
   B. "Yes, there are a few articles that have correlated learning disabilities and diabetes."
   C. "Possibly, due to the hypoglycemic seizures she had in the past."
   D. "There is no scientific evidence to link learning disabilities and diabetes."

4. While reviewing Clarissa's chart, you notice that she is beginning to fall off the growth curve. Why is this important to note with a diabetic child?

A. The chance for hypothyroidism is increased.
B. Children with diabetes are prone to gain weight.
C. Variable blood sugar levels can cause growth hormone deficiency.
D. There is increased chance for hyperthyroidism.

5. When reviewing with Clarissa's teachers and school nurse regarding her diabetes management, what would be your primary focus?

A. Mandating the ability to check her blood sugar at lunch and give an additional insulin shot for more control.
B. Blood sugar monitoring, insulin therapy, exercise and diet management, signs and symptoms of hypoglycemia and hyperglycemia.
C. Signs and symptoms of hypoglycemia and hyperglycemia, especially since Clarissa is having difficulty learning in school.
D. Checking her blood sugar should never be done at school.

6. How important is it for Clarissa to have a snack in the classroom and not allow anyone to make fun of her because of her problems? Clarissa does her own blood sugar tests, but her mom logs the results, makes sure she checks her ketones every morning, and draws up and gives her insulin shots. In planning with her mother for Clarissa to take more responsibility for her own care, what would be the best plan?

A. Allow Clarissa and her mom to plan for when she is psychologically ready to take on more responsibility.
B. Have Clarissa and her mom plan that every year Clarissa will assume an additional task.
C. Have Clarissa make a plan to start at the age of 10.
D. Have the nurse make a plan for Clarissa.

Diagnosis: Idiopathic Growth Hormone Deficiency

History: Michael is a 7-year-old boy who is very bright and very cute. His mother notices that he is extremely short for his age. He is complaining that he wants to take more vitamins in order to grow taller like his classmates. His mother takes Michael to the doctor and asks what she can do to make Michael grow faster.

Plan: To bring Michael to the clinic for testing. Find out if he has growth retardation. Help the parents and the child to deal with the situation.

Nursing problems: Alteration of body image. Teaching parents to accept the child's condition. Assist the parents with anxiety.

1. A 7-year-old boy is shorter than all of his classmates. Diagnostic testing supports a diagnosis of idiopathic isolated growth hormone (GH) deficiency. All of the following are expected clinical findings *except*:

A. Proportional body structure
B. A growth velocity of 3 cm/year
C. Hypertension
D. Delayed skeletal maturation

2. Occasionally, early adolescent girls whose families are tall may be treated to reduce predicted adult stature. This treatment usually consists of which one of the following agents?

A. Glucocorticoid
B. Thyroid hormone
C. Estrogen
D. Gonadotropin-releasing hormone (GnRH)

ANSWERS

Diabetes

1. C. Weight loss is from the hyperglycemia and the body's compensatory mechanisms to find sources of glucose (fat and muscles), plus the diuresis that occurs with hyperglycemia. Bed-wetting is common among children even after they are toilet trained, because of the polyuria. Leg cramping is common, secondary to the muscle wasting, and lethargy can be from hypokalemia.

2. C. In working with families with chronic conditions the health care provider must be sensitive to family, personal, cultural, and financial issues that may interfere with the Western medical model. Once the rationale is explained, the family, patient (if age-appropriate), and health care provider can work together to find the appropriate modality for each family. Shame, guilt, and anger are not appropriate mechanisms in working with children and their families with or without chronic conditions.

3. D. There is no evidence to link learning disabilities and diabetes. Some children do have trouble in school if their blood sugar levels are not within normal parameters (poor control). This may lead to missing school.

4. A. There is scientific evidence to link hypothyroidism with diabetes. It is important to watch these children closely for hypothyroidism.

5. C. There have been studies on what school personnel and teachers should know about children with chronic illnesses. They need to know how diabetes affects their student and, if there is a problem, how to address it. Hypoglycemic reactions are particularly important, especially for Clarissa, because she is more apt to get tired, not be able to concentrate, and have difficulty learning. *A:* This may be an important issue for some children, but it is most important that they can recognize symptoms of hypoglycemic reaction. *B:* These are the categories of diabetes education. *D:* This is not a wrong answer, but it is not the best answer.

6. A. Studies have shown that if you force children before they are psychologically or developmentally ready to take responsibility for their care, there are some negative outcomes psychologically as well as metabolically. This should be a plan that the family and patient make together.

Idiopathic Growth Hormone Deficiency

1. *C.* Hypertension is not associated with idiopathic growth hormone deficiency. However, a common feature of Cushing syndrome is slow growth during childhood. Idiopathic growth hormone deficiency accounts for most cases of GH deficiency, which include the typical features—short stature and pudgy doll-like appearance; slow growth velocity (less than 5 cm/year in older children); and mild truncal adiposity and delayed skeletal maturation. Body proportions are normal in contrast to the immature proportions seen in congenital hypothyroidism.

2. *C.* High-dose estrogen treatments may induce premature epiphyseal fusion and a reduction of final adult stature.

*G*LOSSARY

congenital hyperthyroidism   a condition caused by excessive secretion of the thyroid gland, which increases the basal metabolic rate, causing increased demand for food to support the metabolic activity.

congenital hypothyroidism   a condition caused by deficiency of the thyroid secretion, resulting in a lowered basal metabolism. A lesser degree of cretinism.

cretinism   congenital condition caused by lack of thyroid secretion.

diabetes mellitus (type I)   a disorder of carbohydrate metabolism, characterized by hyperglycemia and glycosuria, and resulting from inadequate production or utilization of insulin; sudden onset prior to age 25, usually difficult to regulate.

diabetes mellitus (type II)   same as type I, except gradual onset is after age 40, so it doesn't affect children.

dwarfism   condition of being abnormally small. May be hereditary or a result of endocrine dysfunction, deficiency disease, renal insufficiency, diseases of the skeleton, or other causes.

pituitary gland   an endocrine gland secreting a number of hormones that regulate many bodily processes, including growth, reproduction, and various metabolic activities.

precocious puberty   onset of puberty at an age much earlier than normal.

thyroid gland   a gland of internal secretion, which acts to control metabolic functions, located in the base of the neck on both sides of the lower part of the larynx and upper part of the trachea.

*B*IBLIOGRAPHY

AMERICAN DIABETES ASSOCIATION 1997. Diabetes Info: Diabetes Facts and Figures. http://www.diabetes.org/ada/c20a.htm.#youth.

BARTLETT, J. G. *Pocket Book of Infectious Disease Therapy.* 7th ed. Philadelphia: Williams & Wilkins, 1996.

BOYTON, R. W., DUNN, E. S., AND STEPHENS, G. R. *Manual of Ambulatory Pediatrics*. 3rd ed. Philadelphia: Lippincott, 1994.

BURNS, C. E., BARBER, N., BRADY, M. A., AND DUNN, A. M. *Pediatric Primary Care: A Handbook for Nurse Practitioners*. Philadelphia: Saunders, 1996.

BUTEL, J., JAWETZ, E., MELNICK, J., ADELBERG, E., BROOKS, G., AND ORNSTON, L. *Medical Microbiology*. 18th ed. Norwalk, CT: Appleton & Lang, 1989.

MARLOW, D. R., AND REDDING, B. A. *Textbook of Pediatric Nursing*. 6th ed. Philadelphia: Saunders, 1988.

MAWSON, A. R., WARRIER, R. P., KUVIBIDILA, S., AND SUSKIND, R. Pediatric AIDS and nutrition. In R. M. Suskind and L. Lewinter-Suskind (eds.), *Textbook of Pediatric Nutrition*. (Pp. 447–453). New York: Raven Press, 1993.

MCCANE, K. L,. AND HUETHER, S. E. *Pathophysiology: The Biologic Basis for Disease in Adults and Children*. 2nd ed. St. Louis: Mosby-Year Book, 1994.

MEDLINENET INC. Diseases and treatments: Hyperthyroidism. http://www.medicinenet.com/art.asp?li=mni&ag=y&articlekey=391. 1995–1997.

MEDLINENET INC. Diseases and treatments: Hypothyroidism. http://www.medicinenet.com/art.asp?li=mni&ag=y&articlekey=914. 1995–1997.

MEDICINENET INC. Diseases and treatments: Influenza. http://www.medicinenet.com/art.asp?li=mni&ag=y&articlekey=365. 1995–1997

PUBLICATION MANUAL OF THE AMERICAN PSYCHOLOGICAL ASSOCIATION. 4th ed. Washington, D.C.: American Psychological Association, 1995.

THOMAS, C. L. (ed.) *Taber's Cyclopedic Medical Dictionary*. 15th ed. Philiadelphia: F. A. Davis, 1985.

UPHOLD, C. R., AND GRAHAM, M. V. *Clinical Guidelines in Family Practice*. Gainesville, FL: Barmarrae Books, 1994.

𝓗ELPFUL INTERNET SITES

PEDINFO: An Index of the Pediatric Internet at http://www.pedinfo. org This is an excellent site that covers nearly all topics within this review. It has a wealth of information and is worth a visit. It is written for health care professionals but others could also use the information.

Virtual Naval Hospital Information for Providers at http://www.vnh. org/Providers.html This site is part of the University of Iowa's health care site and is linked to a large set of databases that can be used by health care providers. The site covers a larger number of links to other sources on health care issues and problems. This is an excellent starting place to discover information on various common diseases and their treatments.

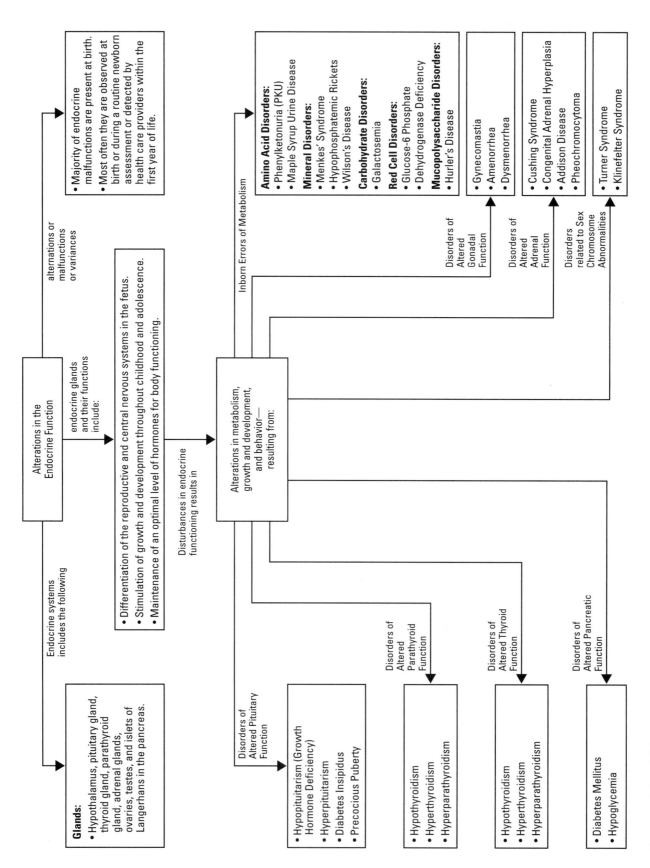

Concept Map 16-1

472

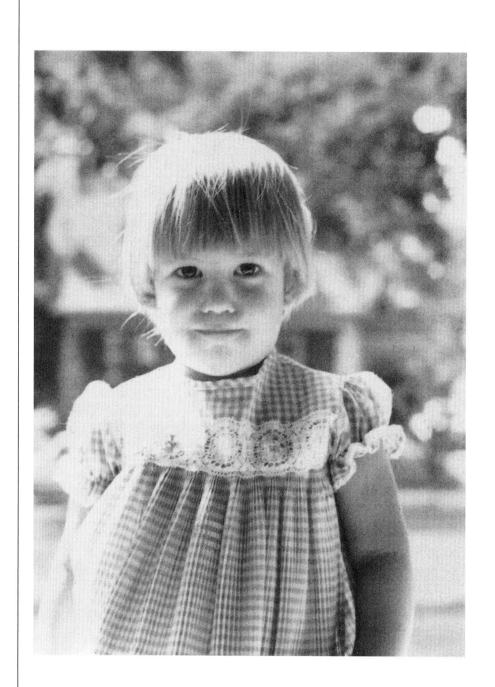

⚿

𝒰RINARY TRACT DISORDERS

𝒥NTRODUCTION

The genitourinary system is responsible for maintaining metabolism and for expelling waste products from the body. The genitourinary system consists of the kidneys, nephrons, distal tubules, collecting ducts, renal pelvis, ureter, bladder, urethra, and sphincters. The genitourinary system is different in males than in females; the male genitourinary system has both excretory and reproductive functions. Genitourinary problems in pediatrics range from the simple to the complex, and from psychological to structural. Therefore, the role of the nurse is not only to diagnose the condition correctly, but also to plan for extended care, as well as to treat the acute phase of these dysfunctions. Figures 17-1 through 17-10 (pages 498–507) illustrate the male and female genitourinary systems.

The kidneys are paired organs located on the posterior abdominal wall outside the peritoneal cavity. Each kidney is approximately 11 cm long and 5 to 6 cm wide. The primary function of the kidney is to maintain balanced metabolism. The kidney balances solute and water transport, excretes metabolic waste products, conserves nutrients, and regulates the acid-base balance in the body. Another function of the kidney is to secrete the hormones renin, erythropoietin, and 1,25-dihydroxyvitamin D for blood pressure regulation, erythrocyte production, and calcium metabolism.

The other structures that are part of the urinary system are the ones that are involved in the formation of urine. Urine is formed by the nephron from the distal tubules and collecting ducts. From the renal pelvis, urine is funneled into the ureter. The lower end of the ureter passes obliquely through the posterior part of the bladder wall. The bladder is a bag composed of a basketweave of smooth muscle fibers. The bladder has a profuse blood supply. The urethra extends from the inferior side of the bladder to the outside of the body. The muscles that control the excretion of urine are called sphincters. The enervation of the bladder and internal urethral sphincter is supplied by parasympathetic fibers of the autonomic nervous system. The urine is collected in the bladder, and when it reaches 250 to 300 cc, the bladder contracts, and the internal urethral sphincter relaxes. At this time the person feels the urge to void.

The genitourinary disorders in children are divided into upper and lower tract disorders.

Upper urinary tract disorders

Hematuria

Hematuria. Blood in the urine.

Hematuria is caused by several conditions. In children, **hematuria** is usually caused by urinary tract infections, usually cystitis. The conditions that are associated with hematuria could be acquired or congenital. The congenital conditions associated with hematuria are hypercalcinuria, benign familial hematuria, and structural defects of the urinary system: benign recurrent hematuria and hereditary nephritis. The acquired conditions are poststreptococcal glomerulonephritis, urinary calculi, systemic conditions, hemolytic-uremic syndrome, systemic lupus erythematosus, polyarteritis nodosa, necrotizing vasculitis, and Goodpasture syndrome. Renal trauma conditions are contusions, minor lacerations, major lacerations, and vascular injury.

Children with painful hematuria should be investigated for direct or indirect causes. Usually, back pain is related to pyelonephritis, and colicky flank pain associated with the presence of red blood always accompanies the passage of a stone. Bright red blood or clots in the urine occur with bleeding disorders or trauma. Abdominal masses suggest the presence of obstructions, cystic disease, or tumors.

Asymptomatic hematuria is the biggest challenge because the examination is geared to the discovery of determining the cause of the hematuria and not to the treatment of hematuria.

Acute poststreptococcal glomerulonephritis is often seen in children. Antigen-antibody complexes induced by the infection are formed in the bloodstream and deposited in the glomeruli. It is believed that these glomerular inflammations activate the bleeding. The diagnosis is based on the evaluation as to where the hematuria originated. A mid-stream urine specimen is usually obtained to confirm the diagnosis. If the urinary specimen fails to reveal evidence of infection, a calcium-to-creatinine ratio is obtained. After infection and hypercalcinuria have been ruled out, the parents' urine specimens may be obtained to rule out the presence of familial hematuria. If these evaluations remain negative, the child must be referred to a pediatric urologist.

The appropriate treatment of hematuria is based on the treatment of the underlying cause. One of the roles of the nurse is that of educator, reassuring the parents that hematuria is rarely associated with a terminal disease. The condition of the child is the guidepost as to the information the nurse gives to the parents. For example, if the child has hematuria because of a streptococcal infection, parents should be taught about prevention, compliance with medications, and follow-up visits with the pediatrician. Hematuria associated with urinary tract infection (UTI) should be followed up after appropriate therapy (7 to 14 days). A repeat urinalysis should be done in order to evaluate if the underlying condition has been resolved.

Children with idiopathic hematuria should be assessed every year for evidence that the disease is completely eradicated.

Proteinuria

Proteinuria is the presence of protein in the urine. Proteinuria can be persistent or intermittent. The diagnosis is made through the urinary dipstick. A dipstick reading of 2 or greater indicates significant proteinuria. Proteinuria can be a symptom of a disease or a self-limiting condition. Persistent proteinuria may be secondary to nephrotic syndrome, glomerulonephritis, or acute or chronic renal failure.

The most common type of proteinuria in children is orthostatic proteinuria. The child with this condition excretes an abnormal amount of protein when upright but a normal amount when lying down. Other forms of proteinuria are exercise-induced proteinuria, which is seen after the child has exercised vigorously, and febrile proteinuria, which accompanies the disease any time the child has an elevated temperature because of a viral or infectious process.

Proteinuria. Protein, usually albumin, in the urine.

Acute Glomerulonephritis

Acute glomerulonephritis is an immune complex disease that can be a manifestation of a systematic disorder or a primary disorder. The disorder can be minimal or severe. The symptoms are oliguria, edema, hypertension, circulatory congestion, hematuria, and proteinuria. Acute glomerulonephritis is associated with postinfection of pneumococcal, streptococcal, and viral infections, which, in turn, result in the formation of glomerular deposition.

Acute glomerulonephritis after streptococcal infection is the most common of the noninfectious renal diseases in children. It can occur at any age but is most common in children 3 to 7 years of age. Most of the streptococcal infections do not cause the disease, but the onset of clinical manifestation is between 10 and 14 days. Secondary to streptococcal pharyngitis, it is most prevalent in the winter and the spring. On the other hand, it can be secondary to impetigo, which is more prevalent in warm climates or during the summer or early fall. The initial sign of the disease is edema, which is more prevalent in the morning, but spreads during the

Acute glomerulonephritis. A form of nephritis in which the lesions involve primarily the glomeruli.

day to the extremities and abdomen. The urine is cloudy, smoky brown in color, and scanty in volume.

Older children complain of headaches, abdominal discomfort, and dysuria. The child is pale and irritable. On examination, the blood pressure is slightly elevated. The acute phase of glomerulonephritis is characterized by the presence of edema, which usually persists for 10 days, but can last for up to 3 weeks. This phase is delicate because blood pressure can reach dangerous levels. The child usually is anorexic, and the urine remains thick and smoky.

The confirmation that the child is improving is evidenced by weight loss and a small increase in the urine output. Once the child has started this improvement, it is followed by 48 hours of diuresis, which allows the child to feel better. Blood pressure decreases, and the child has improvement in appetite. The color of the urine is clear because of the decrease of gross hematuria, but microscopic hematuria can persist for weeks or months. The blood urea nitrogen (BUN) decreases but proteinuria may persist for weeks.

The prognosis is good if the disease is diagnosed and treated early, and after the process of the disease is complete, children develop immunity. In the acute phase, the danger is in the development of hypertensive encephalopathy, acute cardiac decompensation, and acute renal failure. The diagnosis is confirmed with the presence of hematuria, proteinuria, and an increase in the specific gravity of the urine. Microscopic examination of the urine reveals the presence of red blood cells, leukocytes, and epithelial cells. Urine cultures are always negative.

No specific treatment is available, and recovery is spontaneous. Management is supportive and early treatment is geared to avoid complications. Bed rest is recommended in the acute phase. Regular monitoring of vital signs is essential since the blood pressure is the measurement that determines the progression of the disease. Dietary restrictions depend on the stage and severity of the condition. Regular diet is usually given, but with sodium restrictions. Antibiotic therapy is indicated only for those children with evidence of infection.

The major nursing intervention is the assessment of the progression of the disease, the alertness to prevent complications, and the supportive care for the child and the family, especially during the acute phase.

Nephrotic Syndrome

Nephrotic syndrome. Disease of the basement membrane of the glomerulus that causes severe proteinuria, hypoalbuminemia, generalized edema, lipiduria, and hyperlipidemia. Blood pressure remains normal.

Nephrotic syndrome is caused by kidney malfunction. It presents massive proteinuria, hypoalbuminemia, hyperlipidemia, and edema. The main mechanism of the massive protein loss is an increase in glomerular permeability. The loss can be selective or nonselective, and the distinction is very important in the diagnosis. Because of the protein loss, the liver increases its synthesis of protein, which causes hyperlipidemia and lipiduria. Nephrotic syndrome is classified as primary and secondary. In primary, the syndrome is restricted to glomerular injury; in secondary, it develops as part of a systematic illness.

Nephrotic syndrome occurs as a result of immune, systemic, nephrotoxic, allergic, infectious, malignant, vascular, or idiopathic processes. The incidence is greater in children than in adults; two-thirds of the cases are in children. Onset occurs between 1 and 5 years of age, with peak incidence at 2 to 3 years of age.

The clinical picture of children with nephrotic syndrome is puffy eyes, low urine production, anorexia, diarrhea, and vomiting. The child is easily fatigued and irritable but does not appear gravely ill. The diagnosis is made on the basis of history of periorbital edema in the morning, and changes to swelling of the abdomen and lower extremities in the evening; hypertension and muscle wasting are also present; and if the disease progresses the child exhibits respiratory difficulty or ascites with labial edema. Laboratory studies reveal massive proteinuria. Urine analysis and microscopic examination reveals protein greater than or equal to 2, hyaline granular casts, microhematuria 33%, and elevated specific gravity. Hemoglobin and hematocrit are usually normal and the platelet count is elevated as a result of hemoconcentration. Renal biopsy may be obtained in order to establish if the edema is renal in origin and also to distinguish minimum change nephrotic syndrome from other glomerulonephritis with nephrotic syndrome as a manifestation.

The medical treatment consists of both general and specific measures. For the most part, treatment is supportive. Diet, if the child is in remission, is regular with sodium restrictions. Corticosteroid therapy is started as soon as the diagnosis has been confirmed. Medication is given until the urine is free from protein and remains normal for 2 weeks. Children usually respond to therapy and are recovered within 7 to 21 days after the steroid treatment has been given. If the child does not respond to steroids after 28 days of treatment, the probability of subsequent response diminishes greatly.

Children with nephrotic syndrome are often described according to their response to corticosteroid therapy. Twenty to 40% of the children respond to a single short course of steroid therapy without relapsing. After the treatment is discontinued, those children are classified as steroid-sensitive. Frequent relapses are 2 or more relapses in a 6- to 12-month period. Steroid-resistant children are those who never respond to steroid or become resistant. The main problem with children who have frequent relapses or who do not respond to steroid therapy is that they are prone to infections and growth retardation, and are susceptible to many complications. The last hope for children when they do not respond to steroid therapy is immunosuppressant therapy. The drug of choice is Cytoxan along with prednisone. Both drugs are given for a period of 3 months. The use of these drugs causes leukopenia, which should be discussed early with parents.

The most salient characteristic of the edema of nephrotic syndrome is that it does not respond to diuretic therapy. If the edema interferes with respiration, or creates hypotension or hyponatremia, loop diuretics are usually given. At this point, the prognosis is good because the disease is self-limiting. The aim is to recognize the disease early, and to institute early treatment in order to eradicate proteinuria.

Nursing care is based on continuous assessment in order to meet the specific and complex problems that this disease presents. Nursing intervention during hospitalization is directed to maintaining nutrition and rest, monitoring fluid intake and output, preventing infection—since corticosteroid therapy is a constant source of danger for infections—and being a source of information and support for the child and his/her family.

Acute Renal Failure

Acute renal failure. Acute failure of the kidney to perform its essential functions. May be due to trauma or any condition that impairs the flow of blood to the kidneys.

Acute renal failure is an abrupt decline in the renal regulation of water, electrolytes, and acid-base balance, which results in the retention of nitrogenous waste. Although the condition can be reversed, it can also be fatal. Therefore, the diagnosis has to be made early and the therapy is geared to the prevention of complications. Some medical authorities divide the process of acute renal failure into three phases:

Phase One: The initiation phase, in which the toxin produces an injury to the tubular epithelial cells.

Phase Two: The maintenance phase, during which the glomerular filtration remains relatively low for several days or weeks.

Phase Three: The recovery phase, in which there is gradual restoration of the tubule function.

Diagnostic evaluation is based on the acute decrease of urine output and paralysis of tubular function. There is also an increase in BUN and the serum creatinine concentrations. The urine that is produced has a high level of urine sodium, and is isotonic compared to plasma. The clinical conditions associated with the development of acute renal failure include hypotension, shock, renal ischemia, nephrotoxicity, drug toxicity, hyperuricemia, asphyxia, and sepsis. In children, this condition is associated with glomerulonephritis and hemolytic-uremic syndrome.

Once the child is diagnosed with acute renal failure, all aspects of nursing care must be monitored closely. If the child does not develop complications or if the cause of the failure cannot be corrected, most children's renal functions return to normal within 1 to 3 weeks.

The treatment is based on careful assessment of the volume status, treatment of the underlying cause, and management of complications. Nurses taking care of these children need to be very knowledgeable about the signs and symptoms of hyperkalemia. Serum potassium does not reflect total body potassium content adequately, because potassium can move into or out of cells in exchange for hydrogen ions. Therefore, serum potassium must be interpreted on the basis of the child's acid-base status. Hyperkalemia is a life-threatening complication and must be treated promptly to avoid cardiac toxicity. The treatment is based on the management of fluid intake and urine output. Another treatment is the institution of dialysis. There are 6 indications for dialysis: volume overload with indication of pulmonary edema, hyperkalemia, metabolic acidosis, BUN above normal, neurologic problems secondary to uremia, and hypocalcemia. Both peritoneal and intermittent dialysis have been used successfully in children.

Lower Urinary Tract Disorders

Urinary Tract Infections

A **urinary tract infection** (UTI) occurs when there is an invasion of bacterial microorganisms into the urinary tract structures. This invasion can occur in the upper part of the urinary system, renal pelvis, calyces, or renal parenchyma, or in the lower part of the urethra or the bladder.

The predisposing factors that cause incomplete drainage and stasis of urine can be functional and/or anatomic in nature. The infected urine may reach the renal parenchyma and cause damage, which contributes to UTI. The anatomic factors can be reflux, ureter with anatomic abnormalities, or neurologic bladder. The functional obstruction in children can be constipation and infrequent voiding. Female children may have problems with cleaning themselves after defecating or may be bathed with bubble baths. UTI also occurs in male children who have not been circumcised. Other causes of UTI are diabetes, nephrocalcinosis, malnutrition, trauma, and sexual abuse.

The most common bacterial pathogens are *Staphylococcus saprophyticus*, which is commonly seen in sexually active adolescents. In younger children, the most common pathogens are *Escherichia coli, Proteus,* and *Klebsiella.* The most common viral pathogen is the adenovirus. UTI is rarely seen in full-term newborns, but the incidence is higher in premature neonates. The incidence is higher in females, with a peak between 2 and 6 years of age. The diagnosis is based on urinalysis and urine cultures. The nurse usually collects a mid-catheter urine specimen. Sometimes it is necessary to catheterize the child, which should be done with extreme care and psychological preparation of the parents and the child prior to the catheterization.

The management of the disorder is geared toward elimination of the infection. The main nursing intervention is teaching parents how to prevent recurrent infections. Teaching should include compliance with medication, the importance of forcing fluids to the child, teaching the child and the parents about appropriate hygiene, teaching the child how to empty the bladder, and compliance with follow-up cultures in order to determine if the infection has been eradicated. If the child has more than 3 UTIs in the period of a year, he/she should be placed in prophylactic therapy and should be monitored closely.

Urinary tract infection. An infection of the organs and ducts participating in secretion and elimination of urine.

Vesicoureteral Reflux

Vesicoureteral reflux (VRI) is the flow of bladder urine into the ureter, which increases the chance of infection because void urine is swept up to the ureter and then allowed to empty after voiding. The degree of the reflux is primary or secondary.

Vesicoureteral reflux. Backward flow of urine in the urinary bladder and a ureter.

Primary reflux results from a congenital anomaly affecting the uretero-vesical junction. Abnormal tunneling of the intramural ureteral segment and defects of formation of the ureteral orifice are associated with primary reflux. Primary reflux is associated with a familial pattern. Secondary reflux occurs as a result of an acquired condition. The presence of UTI sometimes produces a transient form of reflux. Children with this condition are at a greater risk for recurrent UTI. Also, neuropathic bladder dysfunction with bladder obstruction may produce reflux.

Reflux with infection often leads to kidney damage, since the urine is refluxed into the nephron, allowing the microorganisms to access the renal parenchyma and therefore to start to scar the kidneys. Most renal scars associated with reflux occur at an early age and are present at the time of diagnosis. VRI is an important cause of renal damage. Therefore, its diagnosis needs to be made carefully. Careful follow-up is also important in the management of children with UTI and children with reflux. The management is conservative, and it aims to control infection.

Therapy consists of continuous low-dose antibacterial therapy. The efficacy of the antibacterial therapy is monitored by continuous urine cultures, which can be done at home. If the reflux has not been corrected with conservative measures, the condition needs to be corrected surgically. Antireflux surgery consists of reimplantation of the ureter. The postsurgical care entails antibiotic therapy for up to 3 years to ensure that there is no more bacterial growth in the renal area. The primary nursing goal is to ensure compliance with the medical regime and with the medications. In teaching the parents the nurse needs to focus on stressing the differences in the anatomy of female and male children. The main point to stress about the anatomy of female children is that the female urethra is close to the vagina and to the anus; therefore, perineal hygiene is most important in the management of female children. Female children need to clean themselves from front to back, in order to avoid fecal contamination. Also, they need to avoid tight underwear and clothing; the underwear needs to be cotton. For both sexes, parents need to be told not to teach children to hold their urine, encourage children to ask for help to go to the bathroom as needed, and allow children to take all the time they need to empty the bladder. Encourage parents to give their children all the fluid they want, and if the urine is concentrated, encourage the consumption of juices that will help the acidification of the urine.

Hydrocele

Hydrocele. The accumulation of serous fluid in a saclike cavity, especially in the tunica vaginalis testis.

Hydrocele represents the persistent patency of the processus vaginalis, which normally obliterates before birth. **Hydrocele** is a scrotal swelling or inguinal swelling that includes abdominal contents in an inguinal hernia. This condition allows communication of fluid between the scrotum and peritoneum, which accounts for the increase in size of the scrotal sac. A hydrocele can be communicating or noncommunicating. A communicating hydrocele happens when the processus vaginalis remains patent, so that the fluid moves from the abdomen to the scrotum; it is associated with hernia. A noncommunicating hydrocele is rare in children; it represents partial obliteration of the processus vaginalis, leaving the sac of fluid about the testicle, but not communicating with the peritoneum. Communicating hydrocele should be repaired promptly so that incarceration of the bowel does not occur. The management depends on the kind of hydrocele. In a noncommunicating hydrocele, fluid generally absorbs, and no treatment is indicated unless the hydrocele is so large that it is uncomfortable and persists longer than a year. Communicating hydrocele can resolve, but is more likely to develop into a true hernia requiring surgical repair; surgery is usually done.

The major nursing intervention is parent education. Parents are taught to observe the child for any changes that may require emergency surgery. The surgery is usually done on an outpatient basis and children recuperate quickly.

Phimosis

Phimosis is the narrowing of the foreskin in males that prevents retraction over the glans penis. There is no clear reason why some children are born with this condition, but what should be emphasized is that the foreskin should not be forced to retract, which can cause scarring and paraphimosis. The adhesions will disappear by the time the child is 3 years of age.

The treatment depends on the severity of the condition. If the narrowing of the skin is almost complete, an emergency circumcision must be performed. Parents need to learn about proper hygiene and external cleansing.

Phimosis. Stenosis or narrowness of preputial orifice so that the foreskin cannot be pushed back over the glans penis.

Testicular Torsion

Testicular torsion is an acute, painful condition in which the spermatic cord is twisted just above the testicle, blood flow is compromised to the testicle, and the child exhibits cremasteric muscle spasms. Torsion occurs at any age but is most prevalent in adolescence, with a peak at about 14 years of age. The diagnosis is made by using Doppler ultrasound. The condition is treated as an emergency in order to avoid testicular atrophy and loss of the testis. Ideally, surgery should be done within 6 hours after the torsion has occurred.

Testicular torsion. Painful twisting of a testicle.

Exstrophy of the Bladder

Exstrophy of the bladder is classically a rare anomaly of the lower abdominal wall in which a persistent cloacal membrane prevents the medial ingrowth of mesenchyme. The deeper layers of ectoderm and mesoderm do not fuse. When rupture of the membrane occurs, there is a

Exstrophy of the bladder. A congenital turning inside out of the bladder.

separation of the midline structures, including the lower abdominal wall, rectus abdominis muscle and fascia, bladder, pubis, urethra, and genitalia. The degree of exstrophy depends on the size of the cloacal membrane and the time of its rupture. Most commonly the bladder is open and exposed on the lower abdominal wall. The rectus muscles and fascia diverge to rest on the laterally displaced pubic bones. The external genitalia are splayed. In the female the clitoris is bifid, the labia lateral, and the vagina anterior. In the male, the penis is short and wide with a dorsal urethral strip.

Diagnosis is obvious at birth, and prompt supportive care should be instituted. At this time, there is no recognized pattern of involvement with other organs in this defect. The goal of treatment is to provide a functioning bladder capable of social continence. The initial surgical procedure is the closure of the bladder and abdominal wall, leaving an open incontinent epispadiac bladder neck. The procedure is done preferably 48 to 72 hours postbirth. If it is not done, the child has an iliac osteotomy just before bladder closure. Surgery is aimed to allow the bladder to drop into the abdominal cavity and facilitate closure of the anterior abdominal wall. Successful results are reported in 90% of these children.

$\mathcal{G}$YNECOLOGICAL CONDITIONS

Gynecological conditions of the reproductive system can be classified as menstrual problems, inflammatory conditions, infections, and reproductive problems. The structure and function of the reproductive system depend on sex hormones, the most important of which is testosterone, in the embryonic development. At the age of 8 weeks' gestation, the reproductive structures of males and females are similar. During development the paramesonephric ducts degenerate and the mesonephric ducts and vas deferens are formed. In the female fetus, the lower ends of the paramesonephric ducts become the uterus and the upper portions become the fallopian tubes. Therefore, at the end of 8 weeks of gestation both sexes have different genital tubercles. By the ninth month, internal and external genital structures are all present.

Amenorrhea

Amenorrhea. Absence or suppression of menstruation.

Menstrual disorders are common concerns during adolescence. **Amenorrhea** or absence of menses is a very worrisome symptom that makes the concerned teenager go to see a gynecologist for evaluation. Amenorrhea is primary or secondary. Primary amenorrhea is defined as the absence of menses by age 16 in the presence of good health. Secondary amenorrhea is the absence of menses for at least 6 months after the menstrual cycle has been established.

There are multiple causes for amenorrhea, including stress, systematic illness, extreme exercise or weight loss, eating disorders, endocrine disorders, or structural abnormalities. Evaluation of the adolescent should encompass a carefully elicited, complete history and physical examination. In doing the tests, the nurse should never discard the possibility of pregnancy. Whatever the cause of amenorrhea, the nursing intervention is geared toward relieving the patient and her parents of their concerns. The nurse should educate the parents about the need for counseling and treatment of the underlying cause of the amenorrhea.

Dysmenorrhea

Dysmenorrhea, or dysfunctional vaginal bleeding, should alert the nurse to the possibility of abnormal ovulation in adolescent females. The excessive bleeding includes the use of 10 sanitary napkins per day for a period of 8 days. The evaluation is very important because it helps to determine the amount and the severity of the blood loss.

Dysmenorrhea. Pain in association with menstruation.

Therapy is directed toward the underlying condition. There are different treatments, including the use of progesterone or oral contraceptives in high doses. Therapy is given for several months in order to build up the endometrial lining. For adolescents who have had dysmenorrhea for an extended period of time, iron supplements are recommended.

Vaginitis/Cervicitis

Vaginitis/cervicitis is a lower genital tract infection in females, involving the urinary tract, cervix, vulva, and/or vagina, which can produce a variety of symptoms including pruritus, dispareunia, dysuria, and an alteration of the vaginal discharge. The three most common types of vaginitis are bacterial vaginitis, *Trichomonas vaginalis* vaginitis, and *Candida* vaginitis.

Vaginitis. Inflammation of the vagina.

Cervicitis. Inflammation of the cervix and uterus.

Careful evaluation should include examination of vaginal fluid, endocervical culture, and Papanicolaou smear.

Candida vaginitis includes vaginal and vulvar erythema, vulvar edema, pruritus, and the presence of thick, cottage cheese–like discharge. The diagnosis is made by microscopic findings. The treatment is done with topical vaginal clotrimazole or miconazole, which usually results in the relief of the symptoms.

Trichomonal vaginitis is characterized by a vaginal discharge with a foul odor and is described as yellow-green and frothy. The vagina and cervix may be erythematous, and occasionally strawberry spots are seen on the cervix. The only treatment is metronidazole, which can be given in 1 dose of 2 g or can be given over a period of days.

Bacterial vaginosis is the most common cause of an abnormal vaginal discharge. The diagnosis is based on the finding of a gray homogeneous discharge. The treatment of choice is metronidazole, 500 mg bid for 7 days.

Pelvic Inflammatory Disease

PID. Pelvic inflammatory disease; ascending infection from the vagina or cervix to the uterus, fallopian tubes, and broad ligaments.

Pelvic inflammatory disease (**PID**) is the syndrome that results from the ascending spread of microorganisms from the vagina and cervix to the endometrium. About 1 million women are treated for this disease each year. PID has been called the disease of young women, primarily of adolescents. The organisms most commonly identified with PID are *Chlamydia trachomatis*, *Neisseria gonorrhoeae*, and a variety of anaerobic bacteria. The diagnosis of PID is difficult; it can be confused with appendicitis or pyelonephritis. The suggested criteria for the diagnosis of PID are history of abdominal pain, presence of direct lower abdominal pain, and cervical motion tenderness.

The treatment is aimed at the prevention of infertility and the treatment of chronic residual infection. Several treatments exist for the management of PID. The most widely used are intravenous cefatoxin and doxycycline because of its comprehensive coverage for *N. gonorrhoeae*, and *C. trachomatis*.

Gonorrhea

Gonorrhea. A specific, contagious, catarrhal inflammation of the genital mucous membrane of either sex.

Gonorrhea is a sexually transmitted disease. The most common cause of lower genital tract infections involving the cervix occurs via urethral, cervical, anal, pharyngeal, and conjunctival contact. It is believed that *N. gonorrhoeae* is transmitted more from males to females, the highest incidence being in the late teen years. The incubation period is from 3 to 10 days, but there is frequently asymptomatology, which contributes to the seriousness of the sequelae of this infection. In males, the organisms typically invade the anterior urethra and they exhibit mucous urethral discharge and dysuria. In females, the organisms may invade the endocervical columnar epithelium, and may involve the Bartholin's glands or the urethra. Besides genital contact, the infection also can be spread to an unborn baby if the child is born vaginally.

The diagnosis is made by a serologic test for syphilis, and by Thayer-Martin culture to confirm the diagnosis. The treatment is to give penicillin as the first drug of choice. Penicillin is given with probenecid, which blocks penicillin excretion from the body. The most important nursing intervention, however, is counseling the adolescent that his/her partner also needs treatment; otherwise he/she will become reinfected.

SUMMARY

The genitourinary system is responsible for maintaining metabolism and for excreting waste products from the body. The genitourinary system consists of the kidneys, nephrons, distal tubules, collecting ducts, renal pelvis, ureter, bladder, urethra, and sphincters. This chapter reviews the main genitourinary disorders identified in children, including nursing diagnostic procedures and interventions. Chronic, congenital, and acquired disorders are reviewed.

Critical Points in the Care of Urinary Tract Disorders

Urinary tract infections are second only to upper respiratory infections as a source of morbidity from bacterial infections in childhood. The recognition and assessment of these conditions require a thorough workup by the nurse, including history taking, physical examination, and diagnostic procedures, based on the assessment of collected data. The aim of the nurse should be to aid in the prevention of disease and to place at-risk children in programs designed to alleviate severe recurrences.

Most of the treatment of children with genitourinary problems is symptomatic and is driven by social as well as medical factors. The main goal of nursing in the care of these conditions is to prevent serious deterioration of the system and avoid any permanent damage. For example, in the case of the child with a urinary tract infection, the nurse will utilize all his/her knowledge to categorize the child in an appropriate risk category. If the assessment is not based on sound nursing knowledge, the child could be placed in a situation in which the UTI will develop again with even more complications. In doing a thorough assessment, the nurse should avoid hasty conclusions and base the diagnosis on solid documentation. Also, the nurse is the person who collects the specimens. He/she must do so properly, based on knowledge of anatomy and physiology.

A solid teaching plan for the parents should be developed by the nurse, in which prevention activities are based on hygienic principles and on helping parents comprehend the common symptoms associated with the condition. Revision of instructions, including medications, dosages, side effects, collection for urinalysis (which can be done in the home), and evaluating fever of unknown origin, should be addressed in the teaching plan.

In the treatment of glomerulonephritis, the nurse has to have a clear understanding of fluid and electrolyte balance along with a clear understanding of how to evaluate the child with this disease. The nurse should manage the condition by including the care of any underlying conditions. One vital area to be considered would include the type of psychological care provided by the nurse to anxious parents of an ill child who has blood in the urine, or who is gravely ill.

The key points in the management of any genitourinary condition are the knowledge of the physiologic conditions and the ability to integrate psychological care with medical management.

QUESTIONS

Diagnosis: Testicular Torsion

> History: 14-year-old Juan comes home from school crying. He tells his mother that when he was leaving school he had a terrible pain in his scrotum, and he wanted to die because it hurt so much. His mother asks how he is now. He tells her that he is hurting badly and he wants her to take him to the hospital. At the emergency room the doctor tells Juan's mother that Juan has a testicular torsion. His mother turns to the nurse and tells her that she wants to talk to her.
>
> Plan: Juan is to go home with his parents. The management of his condition is based on its seriousness.
>
> Nursing problems: Crisis intervention for the parents. Preoperative care for Juan. Use of medications for pain. Teaching parents and Juan about the disorder.

1. Juan's mother asks the nurse what treatment is indicated for children with testicular torsion. The nurse responds:

    A. Immediate surgery
    B. Complete bed rest
    C. Follow-up in 1 week
    D. Observation for 1 week

2. The nurse tells Juan's mother that because of the severity of his condition, the aim of surgery is to distort rather than fixate the testis in the abdomen. This is done to:

    A. Prevent future torsion
    B. Prevent future swelling
    C. Remove underdeveloped tissue
    D. Aid in the development of the testis

3. The nurse knows that the differential diagnosis with regard to pyuria and not to scrotal position is:

    A. Trauma
    B. Orchitis
    C. Epididymitis
    D. Incarcerated hernia

4. The nurse knows that the diagnosis of testicular torsion must be differentiated from epididymitis and torsion of the testicular appendage. An appropriate procedure to assess blood flow is:

    A. Surgical exploration
    B. Doppler examination
    C. Nuclear technetium
    D. Radionucleotide scanning

Diagnosis: Phimosis

History: Henry, a 3-year-old boy, came to the hospital because he was having a small amount of bleeding from his penis. In doing the physical exam, the nurse realizes that he has a serious case of phimosis, but otherwise he is well developed and has no other physical problems. The nurse realizes that Henry's parents live far away from the city and have no means of transportation. The nurse confers with the pediatrician, and after careful consideration, the pediatrician decides that it is best to do a circumcision immediately in order to prevent future problems.

Plan: Henry will have surgery in the morning.

Nursing problems: Parent education. Preparation for Henry to have the circumcision and for discharge.

Chief concern: The nurse realizes that at this time the most important nursing intervention is teaching the parents and clarifying questions and fears they may have.

1. Based on their economic status and their access to immediate medical care, Henry's parents are told that the medical personnel believe that he will need a circumcision and that it would be best to do it now while they are in the hospital. The rationale for surgery is to:
   A. Diminish the swelling
   B. Remove additional glands
   C. Redirect the urinary canal
   D. Enlarge the preputial opening

2. The nurse knows that in making the diagnosis the doctor had to consider what other differential diagnosis?
   A. Hypospadias
   B. Paraphimosis
   C. Cryptorchidism
   D. Blanoposthesis

3. Henry had surgery and he had no problems. A day later he was discharged from the hospital, but before being discharged his mother asked what additional instructions she needed before taking him home.
   A. Exercise and diet
   B. Adequate oral intake
   C. Prevention of infection
   D. Hygiene and external cleansing

Diagnosis: Urinary Tract Infections

History: Raquel Gomez, a 5-year-old, has been brought to the clinic by her mother because she has been complaining of lower abdominal pain and frequency of urination. Raquel is afebrile. Ms. Gomez tells the nurse that she noticed discoloration in Raquel's urine for the last few days but has given no medication. The child has no allergies.

Plan: Raquel is to go back home with her mother. Ms. Gomez will be taught the management of Raquel's condition.

Chief concern: The nurse realizes that the most important nursing intervention is teaching Ms. Gomez management of the disease and the importance of compliance and prevention of future infections.

1. What should be the initial approach in the care of Raquel?
   A. Rule out urethritis.
   B. Rule out trauma.
   C. Request an analgesic.
   D. Help localize the site of infection.

2. Raquel had a series of urine cultures obtained 72 hours after admission. Knowing this, the nurse realizes that the diagnosis will be made on the basis of:
   A. pH of the urine
   B. Dipstick of protein
   C. Dipstick of red blood cells
   D. Leukocyte esterase test

3. Raquel's tests have come back and the results from the leukocyte esterase test show a strong WBC, RBC, and mila protein. Given the history, the diagnosis is:
   A. Cystitis
   B. Ureteritis
   C. Kidney stones
   D. Ureter stricture

4. Raquel was placed on Septra 40 mg/kg/c for 10–14 days. The rationale for the 14-day regimen is:
   A. To prevent drug tolerance.
   B. New pathogens could develop.
   C. Antibiotics take longer to exert a positive effect.
   D. Children need more time to resolve infections.

Diagnosis: Acute Poststreptococcal Glomerulonephritis

History: A young mother comes to the clinic, concerned because her 4-year-old daughter is complaining of headache, vomiting, and lethargy. The mother reports that the urine is the color of dark tea.

Plan: Child is to go home with her parents after the acute phase of the disease has subsided, and the management of the disease will be based on the progression of her recovery.

Nursing problems: Compliance with treatment. Prevention of complications. Teaching of prevention measures.

Chief concern: For the child, the resolution of the disease and return to normal health. For the family, compliance with the regimen and the implementation of preventive measures. For the child, compliance with follow-up visits to the doctor's office.

1. In the initial history and physical examination, which of the following findings would help the nurse to arrive at a diagnosis of glomerulonephritis?

   A. Edema
   B. Nausea
   C. Lethargy
   D. Dark tea-colored urine

2. What tests would be ordered in addition to urinalysis?

   A. B-titers
   B. Serum ASA
   C. WBC count
   D. Streptococcus screen

3. The history and initial findings support the diagnosis of acute poststreptococcal glomerulonephritis. The most important laboratory findings to confirm the diagnosis are:

   A. Serum ASP pepresed
   B. Leukocyte casts
   C. Granular casts
   D. Depressed serum concentrations of C_3

4. Eight weeks after the diagnosis, the C_3 concentration remains low, and it is suspected that the patient may have another type of nephritis. The next test that should be ordered is:

   A. ASO
   B. C_3 level
   C. C_4 level
   D. Renal biopsy

5. After all the lab studies were done, the nurse decides that the best intervention is:

   A. Supportive therapy
   B. Prednisone therapy
   C. Massive antibiotic therapy
   D. Complete bed rest for 2 weeks

Diagnosis: Pelvic Inflammatory Disease

History: 18-year-old Melissa comes to the clinic because she has had abdominal pain for the last 3 months. She says that a friend told her that she had the same pain, and that she ended up with PID. Melissa is afraid of having the disease, but wants to make sure that she is okay.

Plan: Melissa is to go back and live a normal life without PID, but this time she will know what she needs to know in order to get better and never get infected again.

Nursing problems: Compliance with medication. Counseling about sex practices. Use of prophylactics. Prevention of future infections.

Chief concerns: For Melissa, the resolution is curing of the infection and return to normal health, compliance with medication, and adherence to the medical regimen. For her partner, treatment because he is also infected.

1. What are the important clinical elements in the diagnosis of PID?
   A. History of abdominal pain, direct lower abdominal tenderness, cervical motion, tenderness, adnexal tenderness
   B. Direct lower abdominal pain, adnexal tenderness, cervical tenderness, temperature of 100.2°F
   C. Direct lower abdominal pain, adnexal tenderness, cervical pain, cervical discharge
   D. Direct lower abdominal pain, low-grade fever, leukocytosis, adexnal tenderness

2. While doing the diagnosis the nurse knows that the differential diagnosis that should be recognized before making the final diagnosis is:
   A. Appendicitis
   B. Septic abortion
   C. Renal calculus
   D. Ruptured ovarian cysts

3. Melissa was initially started on cefatoxin and doxycycline. What is the nursing intervention?
   A. Advise partner treatment
   B. Obtain CBC and platelet count
   C. Obtain blood cultures 72 hours after treatment is started
   D. Obtain blood cultures at the termination of treatment

4. Which long-term sequela must be prevented through education and guidance?
   A. Phosalphinx
   B. Dispareunia
   C. Chronic pelvic pain
   D. Involuntary infertility

Diagnosis: *Candida* Vaginitis

History: 15-year-old Theresa comes to the clinic and complains of vaginal discharge and discomfort in the lower abdomen. After examination, the nurse suspects that Theresa has vaginitis. She realizes that the treatment is based on what kind of vaginitis Theresa has.

Plan: Theresa is to go home knowing how to care for herself and avoid becoming infected again.

Nursing problems: Compliance with prevention. Use of prophylactics.

Chief concern: For Theresa, to know more about her disease and to know how to prevent becoming infected again.

1. In making Theresa's diagnosis, which medical test helped to identify the type of vaginitis she had?

   A. Whiff test
   B. pH of vaginal discharge
   C. Culture of vaginal discharge
   D. Examination of vaginal discharge

2. Theresa's history and physical examination reveal vaginal and vulvar erythema, vulvar edema, pruritus, thick cottage cheese–like discharge. This is an indication that the diagnosis is:

   A. *Candida* vaginitis
   B. *Trichomonas* vaginitis
   C. Bacterial vaginosis
   D. *Gardnerella* vaginitis

3. Which finding is the most important in making the diagnosis?

   A. Positive Whiff test
   B. Vaginal pH greater than 4.5
   C. Microscopic findings on a saline preparation
   D. Microscopic findings on a potassium hydroxide preparation

Diagnosis: Gonorrhea

History: 15-year-old Mary showed localized infection of the cervix, urethra, and Skene glands. After the physical exam the nurse suspects that Mary has gonorrhea.

Plan: To ensure that the diagnosis will be correct.

Nursing problems: Rule out differential diagnosis.

Chief concerns: The resolution of the infection.

1. In order to confirm the diagnosis that Mary has gonorrhea, a more detailed physical examination is done. The decision is based on the possibility that Mary may have:

   A. Endocarditis
   B. Pharyngitis
   C. Anorectal infections
   D. Fitz-Hugh-Curtis syndrome

2. In order to eliminate Mary's infection as effectively, economically, and safely as possible, the best therapy is:

   A. Ceftriaxone for 14 days
   B. Streptomycin, 4 g, and a 3-day course of tetracycline
   C. Doxycycline, 100 mg, 1 dose, followed with ceftriaxone for 14 days
   D. Doxycycline, 1 dose, followed by a 7-day course of tetracycline

𝒜NSWERS

Testicular Torsion

1. *A.* Testicular torsion is a surgical emergency. The surgery must be performed within 6 hours to ensure fertility and to prevent abscess and atrophy.

2. *A.* The aim of the surgery is to distort the testis and prevent future torsion.

3. *A.* Because of the severity of the pain trauma is always ruled out.

4. *B.* Laboratory studies are always useful in the diagnosis of testicular torsion, because of the similarity of the symptoms of epididymal appendage and torsion of the testicular appendage. Doppler examination is needed in 70% of the cases.

Phimosis

1. *D.* By age 3, the preputial opening should be large enough to allow easy retraction of the prepuce.

2. *B.* In phimosis, the skin is too tight to be retracted over the glans penis. Paraphimosis is the opposite: a retracted foreskin that cannot be reduced.

3. *D.* Normal cleansing should be done with gentle stretching of the foreskin.

Urinary Tract Infections

1. *D.* The workup for children with UTI requires sufficient information to place children in categories of risk or nonrisk.

2. *D.* Leukocyte esterase chemical tests detect pyuria.

3. *A.* Cystitis is an inflammation resulting from infection that occurs at any point of the urinary tract.

4. *B.* The goals of the treatment are the eradication of infection and the prevention of recurrence.

Acute Poststreptococcal Glomerulonephritis

1. *D.* The urine is described as smoky and tea-colored, due to hematuria.

2. *C.* Microscopic hematuria is always present with leukocyturia.

3. *B.* Leukocyte casts as well as hyaline and glandular casts are often seen.

4. *B*. One of the most important diagnostic laboratory findings is a depressed serum concentration of C_3.

5. *A*. No specific therapy is effective. In ameliorating the inflammatory process, all therapy is supportive and directed toward treating the clinical manifestations.

Pelvic Inflammatory Disease

1. *A*. The suggested criteria for the diagnosis of PID are the presence of direct lower abdominal tenderness, cervical motion tenderness, and adnexal tenderness.

2. *A*. Appendicitis mimics PID.

3. *A*. Treatment of any sexual partner is a must. The patient should be advised that no intercourse should take place until the sexual partner has been treated, in order to prevent reinfection.

4. *D*. Infertility is the number one complication of PID.

Candida Vaginitis

1. *D*. The diagnosis is confirmed by a microscopic examination of vaginal discharge.

2. *A*. Along with vaginal and vulvar erythema, the patient has a thick cottage cheese–like discharge.

3. *D*. The diagnosis is confirmed by microscopic finding of the yeasts on a potassium hydroxide preparation.

Gonorrhea

1. *C*. Anorectal infections from gonorrhea are common in women, even in the absence of rectal intercourse.

2. *D*. To address the many concerns associated with this disease the best treatment is a single dose of treatment followed by a 7-day course regimen.

GLOSSARY

acute glomerulonephritis   a form of nephritis in which the lesions involve primarily the glomeruli.

acute renal failure   acute failure of the kidney to perform its essential functions. May be due to trauma or any condition that impairs the flow of blood to the kidneys.

amenorrhea   absence or suppression of menstruation.

cervicitis   inflammation of the cervix and uterus.

dysmenorrhea   pain in association with menstruation.

exstrophy of the bladder   a congenital turning inside out of the bladder.

gonorrhea   a specific, contagious, catarrhal inflammation of the genital mucous membrane of either sex.

hematuria   blood in the urine.

hydrocele   the accumulation of serous fluid in a saclike cavity, especially in the tunica vaginalis testis.

nephrotic syndrome   disease of the basement membrane of the glomerulus that causes severe proteinuria, hypoalbuminemia, generalized edema, lipiduria, and hyperlipidemia. Blood pressure remains normal.

phimosis   stenosis or narrowness of preputial orifice so that the foreskin cannot be pushed back over the glans penis.

PID   pelvic inflammatory disease; ascending infection from the vagina or cervix to the uterus, fallopian tubes, and broad ligaments.

proteinuria   protein, usually albumin, in the urine.

testicular torsion   painful twisting of a testicle.

urinary tract infection   an infection of the organs and ducts participating in secretion and elimination of urine.

vaginitis   inflammation of the vagina.

vesicoureteral reflux   backward flow of urine in the urinary bladder and a ureter.

$\mathcal{B}$IBLIOGRAPHY

BEHRMAN, R., AND KLIEGMAN, R. *Nelson Essentials of Pediatrics.* 2nd ed. Philadelphia: Saunders, 1994.

CIRCANOWICZ, M. M. *Nurse Review.* Springhouse, PA: Springhouse Corp., 1991.

MCCANCE, K., AND HUETER, S. *Pathophysiology: The Biologic Basis for Disease in Adults and Children.* St. Louis: Mosby-Year Book, 1994.

MILLONIG, V. S., ed. *Pediatric Nurse Practitioner Certification Review Guide.* 2nd ed. Potomac, MD: Health Leadership Associates, 1994.

PASCOE, D., AND GROSSMAN, M. *Quick Reference to Pediatric Emergencies.* 3rd ed. Philadelphia: Lippincott, 1984.

RUSSO, R., AND VYMUTT, G. *Practical Points in Pediatrics.* 4th ed. New York: Medical Examination Publishing Company, 1986.

THOMAS, C. L. (ed). *Taber's Cyclopedic Medical Dictionary.* 15th ed. Philadelphia: F. A. Davis, 1985.

WHALEY, L. F., AND WONG, D. L. *Nursing Care of Infants and Children.* 4th ed. St. Louis: Mosby-Year Book, 1991.

$\mathcal{H}$ELPFUL INTERNET SITES

PEDINFO: An Index of the Pediatric Internet at http://www.pedinfo. org   This is an excellent site that covers nearly all topics within this review. It has a wealth of information and is worth a visit. It is written for health care professionals but others could also use the information.

Bladder Exstrophy—The Association for Bladder Exstrophy Children at http://www.bladderexstrophy.com   The site is dedicated to issues and problems surrounding bladder exstrophy in children.

Virtual Naval Hospital Information for Providers at http://www.vnh. org/Providers.html   This site is part of the University of Iowa's health care site and is linked to a large set of databases that can be used by health care providers. The site covers a larger number of links to other sources on health care issues and problems. This is an excellent starting place to discover information on various common diseases and their treatments.

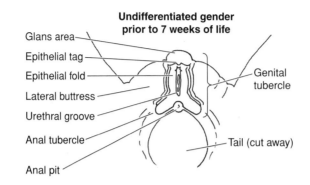

**Undifferentiated gender
prior to 7 weeks of life**

Glans area
Epithelial tag
Epithelial fold
Lateral buttress
Urethral groove
Anal tubercle
Anal pit
Genital tubercle
Tail (cut away)

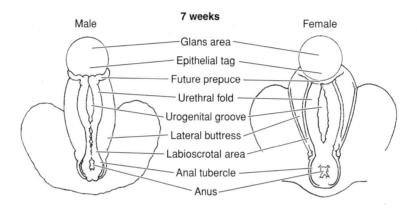

7 weeks

Male   Female

Glans area
Epithelial tag
Future prepuce
Urethral fold
Urogenital groove
Lateral buttress
Labioscrotal area
Anal tubercle
Anus

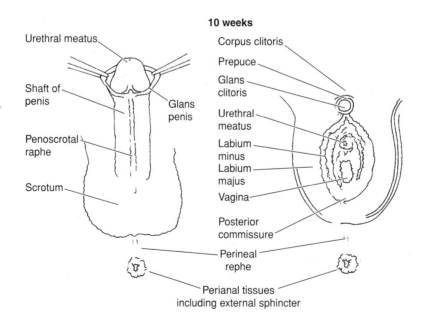

10 weeks

Urethral meatus
Shaft of penis
Penoscrotal raphe
Scrotum
Glans penis

Corpus clitoris
Prepuce
Glans clitoris
Urethral meatus
Labium minus
Labium majus
Vagina
Posterior commissure
Perineal rephe
Perianal tissues including external sphincter

FIGURE 17-1 External genitalia development.

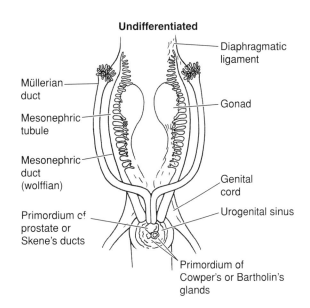

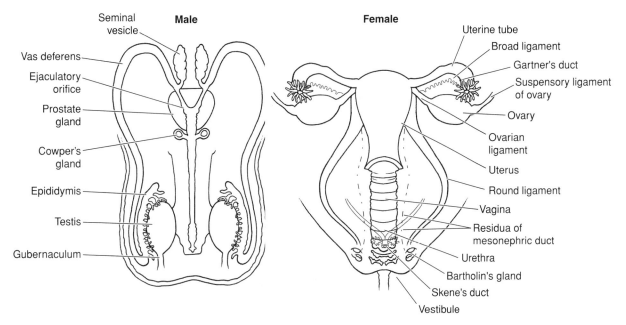

FIGURE 17-2 Internal genitalia development.

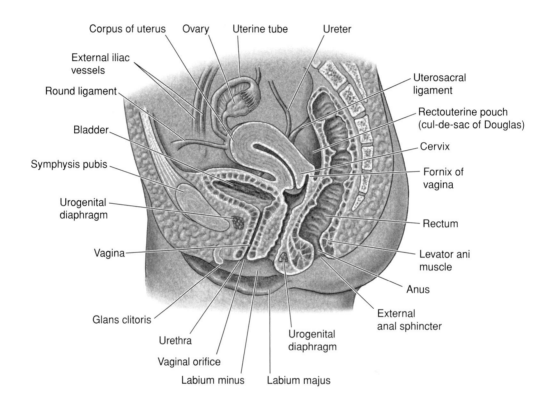

FIGURE 17-3 Female reproductive system: function and structure.

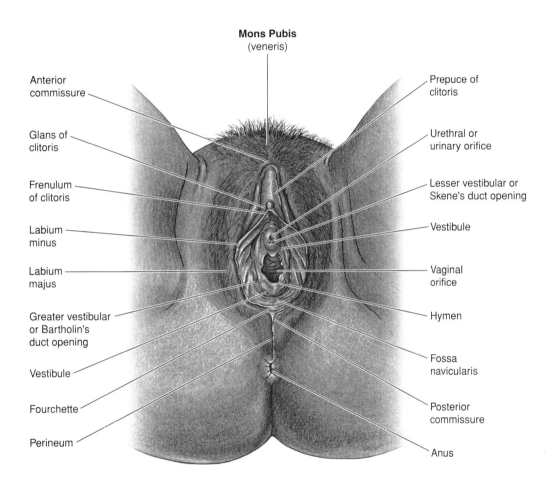

Mons Pubis
(veneris)

Anterior
commissure

Glans of
clitoris

Frenulum
of clitoris

Labium
minus

Labium
majus

Greater vestibular
or Bartholin's
duct opening

Vestibule

Fourchette

Perineum

Prepuce of
clitoris

Urethral or
urinary orifice

Lesser vestibular or
Skene's duct opening

Vestibule

Vaginal
orifice

Hymen

Fossa
navicularis

Posterior
commissure

Anus

FIGURE 17-4 External female genitalia.

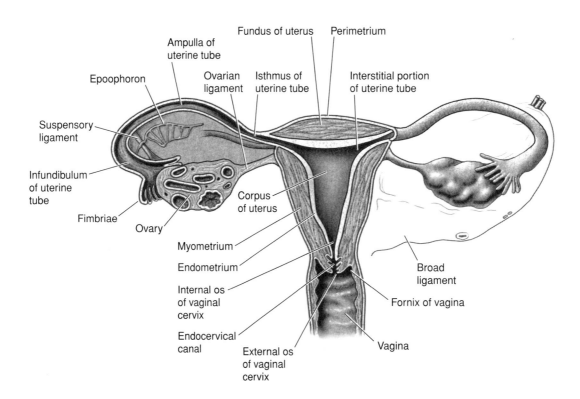

FIGURE 17-5 Cross section of uterus, fallopian tubes, and ovaries.

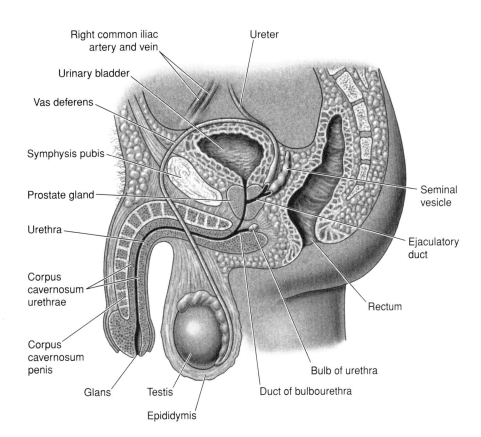

FIGURE 17-6 Sagittal section of the penis.

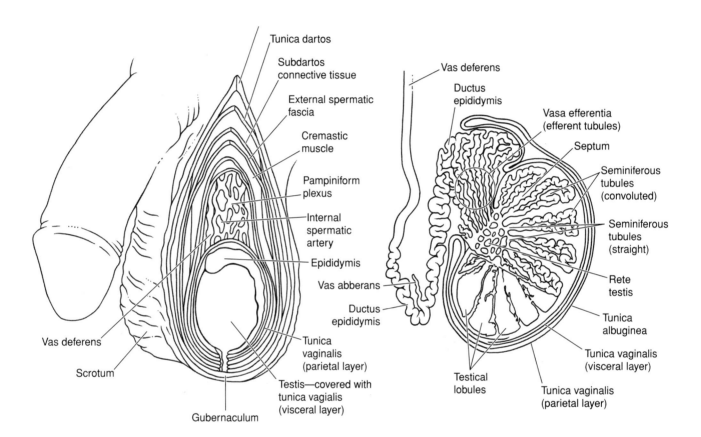

FIGURE 17-7 The testes. External and sagittal views showing interior anatomy.

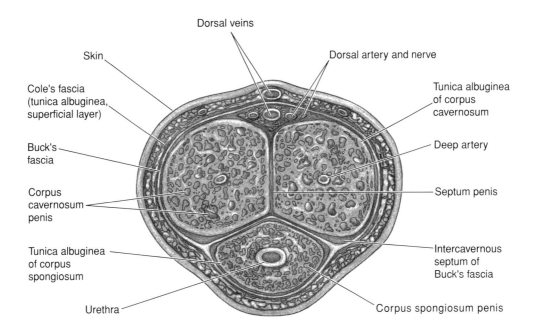

FIGURE 17-8 Cross section of the penis.

**Formation of
inguinal canal**

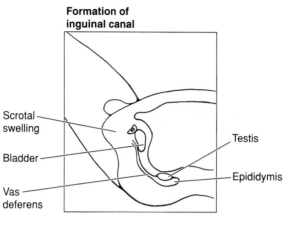

Scrotal
swelling

Bladder

Vas
deferens

Testis

Epididymis

Inguinal canal

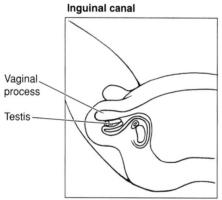

Vaginal
process

Testis

Tunica vaginalis

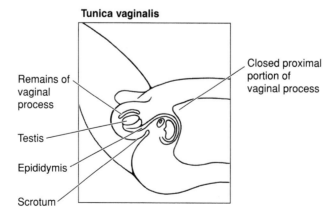

Remains of
vaginal
process

Testis

Epididymis

Scrotum

Closed proximal
portion of
vaginal process

FIGURE 17-9 Descent of a testis. The testes descend from the abdominal cavity to the scrotum during the last 3 months of fetal development.

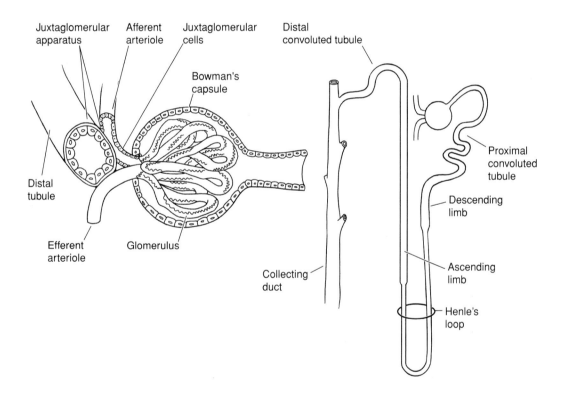

FIGURE 17-10 Components of the nephron.

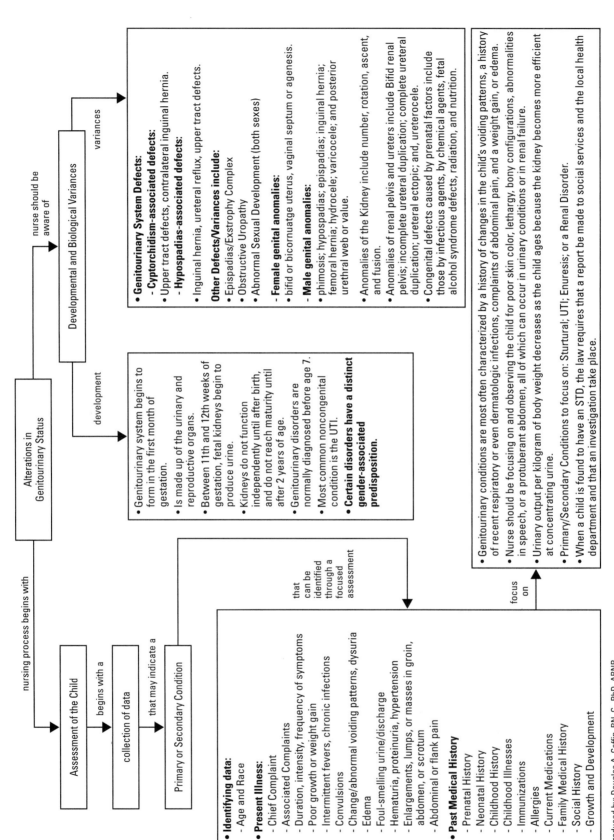

Alterations in Genitourinary Status

nursing process begins with →

nurse should be aware of →

Developmental and Biological Variances

variances →

Genitourinary System Defects:
- **Cyptorchidism-associated defects:**
  - Upper tract defects, contralateral inguinal hernia.
- **Hypospadias-associated defects:**
  - Inguinal hernia, ureteral reflux, upper tract defects.

Other Defects/Variances include:
- Epispadias/Exstrophy Complex
- Obstructive Uropathy
- Abnormal Sexual Development (both sexes)
  - **Female genital anomalies:**
    - bifid or bicornuatge uterus, vaginal septum or agenesis.
  - **Male genital anomalies:**
    - phimosis; hypospadias; epispadias; inguinal hernia; femoral hernia; hydrocele; varicocele; and posterior urethral web or value.
- Anomalies of the Kidney include number, rotation, ascent, and fusion.
- Anomalies of renal pelvis and ureters include Bifid renal pelvis; incomplete ureteral duplication; complete ureteral duplication; ureteral ectopic; and, ureterocele.
- Congenital defects caused by prenatal factors include those by infectious agents, by chemical agents, fetal alcohol syndrome defects, radiation, and nutrition.

development →

- Genitourinary system begins to form in the first month of gestation.
- Is made up of the urinary and reproductive organs.
- Between 11th and 12th weeks of gestation, fetal kidneys begin to produce urine.
- Kidneys do not function independently until after birth, and do not reach maturity until after 2 years of age.
- Genitourinary disorders are normally diagnosed before age 7.
- Most common noncongenital condition is the UTI.
- **Certain disorders have a distinct gender-associated predisposition.**

Assessment of the Child

begins with a →

collection of data

that may indicate a →

Primary or Secondary Condition

that can be identified through a focused assessment →

focus on →

- Genitourinary conditions are most often characterized by a history of changes in the child's voiding patterns, a history of recent respiratory or even dermatologic infections, complaints of abdominal pain, and a weight gain, or edema.
- Nurse should be focusing on and observing the child for poor skin color, lethargy, bony configurations, abnormalities in speech, or a protuberant abdomen, all of which can occur in urinary conditions or in renal failure.
- Urinary output per kilogram of body weight decreases as the child ages because the kidney becomes more efficient at concentrating urine.
- Primary/Secondary Conditions to focus on: Sturtural; UTI; Enuresis; or a Renal Disorder.
- When a child is found to have an STD, the law requires that a report be made to social services and the local health department and that an investigation take place.

- **Identifying data:**
  - Age and Race
- **Present Illness:**
  - Chief Complaint
  - Associated Complaints
  - Duration, intensity, frequency of symptoms
  - Poor growth or weight gain
  - Intermittent fevers, chronic infections
  - Convulsions
  - Change/abnormal voiding patterns, dysuria
  - Edema
  - Foul-smelling urine/discharge
  - Hematuria, proteinuria, hypertension
  - Enlargements, lumps, or masses in groin, abdomen, or scrotum
  - Abdominal or flank pain
- **Past Medical History**
  - Prenatal History
  - Neonatal History
  - Childhood History
  - Childhood Illnesses
  - Immunizations
  - Allergies
  - Current Medications
  - Family Medical History
  - Social History
  - Growth and Development

508

Produced by: Douglas A. Coffin, RN, C., PhD, ARNP

Concept Map 17-1

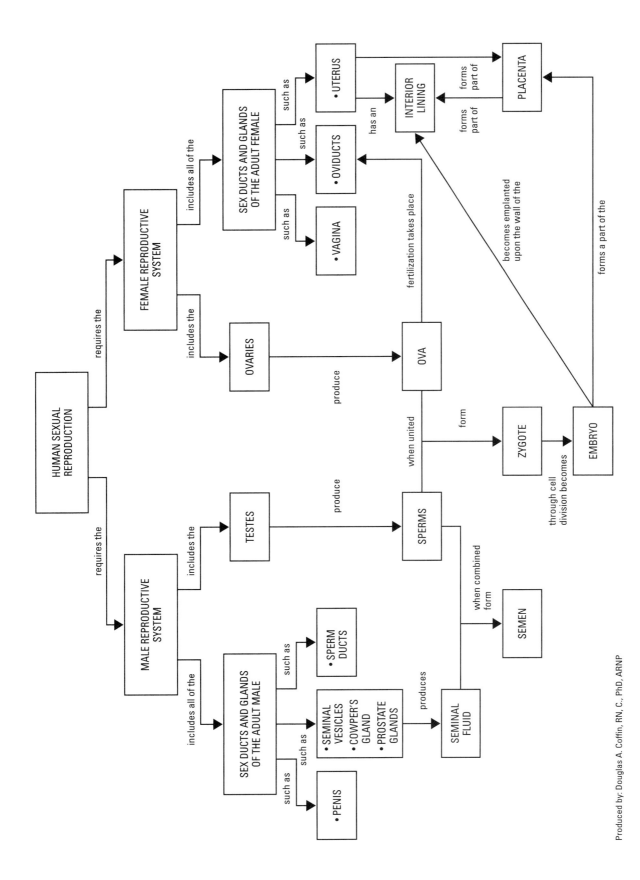

Produced by: Douglas A. Coffin, RN, C., PhD, ARNP

Concept Map 17-2

PEDIATRIC NURSING TODAY

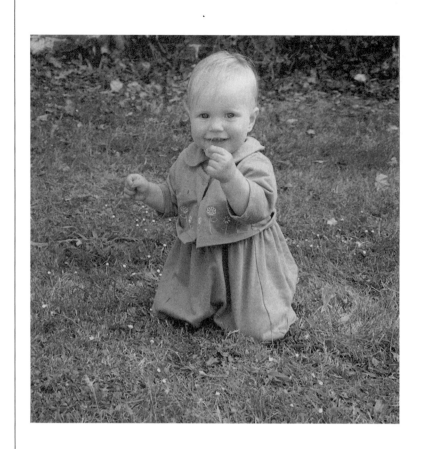

꽃

CURRENT ISSUES
IN PEDIATRICS

𝒥NTRODUCTION

Children are our future. Because of **societal changes**, and more precisely, because of new changes in health practices and changes in the composition of the family, the field of pediatrics has had to focus on prevention and education in order to anticipate threats to the pediatric population. In the 1990s, according to published literature, the overall health of children has improved and the rates of morbidity and mortality have decreased markedly. Yet, when one considers that the habits and practices established in childhood have a profound effect on health and illness throughout life, one must consider the current health practices of young parents. In so doing, health professionals need to refocus all efforts into creating a population of young parents capable of directing the future of their children based on solid health care choices and capable of critical thinking about the **hazards** that can affect their child's health today and throughout life.

Prevention and counseling are the basic tools of pediatrics, yet most of the efforts of today's health care system are geared toward acute care, not toward education and prevention. In one of the richest nations of the world, the United States, 25% of the children live in poverty, and those children have a higher incidence of disease. Entering the new millennium, there is no coordinated system of health services to which all people have access. The most obvious example of this lack of access is the record of children's immunizations in this country. Immunization is preventive care, yet only two-thirds of American preschool children have had all their immunizations.

Societal changes. Changes that occur in society as a result of changes in the world.

Hazards. Any situation handled in such a way that people can suffer personal injury.

Children are our richest resource. Far too many children, however, are being sacrificed because of their lack of access to a health care system. If we are to have solid leaders and responsible adults in the next century, our efforts as health care professionals must be directed toward learning more about the changes that affect the outcome of the health status of our richest resource, our children.

AUTO SAFETY

We read that a child is safe traveling in a car and the incidence of vehicular injuries has declined tremendously. Mandatory auto safety seats and mandatory seat belt laws have helped in the decline of vehicular injuries in all 50 states. The American Academy of Pediatrics (AAP) stresses that the back seat is the safest place for children of any age to ride and urges that all infants (from the time they are newborns, discharged from the hospital) and children ride in the child restraint appropriate to their age and weight. Infants less than 20 pounds and up to 1 year of age ought to ride in rear-facing seats. Low-birth-weight infants should be supported in rear-facing infant-only seats with ample padding. Children more than 20 pounds and 1 year of age can ride in forward-facing seats. Children more than 40 pounds should ride in booster seats until they are big enough to use lap and shoulder belts properly and comfortably. The AAP continues to recommend the use of lap and shoulder belts for older children in both front and back seats of the car. Never use a rear-facing car safety seat in the front seat of a car equipped with a passenger-side air bag. And an infant should never ride in the lap of an adult or while being held by an adult.

CHOLESTEROL TESTING

Hyperlipidemia is an excessive amount of cholesterol, cholesterol esters, phospholipids, or triglycerides in the blood. Cholesterol is a fatlike steroid alcohol, part of the lipoprotein complex in the plasma. It is essential for cellular metabolism and required by most cells for the manufacture and repair of plasma membranes. Triglycerides are natural fats synthesized from carbohydrates for energy. Dietary fat is formed in the small intestines into what are known as chylomicrons. Chylomicrons are required for absorption of fat. They function by transporting the exogenous lipids from the intestines to the liver and peripheral cells, and into fatty tissue or muscle, to be used for energy. The chylomicron remnants, mostly made up of cholesterol, are then taken up by the liver. A series of chemical reactions in the liver results in the production of several types of lipoprotein that include very low density lipids (VLDL), low density lipids (LDL), and high density lipids (HDL).

The factors that contribute to hyperlipidemia include systemic diseases and **exogenous factors**. The systemic diseases are pancreatitis, diabetes, and hypothyroidism; the exogenous factors are oral contraceptives, high dietary fat and caloric intake, obesity, sedentary life-style, and stress. There is also a group of lipoprotein disorders known as primary or genetic hyperlipidemia, which are seen in only a very small percentage of the population, but contribute to premature coronary atherosclerosis and ischemic heart disease. These disorders have been classified into 6 categories with a description of the specific genetic defect to the protein, cell, or organ function. A **genetic predisposition** to one of these disorders lends a strong familial link to early coronary heart disease, which occurs in approximately 5% of the general population. Familial hypercholesterolemia is one of these primary lipoprotein disorders, known as type IIa. Coronary heart disease usually develops by age 45 in men who have familial hypercholesterolemia. These families also account for more than 50% of the cases of coronary disease occurring before the age of 55.

Serum cholesterol levels are one of the most predictive risk factors for coronary heart disease today. It is thought that cholesterol levels in childhood appear to be a major population predictor for adult cholesterol levels.

Hypercholesterol screening in the pediatric population has caused a great deal of controversy. One side of the debate suggests that cholesterol screening should be a part of the routine pediatric exam. The other side recommends targeted screening, testing only those children who meet high risk factor criteria. It should be noted that the age group for initial hypercholesterol screening is being debated and remains controversial. High risk factors include: (1) a family factor of heart disease—parents or grandparents with a history of coronary or peripheral vascular disease before age 55, or parents with blood cholesterol level greater than 240 mg/dL; (2) a diet high in fat and cholesterol; (3) obesity; (4) a sedentary life-style; (5) smoking; (6) hypertension; and (7) diabetes mellitus.

The diagnosis is made by careful screening. The child should fast for 12 hours prior to blood draw. Blood samples should be collected after the child has been still for 5 minutes and the tourniquet should be applied immediately before the venous puncture; posture and vascular stasis may affect the results. Two fasting blood samples should be analyzed and their average values should be used for diagnosis. If the total cholesterol level is greater than 200 mg/dL, a lipoprotein analysis needs to be performed.

Initial therapy for any lipoprotein disorder is dietary restriction of fat and cholesterol along with a program of regular exercise. Children who have a low-risk lipid profile (LDL-C < 110 mg/dL) need to be counseled on diet, exercise, and healthy life-style. Children who have a moderate-risk lipid profile (LDL-C 110–129 mg/dL) need dietary counseling and follow-up lipid profile in 1 year. Children who have a high-risk lipid profile (LDL-C > 130/dL) need a lipoprotein profile of their parents and a step I diet: A dietary consult to assist the patient in eating a diet consistent with less than 10% of total calories being saturated fats, 30% of total calories being fats, and only 300 mg of cholesterol per day. Calories should be adequate to support growth and development. The diet should be able to assist the patient in reaching and maintaining a desirable body weight. If dietary

Exogenous factors. Outside factors, such as high dietary and caloric intake, sedentary life, stress.

Genetic predisposition. Susceptibility to a disease due to heredity.

modifications fail to achieve satisfactory levels of LDL after 3 months, the step II diet is initiated. The step II diet consists of less than 7% of total calories being saturated fat with no more than 30% of calories as fat, and only 200 mg of cholesterol per day. For children who fail to respond to dietary modifications, drug therapy may be necessary: bile acid sequestrates of resins, cholestyramine resin (Questran), colestipol hydrochloride (Colestid). The average dose is 4 grams tid or 6 grams bid. Constipation is the major complaint with these medications. Parents should be advised to give the child 1 multivitamin with iron per day because cholestyramine may interfere with the absorption of the fat-soluble vitamins.

Niacin is generally administered to older children who do not tolerate the bile acid resins. Some children may also require both treatments. Niacin decreases the LDL and increases the HDL. The initial dose in time-release or long-acting preparation is 125 to 150 mg bid, which can be increased to 30 mg/kg/day. Adverse side effects are reported to be flushing episodes, itching, and gastrointestinal upset. Flushing can be avoided by premedicating with aspirin 160 mg/day one-half hour before the dose of niacin. If age-appropriate, the patient needs to be referred to a stop smoking program. And if applicable, the patient needs to be counseled on the use of alcohol and suggestions need to be made for healthy life changes.

Children placed on cholesterol-lowering diet therapy need total cholesterol levels drawn 4 to 6 weeks upon initiation of therapy and every 3 months thereafter. Liver function profiles need to be monitored every 3 months because niacin can elevate liver enzymes and bilirubin. At each visit the whole family should be encouraged to participate in basic dietary changes and healthy life-style changes. The AAP continues to endorse selective cholesterol screening of children older than 2 years of age. Optional **cholesterol testing** may be appropriate for children who are judged to be at higher risk for coronary heart disease.

Cholesterol test. Test that measures cholesterol esters, phospholipids, or triglycerides in the blood.

CIRCUMCISION

The AAP states that circumcision has potential medical benefits and advantages, as well as inherent disadvantages and risks. Therefore, the AAP recommends that the decision to circumcise is one best made by parents in consultation with the pediatrician. **Circumcision** is the surgical removal of the foreskin of the glans penis. In the last 2 decades there has been much controversy about this practice. In the 1970s, the AAP opposed the practice of routine circumcision, but in the1980s they reversed their position and are now in favor of leaving the decision up to the judgment of parents and their pediatricians. Although this argument is still in debate, the reality is that circumcision is also linked to culture and religion. In the Jewish culture, circumcision is performed during a significant ceremony called a Brith, which takes place on the eighth day after birth. The ceremony is performed by a highly trained professional called a mohel. Orthodox Jews do not perform the ceremony with sterile technique

Circumcision. Surgical removal of the foreskin of the glans penis.

and bleeding is controlled by using a tight bandage around the penis. The circumcision can also be done by one of two other techniques. In the Gomco technique, the foreskin is clamped and removed; the clamp crushes the nerve endings and the vessels, promoting homeostasis. In the Plastibell procedure, the foreskin is removed using a plastic ring and a string tied around the foreskin like a tourniquet; the excess foreskin is trimmed. In about 5 to 8 days the plastic ring separates and falls off.

The main focus for the nurse is in the education of the new parents and also to help them to arrive at a clear decision as to whether the child should have a circumcision or not. This procedure requires the completion of an informed consent form before being performed. The care of the circumcision depends on which procedure was used. With the Gomco procedure, the nurse needs to place a Vaselined gauze around the penis to avoid adherence to the diaper; the penis should be inspected for bleeding and swelling. With the Plastibell procedure no gauze is necessary. Parents and child should be united as soon as possible after the procedure.

CONTRACEPTION AND ADOLESCENTS

One of the major crises in the lives of adolescents relates to sex and **contraception**. Often, adolescents believe that they are sophisticated when it comes to knowing about sex and sexual practices, but the reality is that the problem arises from a cluster of factors that are beyond the control of their young years and lack of knowledge and experience.

Pregnancy prevention for adolescents has become a national problem, because of the large number of pregnancies reported in teenagers. Usually, the first time that a high-risk teen visits a health care facility is for a prenatal visit, not for prevention information. The pregnant adolescent starts to live her first developmental crisis: becoming a responsible adult before completing the developmental tasks of adolescence. At this point, the adolescent parent-to-be has placed herself at risk for nonachievement of her full developmental potential in education and achievement. Adolescent mothers have increased stress and lower psychosocial support. Children of adolescents are usually born prematurely; their mortality is high; and if they do survive, they are at risk for low achievement in school and may develop an array of behavioral problems throughout their school-age years. Parenting for adolescents becomes a nightmare plagued by guilt, anxiety, and fear. They tend not to see parenting as a responsibility but rather as an achievement. Therefore, they see the child as something that belongs to them and as a source of love for them. The adolescent parent tends to be less sensitive and lacks knowledge about infant care. They see the child as a demanding being who needs discipline. Research reports a tremendous amount of child abuse and neglect among these mothers. It is estimated that 80% of teen pregnancies are unplanned. In view of all of these problems, family planning services have developed many programs targeting teenagers in recent years.

Contraception. Pregnancy prevention.

The AAP states that teens are concerned about the lack of confidentiality at a health care facility, and therefore do not seek contraceptive information. The nurse must realize that confidentiality is a grave issue with the adolescent. The nurse must ensure the confidentiality of the teen will not be violated. On the other hand, other health professionals feel strongly that parent involvement in this issue should be obtained.

The choice of contraceptive method is usually tailored to the needs of the patient after physical assessment and in-depth discussion. The factors associated with contraception are education, availability, cost, parental education, and discussion about the real issues of pregnancy and parenting. The biggest problem with teenagers and contraception reported in the literature is the teenagers' lack of compliance and delay in seeking contraceptive information. Many health care providers believe that contraception should be part of ongoing sex education and not isolated to when the child becomes a teenager. It is very important that the child learn about sex, relationships, and conception from a responsible adult. Therefore, what is required are good communication skills. If compliance is to be maintained the teen needs a close follow-up to ensure effectiveness of the treatment and to form a relationship with someone he/she can trust. Nursing is placed in an important role in relation to this problem. The current position of the AAP in relation to contraception is that health care professionals ought to counsel teens about the dangers of pregnancy and STDs (sexually transmitted diseases); they should teach teens responsible sexual decision making, beginning with abstinence. However, pediatricians also should encourage the use of contraceptive services to adolescents who are sexually active.

ℬREAST-FEEDING

Historically, breast milk has served as a vital link for nutrition and survival of the human species. During times of adversity and challenge, breast-feeding provided nurturing, nutrition, and immunities to the newborn, infant, and young child. Today, out of the entire world population of 570 million, the percentage of babies who are exclusively breast-fed (no supplementation) ranges from 1% to 90%. The sub-Saharan African country of Rwanda has the most significant breast-fed population on the planet: 90%; but on the same continent, Niger has the lowest: 1%. In the Middle East and North Africa the range is from 12% to 65% and in the Americas, from 3% to 53%. The countries of Asia and the Pacific also have a below-projected percentage of breast-feeding practices, according to the United Nations International Children's Emergency Fund (UNICEF).

Presently, millions of infants worldwide die every year from poor health, caused by preventable diseases and malnutrition. The magnitude of this global problem is enormous. The number of children who die before the age of 5 was estimated to be 12.9 million in 1992 (Time, 1995). Although a decline has been noted, the world statistics of 65 deaths per

1000 births are staggering (Time, 1995). When viewing U.S. statistics on childhood mortality, death and disease are only slightly greater in the developing countries of the world than in the United States. There are no comprehensive national programs in the United States that focus on this problem plaguing our world society.

Annually, the World Alliance of Breast-feeding Action (WABA), a non-governmental organization that spans all continents, focuses on the issue of breast feeding. The International Lactation Consultant Association, with members in some 30 countries, has developed an action kit directing the advancement of breast feeding at the community level. La Leche League International, present in 60 countries, is coordinating their sixth "World Walk for Breast-Feeding." These international nongovernmental organizations are in official relationships with the World Health Organization (WHO).

In Dade County, Florida, mothers agreed that breast-feeding was better than bottle feeding, but many did not choose to breast-feed their children. Cuban Americans (77%) felt that they did not have enough breast milk. Haitian Americans (73%) chose bottle feeding because of the need for employment outside of the home (Thomas & DeSantis, 1995). Both groups thought their babies would be fat or healthy and quiet or pacified if bottle fed, which was desirable (Thomas & DeSantis, 1995). As the demographics of the country change, as reflected in the 1990 census, it is expected that the minority groups will constitute a majority of the studies.

Leininger's Sunrise model was conceptualized to discover cultural and transcultural nursing. The goal of the model is to achieve culturally congruent nursing care, which consists of creatively designed nursing decisions and actions that fit the lives of individuals, families, or groups so as to provide care that is meaningful, satisfying, and beneficial. It is expected that this model will be reached through preservation/maintenance, accommodation/negotiation, and repatterning/restructuring.

Leininger clarifies and defines preservation/maintenance as a sensitive and supportive enabling of the health care professional to preserve health. Accommodation/negotiation helps clients of a cultural group adapt to or negotiate for beneficial or satisfying health. Cultural repatterning or restructuring refers to a change in life patterns for a new or different pattern that is culturally meaningful and satisfying or that supports beneficial and healthy life patterns (Bohay, 1991).

The Sunrise model reinforces the value of cultural consideration and congruent caring as a central issue in nursing. This is reached through respect and understanding of the clients' belief system without attempting to enculturate them.

Studies show that early education about breast-feeding influences the decision to breast-feed. With the appropriate provision of care, which includes a good rapport with the client and family, significant results can be obtained. Health care professionals can no longer consider the client as a patient. It becomes more apparent that the client is an intricate part of a working system called the family, especially when introducing a new member into the family.

The only acceptable alternative to human milk is iron-fortified infant formula. Skim or low-fat milk is not recommended in the first 2 years of life because of the high protein and electrolyte content and low calorie density of these milks.

ℒ EAD POISONING

The most serious and irreversible side effect of lead ingestion is seen in the nervous system: increased intracranial pressure causes cortical atrophy and lead encephalopathy (convulsions, mental retardation, coma, and death). Low levels of lead cause neurological and intellectual problems. The most common symptoms seen are when the child is brought to the doctor's office with abdominal pain, vomiting, constipation, anorexia, headache, and halted developmental progress.

Diagnosis is made upon measurement of the blood lead levels. The blood is collected by finger or heel puncture. If the child is suspected of having **lead poisoning**, a subsequent blood specimen is collected via venous puncture.

The treatment varies with each child since the level of lead in the blood determines the kind of treatment required. Usually, the treatment includes the removal of the source of lead, improved nutrition, and in extreme cases the use of chelation therapy. Nurses involved in the care of these children need to be aware of the guidelines formulated by the Centers for Disease Control (1991). Does the child live in a house or frequent a day care or other houses built before 1960 where there is peeling or chipping paint? Has a sister or brother been treated for lead poisoning? Does the child live with an adult whose job or hobbies involve exposure to lead? Does the child live near an active lead smelter, battery plant, or recycling plant that uses lead? Careful history taking by the nurse is the most important tool in the diagnosis of this condition.

Along with the Centers for Disease Control, the AAP supports broad-based routine lead screenings of children, as well as funding for a national program to screen for lead and to remove lead hazards from the environment. This position is not universally accepted. The arguments are based on lack of funds to support the extensive screenings, the diversion of funds that could be used for more serious diseases, and the skepticism about the significance of a 5-point lowering of IQ scores. Nurses are the ones responsible for screening and educational interventions, and they need to be aware of the arguments in order to be sensitive to the many potential problems that a diagnosis of lead poisoning brings.

𝒥 MMUNIZATIONS

The biggest advances in pediatrics over the past 60 years have been the decline in serious diseases due to the availability of vaccines. The recommended primary schedule of immunizations starts at infancy, and with the

Lead poisoning. Poisoning produced by ingestion of objects that contain lead.

exception of **boosters** is completed during early childhood. Vaccines have helped us control deadly diseases, but they also have created fear or misunderstanding about the side effects that they can cause.

The schedule for immunizations in the United States is governed by the Advisory Committee on Immunization Practices (ACIP) of the U.S. Public Health Service Centers for Disease Control and Prevention (CDC) and the Committee on Infectious Diseases of the American Academy of Pediatrics. The recommended age for beginning primary immunizations in infants is at birth.

Other vaccines are recommended for children at high risk. Most of these children have chronic disorders that make them more susceptible to certain infections.

Nurses, because of their unique position in the administration of vaccines, need to be aware of the reasons for withholding immunizations, for avoiding reactions that could be dangerous to the child. Live virus vaccines are generally not given to any child who has a compromised immune system. Another contraindication is a known allergic reaction to a previously administered vaccine. The major precaution in administering vaccinations is to ensure the proper storage of the vaccine to protect its potency.

A new *Haemophilus influenzae* type b (Hib) conjugate vaccine is now available to provide protection against a number of serious infections caused by Hib. The AAP recommends that all children receive Hib conjugate vaccine at 2, 4, and 6 months of age with a booster dose at 12 and 15 months. This has eliminated bacterial meningitis, epiglottitis, bacterial pneumonia, septic arthritis, and sepsis. These conjugate vaccines connect Hib to a nontoxic form of another organism such as meningococcal protein or diphtheria protein.

It is imperative for the nurse to be familiar with vaccines in order to fully inform families of the risks and benefits of vaccines. The U.S. Public Health Service has developed a series of vaccine information pamphlets that are available to all families. However, the literature is detailed and written at higher reading level than is appropriate for many families. Therefore the nurse needs to be aware of the need for providing parents with the appropriate information, and allowing them to ask questions relevant to their fears and anxieties about the vaccines.

Booster. A suspension of infectious agents, given for the purpose of stimulating an immune response in the body by creating antibodies or activating T lymphocytes capable of controlling the organism.

Hib (*Haemophilus influenzae* type b vaccine). A conjugate vaccine that can prevent bacterial meningitis, epiglottitis, bacterial pneumonia, septic arthritis, and sepsis.

*H*OMOSEXUALITY

Adolescence is a critical time in the development of sexual orientation, and because of the societal stigma on homosexuality, adolescents have a hard time exploring their own sexuality. The dangerous lack of opportunities to discuss this issue can place the adolescent in the situation of experimenting with at-risk behaviors in order to obtain answers. The literature reports that at-risk teenagers engage in sex with at least 7 different same-sex partners, while at the same time having heterosexual encounters.

The majority of homosexual encounters for at-risk teens are with people that they pick up in gay bars or public places. Considering the sensitive nature of this problem the nurse needs to prepare for these issues. When he/she is confronted with an adolescent who has questions about homosexuality, the nurse can appreciate the delicate situation that the adolescent is in, and be able to better answer questions to help the teen understand his/her own sexuality. In counseling adolescents, the nurse should stress that abstinence is the key to reducing the incidence of STD. Sexually active teens should be educated about STD and encouraged to limit their number of sexual partners. Since adolescence is a period of feeling misunderstood and confused, positive reinforcement is hard to come by. Reinforcement of appropriate behavior is important, along with the avoidance of being or appearing judgmental.

In doing an assessment, the nurse needs to be extra sensitive when posing questions about homosexuality. The discussion should center on information and not on the prejudices of the nurse. For instance, the nurse should avoid such obvious judgmental comments as, "It's only a passing feeling." On the contrary, adolescents may have decided that they are homosexual, and have the right to be referred to agencies that provide supportive care for their special needs. Most of these adolescents lack support from their families. Health professionals who are involved with these adolescents have the resources and knowledge to guide them through this difficult period in their development.

$\mathcal{M}$EDIA

Media. Means of communication such as television, Internet, radio, newspapers, magazines, etc.

One of the greatest influences of the 1990s on the development of children is the **media** in their daily lives. This includes mainly television and the Internet, whose influence has not only affected their development, but also the influence that the children will have on society in general. Children used to see the world through the eyes of their parents and teachers and their society; today, however, they see the world through the eyes of an industry whose main concern is to make money, not to educate children.

Research reports indicate that some media can actually be a public health risk factor for children and adolescents, leading to bad eating habits, sexual aggression, and negative influences toward the world in general. Nurses must educate parents to realize the influence of the media on their children and help them to find ways to monitor children's exposure to these phenomena. Parents need to realize that the primary goal of the majority of TV commercials is to sell products to children. Young children cannot distinguish between programs and commercials. Quality television programming helps to educate children. However, the passive lure of television tends to distract children from reading or using active learning skills. The AAP recommends that TV viewing by children be limited to 1 or 2 hours a day. The AAP also supports legislative efforts such as the Children's Television Act of 1990, which mandates that television stations provide 3 hours of educational programming for children per week. The AAP also advocates for content-based TV ratings systems.

Television also exposes children to violence. The media tend to glamorize the use of guns and wrongly teach children that the use of firearms is acceptable behavior. Parents need to sit with their children and explain to them the dangers of these behaviors. In a nutshell, what is needed is to teach children **critical thinking** skills and how to arrive at decisions that will not place them in dangerous situations. When children learn to make appropriate choices and learn how to solve problems, instead of having a dangerous world ahead of them, they will see the world as full of choices and as a wonderful place to live.

Critical thinking. A way of thinking about nursing and medicine which must occur in an expected period of time in order to achieve diagnosis and treatment and to promote optimal standards of care.

SUBSTANCE ABUSE

Among the worst menaces to children from 1991 to 1996 is the increase in the use of drugs among students in grades 8 through 12. Alcohol continues to be the substance most abused by adolescents, but tobacco and marijuana use among young people has reached epidemic levels. Among the most prevalent causes for this epidemic is the media, followed by the perception among adolescents that these drugs are not harmful. In the last 3 years, the health care system has witnessed a decrease in school-based substance abuse programs. In order to combat this epidemic, health care professionals need to incorporate the development of programs aimed at reducing substance abuse, with a view toward supporting good health practices. Adolescents have a great sense of autonomy and at the same time a sense of curiosity, which can be beneficial in the development of such programs.

As we enter the new millennium we realize that health promotion for adolescents involves multiple issues, and that the problem cannot be focused only from the medical model, but must be approached from an interdisciplinary framework. Among the behaviors that teens need to address are some of the same ones that adults need to address. However, when asked about their vulnerability, adolescents tend to underestimate the potentially harmful effects that their choices may have later on. This may be due to their lack of experience or to their sense of immortality. A positive step taken by some health professionals has been the availability of confidential services where teens can ask questions and feel safe and guarded against consequences or criticisms. In single-parent homes, adolescents may not want to bother their already overburdened parent with more problems, or they may feel that no one cares about them. Important for nursing intervention is the clear understanding of how complex the problem is and the need for comprehensive care based on respect and not judgment. The main goal of nursing interventions when dealing with teenagers is the reality that nurses must turn problems into opportunities and bad experiences into building blocks to help the teenager grow and prosper.

The position that the AAP has taken in relation to alcohol consumption for pregnant teenagers is that to protect the developing fetus, pregnant women should not drink any alcohol. The AAP also says that there is no safe dose of alcohol when the woman is pregnant. The AAP message is also clear about smoking during pregnancy: Do not smoke when pregnant. The literature is full of studies that link low birth weight with smoking by the mother. Another problem is passive smoking. Children of parents who smoke have more respiratory infections, bronchitis, pneumonia, and reduced pulmonary function than do children of nonsmokers. The AAP supports regulatory and legislative efforts to decrease access to and use of tobacco by children and adolescents.

Glossary

booster   a suspension of infectious agents, given for the purpose of stimulating an immune response in the body by creating antibodies or activating T lymphocytes capable of controlling the organism.

cholesterol test   test that measures cholesterol esters, phospholipids, or triglycerides in the blood.

circumcision   surgical removal of the foreskin of the glans penis.

contraception   pregnancy prevention.

critical thinking   a way of thinking about nursing and medicine which must occur in an expected period of time in order to achieve diagnosis and treatment and to promote optimal standards of care.

exogenous factors   outside factors, such as high dietary and caloric intake, sedentary life-style, stress.

genetic predisposition   susceptibility to a disease due to heredity.

hazards   any situation handled in such a way that people can suffer personal injury.

hib (*Haemophilus influenzae* type b vaccine)   a conjugate vaccine that can prevent bacterial meningitis, epiglottitis, bacterial pneumonia, septic arthritis, and sepsis.

lead poisoning   poisoning produced by ingestion of objects that contain lead.

media   means of communication such as television, Internet, radio, newspapers, magazines, etc.

societal changes   changes that occur in society as a result of changes in the world.

Bibliography

AMERICAN ACADEMY OF PEDIATRICS. Where We Stand. http:/www.aap.org/advocacy/wwestand.htm, 1997.

AMERICAN PSYCHOLOGICAL ASSOCIATION. *Publication Manual of the American Psychological Association.* 4th ed. Washington, D.C.: Author, 1994.

BOHAY, I. Z. Cultural care meanings and experiences of pregnancy and childbirth of Ukranians. In M. Leininger, *Culture Care Diversity and Universality: A Theory of Nursing.* (Pp. 206–207). New York: National League of Nursing Press, 1991.

BURNS, C., BARBER, N., BRADY, M. A., AND DUNN, A. M. *Pediatric Primary Care: A Handbook for Nurse Practitioners.* Philadelphia: Saunders, 1996

CENTERS FOR DISEASE CONTROL GUIDELINES. *Preventing Lead Poisoning in Young Children.* Atlanta: Centers for Disease Control, 1991.

HARRIS, K. Beliefs and practices among Haitian American women in relation to childbearing. *Journal of Nurse Midwifery* 32(3), May/June 1987.

KAISER PERMANENTE'S STUDY ON BREAST-FEEDING AND HEALTH. 1994–1995 http://www.greaststar.com/lois/bfh.html

LA LECHE LEAGUE. 1997 Benefits of Breast-feeding to the Mother. http://www.lalecheleague.org/benefits.html

THOMAS, J. T., AND DESANTIS, L. Feeding and weaning practices of Cuban and Haitian immigrant mothers. *Journal of Transcultural Nursing* (2):34–42, 1995.

TIME MAGAZINE. The World Fact Book 1994: World People [CD-ROM]. Time, 1995.

INDEX

ISBN 0-07-070009-5
90000

9 780070 700093

WHETSELL/PEDIATRIC
NURSING